AF734611

Neurodevelopmental Diseases – Laboratory and Clinical Research Series

BEHAVIORAL THEORIES AND INTERVENTIONS FOR AUTISM

NEURODEVELOPMENTAL DISEASES – LABORATORY AND CLINICAL RESEARCH SERIES

Behavioral Theories and Interventions for Autism
Phil Reed (Editor)
2009. ISBN: 978-1-60741-165-9

Neurodevelopmental Diseases – Laboratory and Clinical Research Series

BEHAVIORAL THEORIES AND INTERVENTIONS FOR AUTISM

PHIL REED
EDITOR

Nova Science Publishers, Inc.
New York

Copyright © 2009 by Nova Science Publishers, Inc.

All rights reserved. No part of this book may be reproduced, stored in a retrieval system or transmitted in any form or by any means: electronic, electrostatic, magnetic, tape, mechanical photocopying, recording or otherwise without the written permission of the Publisher.

For permission to use material from this book please contact us:
Telephone 631-231-7269; Fax 631-231-8175
Web Site: http://www.novapublishers.com

NOTICE TO THE READER

The Publisher has taken reasonable care in the preparation of this book, but makes no expressed or implied warranty of any kind and assumes no responsibility for any errors or omissions. No liability is assumed for incidental or consequential damages in connection with or arising out of information contained in this book. The Publisher shall not be liable for any special, consequential, or exemplary damages resulting, in whole or in part, from the readers' use of, or reliance upon, this material.

Independent verification should be sought for any data, advice or recommendations contained in this book. In addition, no responsibility is assumed by the publisher for any injury and/or damage to persons or property arising from any methods, products, instructions, ideas or otherwise contained in this publication.

This publication is designed to provide accurate and authoritative information with regard to the subject matter covered herein. It is sold with the clear understanding that the Publisher is not engaged in rendering legal or any other professional services. If legal or any other expert assistance is required, the services of a competent person should be sought. FROM A DECLARATION OF PARTICIPANTS JOINTLY ADOPTED BY A COMMITTEE OF THE AMERICAN BAR ASSOCIATION AND A COMMITTEE OF PUBLISHERS.

LIBRARY OF CONGRESS CATALOGING-IN-PUBLICATION DATA

Behavioral theories and interventions for autism / [edited by] Phil Reed.
p. ; cm.
Includes bibliographical references and index.
ISBN 978-1-60741-165-9 (hardcover)
1. Autism--Treatment. 2. Behavior therapy. I. Reed, Phil.
[DNLM: 1. Autistic Disorder--therapy. 2. Behavior Therapy--methods. WM 203.5 V4192 2009]
RC553.A88.B44 2009
616.85'882--dc22

2009006345

Published by Nova Science Publishers, Inc. ✝ New York

CONTENTS

Preface: Behavioral Research and Interventions for Autism – New Directions

For many in the lay community, there is a strong, almost synonymous, relationship between Applied Behavior Analysis (ABA) and Autistic Spectrum Disorders (ASD). This should not be surprising, as, for parents whose child has an ASD, ABA often holds out the best hope of improvements for their child, and that is the only thing that will matter to many of those parents. While the wider community of Behavior Analysts, who are engaged in work that is not directed at ASD, may find this perception to misrepresent their field, there can be no doubt that the relationship to ASD has strengthened immensely the position of Behavior Analysis within the wider field of Psychology. However, the relationship between ASD and ABA has also been an important one symbiotically for both fields. It is undoubtedly true that the study of ASD through Behavior Analytic techniques has immeasurably improved the understanding of that disorder and its treatments. Conversely, the challenges posed to Behavior Analysis by its application to ASD have also illuminated, and in many cases forced, the development of Behavior Analysis into new and exciting directions. It is with this more symbiotic relationship in mind that the current book approaches the area, with the hope that some insights will be shed into both ASD and Behavior Analysis.

Behavioral interventions for ASD are now among the most widely used, and have proved both extremely popular with parents, and controversial with professionals. These ABA techniques are some of the few approaches to the treatment of ASD to be scientifically validated, but this availability of evidence allows both their strengths and weaknesses to be debated. Much debate focuses on the initial claims about the successes of ABA approaches made nearly two decades ago. However, there have been enormous developments and diversifications in the ABA approaches offered to the treatment of ASD since that time, and this text attempts to bring together evidence regarding these contemporary developments. In order to achieve this aim, leading figures in the field have provided accounts of the developments in their area, along with a review of the empirical evidence relating to those developments.

The chapters in the current text can be read to gain a rounded understanding of the way Behavior Analysis approaches ASD. They allow insights into the nature of Behavior Analysis, and also into the key issues that are emerging as the discipline develops. There have been enormous developments in this field over the last twenty years, not only have these developments had an enormous impact on the re-emergence of behavioural psychology in general, and on early educational practice in particular, but such developments have rarely been documented in one place in a manner that would allow easy comparison between them. It is hoped that doing so will be extremely useful to those with an interest in an empirically-based evaluation of teaching interventions for ASD. In particular, there are two groups of readers who may find this text interesting. Firstly, it is aimed at those professionals working in the area, such as researchers, and educational professionals within authorities with a responsibility for deciding on provision for ASD. The research material on the effectiveness of various forms of intervention, the factors that mediate effectiveness, and the likelihood of success of the various approaches, would be valuable for educational professionals. This book would also be useful for those working on home-based teaching interventions, in order to see the current ideas on best practice from the literature. Secondly, students of all levels taking a wide range of courses on learning, developmental psychology, clinical and abnormal psychology, psychology and education, and final year students researching ASD, may all find this approach offers a different perspective from that typically given.

In fact, there are two readings of the chapters contained in this book, one is provided by the linear placement of the chapters into sections that are structured to allow a reader to gain understanding into: (1) the way that ASD problems are conceptualized by behavioral psychologists; (2) the way that these conceptions have led to the development of interventions for ASD; and (3) the factors that are known to modulate the effectiveness of behavioral interventions. The other reading of the chapters is to engage with the themes that emerge across, and that are shared by, these chapters, and which highlight many novel developments in Behavior Analysis. These themes include: (A) the functional nature of the explanations given in Behavior Analysis; (B) the development of a mature and sophisticated behavioral theory of language development; (C) the emergence of behavioral theorizing about developmental processes; and (D) the recognition that the environment includes not only inanimate stimuli and reinforcers, but also interactions with other people whose impact needs to be considered.

To the first end, namely the linear structuring of the material, the book is organized into three sections dealing with conceptualization of ASD problems, the development and analysis of various ABA interventions for ASD, and the factors that modulate the effectiveness of ABA interventions. The chapters in Part 1 of this book deal with the core characteristics of ASD, and their specific treatments, from a Behavior Analytic perspective, including analysis of the deficits often noted in attention (Dube), imitation (Ingersoll and Schreibman), perspective taking (McHugh), as well as the important concomitant behavioral problems displayed by children with ASD (Wacker, Berg, Harding, and Cooper-Brown). This section is followed by four chapters that expand the analysis of ABA approaches to treating ASD, from examining specific core behavioral characteristics, to presenting a number of over-arching behavioral strategies for the development of early interventions for ASD. In this second section, each chapter outlines and reviews the evidence for a different ABA approach to the treatment of ASD. These range from the traditional ABA interventions for ASD that stem from the work of Lovaas (Leader, Healy, and O'Connor), through Verbal Behavior (McGreevy) and CABAS® (Greer and Keohane) approaches, to the application of Positive Behavioral Support, particularly for adults (Grey, McClean, and McCauley). The final section of the book contains chapters that go beyond the child with ASD, and the interventions developed by ABA, to consider the factors that contribute to the success, or otherwise, of such interventions. These factors include an analysis of the role of the family, and especially of parenting stress and styles (Osborne), the impact of parental education on outcomes for children with ASD (Fiske and Harris), and the impact of professional education (Symon, Openden, and Jacoby). The final chapter assesses procedures that might be beneficial to adults with ASD (McClannahan, MacDuff, and Krantz). All of these chapters provide an up to date summary of the field for those with a professional interest (both researchers and practitioners), and for students pursuing training in ASD and Behavior Analysis.

However, in addition to this linear structure, the chapters provide a sample of a number of common themes that characterize contemporary behavioral theorizing both in general, and in relation to ASD in particular. There are many such themes, and they include the functional nature of explanation offered by Behavior Analysis, the role and understanding of language and developmental change, and the recognition of a need for the inclusion of an analysis of a wide range of variables involved in the system under investigation, including the family of the child with ASD. Several of these themes are highlighted below.

In terms of the nature of behavioral theorizing, the chapters in Part 1 of this book all highlight the need to focus on the relationship between behavior and the environment of which it is a product (see especially Wacker et al., and Ingersoll and Schreibman). This type of functional explanation (as opposed to an appeal to unseen cognitive processes) is one that characterizes a key aspect of Behavior Analysis. This approach can also be seen in the chapters that deal with more wide-ranging treatments (those not directed at one behavior in particular), such as is outlined by Grey et al., and by Osborne, in their analyses of more complex systems. In all of these cases, the system, and its interactions, is defined by reference to measurable aspects of behavior, and the way that one set of behaviors is a product (i.e. a function) of another set of behaviors.

Another theme that emerges through a number of these chapters is the development of a sophisticated behavioral theory regarding the relationships that produce and maintain language; an ability often missing in children with ASD, and which is often regarded as a deficit in Behavioral theorizing. However, the current chapters show a range of important developments in identifying the ways in which language is maintained, which includes analysis of the behavior of both the speaker and the listener (see chapters by McGreevy, and Greer and Keohane), and the way such language can generalize, and form the basis of more complex 'cognitive' processes (McHugh).

Many of the chapters also show sophistication in the manner in which behavioral theory tackles the problem of developmental psychology. As with the analysis of language, noted above, developmental psychology often appealed to unseen structures to explain change, pointing to apparently invariant stages in development as being beyond the explanatory scope of simple learning theory. Whether these stages were truly invariant, or not, they often posed a problem for behavioral theory. However, many of the chapters in the current book attempt to show how such 'stages' may be the result of necessary building of one behavior from previously established simpler behaviors. The concepts of behavioral developmental cusps (Greer and Keohane), of a series of necessary relational frames to be established for new relations to be learned (McHugh), and developmental changes in systems over time (Osborne), pervade many of these views on offer in this text.

Finally, many of the chapters examine the behavior of an individual with ASD not only from the perspective of how that individual is confronted with various stimuli in their environment, but attempt to show how many aspects of the environment need to be accommodated in understanding the behavior of the individual. This 'systems' approach to behavior can be seen in the development of treatments, such as the CABAS® method (Greer and Keohane), or the Positive Behavioral Support system (Grey et al.). This role of the larger community of individuals, comprising parents (Fiske and Harris), and professionals (Symon et al.), is also acknowledged in many of the chapters in the final section of the book.

Thus, it is hoped that the current text will allow the reader to develop both a specific knowledge of particular ABA theories and procedures developed for ASD, and, if the chapters are read with reference to one another, a view of a thriving, integrated, and theoretically sophisticated discipline will emerge.

ACKNOWLEDGMENTS

The editors of volumes, such as this, can claim very little credit for their contents, which firmly lies with the various contributors to the project. A very large thank you, therefore, is due to all of the excellent contributors to this volume, who kindly gave their time and work very generously, and who responded patiently to my few suggestions about how to alter their chapters. Thanks are also due to all at Nova Science Publishers for their help and patience in the preparation of this text.

As always, my thanks go to Lisa, whose support and encouragement in any endeavor that I undertake is always complete, and breathtaking: a day with you is a lifetime of memories, and you are my first and last thought each day.

One of the few privileges for the editor, apart from formatting the chapters, is to dedicate the work to people who have been particularly inspirational. In all cases for me, that has to be Lisa, first and abovc all, but I would also like to mention a couple of other sources of inspiration. The male brain has so very little to do with ASD, and, as one non-autistic possessor of such a brain, I have to confess to having very little interest in those systematizing areas which, it is suggested, should characterize me. However, the stereotypical interests of the British male may have shaped my responses to two powerful sources of reinforcement which, along with Lisa, helped me to complete the editing of this book. In that light, I would like to dedicate this book to Bobby Moore and Debbie Harry.

Part 1:
The Characteristics of Autistic Spectrum Disorders and Behavioral Approaches to Their Treatment

In: Behavioral Theories and Interventions for Autism
Editor: Phil Reed
ISBN 978-1-60741-165-9
© 2009 Nova Science Publishers, Inc.

Chapter 1

MATCHING TREATMENT TO THE FUNCTION OF DESTRUCTIVE BEHAVIOR

David P. Wacker, Wendy K. Berg, Jay W. Harding and Linda J. Cooper-Brown
The University of Iowa, USA

Destructive behaviors are so named because they are composed of response topographies that result in (a) injury to the person (self-injury), (b) injury to others (aggression), (c) damage to the physical environment (destruction), and (d) disruption of academic and social development (stereotypy). Although most children engage in problem responses intermittently, children with autism spectrum disorders (ASD) have a higher probability of engaging in high-intensity, high-frequency, and long-duration destructive behavior. Thus, treatment of destructive behavior for children with ASD is often a high priority in early intervention and educational programs.

Iwata, Vollmer, Zarcone, and Rogers (1993) described an approach to the treatment of destructive behaviors in which treatment procedures were matched to the function of behavior rather than to its topography. In contrast to previous approaches to behavioral treatment, this function-based approach provided a conceptual basis for identifying that a treatment procedure might be effective for a given behavior rather than specifying which treatment should be selected. As discussed by Iwata et al. (1993), and as was still the case in 2007, the majority of textbooks and articles describing behavioral treatments focus on the topography of behavior and the direction of desired behavior change. Thus, procedures such as planned ignoring or contingent removal of an individual are described as reductive (i.e., extinction and punishment) because the intent is to decrease the occurrence of a specific topography of behavior. The term "reductive procedures" is, of course, an arbitrary classification because we must infer that being ignored or being removed disrupts the targeted response-reinforcer relation. As an example of the application of arbitrary reductive/punishment procedures, consider a classroom teacher placing a student with ASD in a "time-out" area in an attempt to reduce destructive behavior during individual seat work. In this scenario, the selection of time-out as a reductive procedure requires the inference that the destructive behavior is maintained by positive reinforcement (e.g., attention). If that is indeed the case, then removing the student via a time-out procedure may be successful in reducing problem behavior. If, however, destructive behavior is maintained by negative reinforcement (e.g., escape from academic tasks), then removing the student may increase the future probability of the occurrence of destructive behavior because time-out provides brief escape from demands.

In contrast, a functional approach first identifies the response-reinforcer relation, which then establishes a menu of treatment options that (a) disrupt ongoing reinforcement for destructive behavior, (b) provide the same reinforcement for socially acceptable behavior, and (c) identify antecedent conditions (such as states of deprivation or satiation) that influence the probability that destructive behavior will occur in the future.

Using our previous example, the identification of the functional reinforcer for the student's destructive behavior during seat work provides information that can be used directly in developing an internally consistent treatment program. Identifying that destructive behavior is maintained by escape from academic tasks (i.e., negative reinforcement) suggests an array of function-based interventions. Antecedent components might include making changes to the type or difficulty level of academic tasks so that the student is not motivated to engage in destructive behavior. As a reinforcer component, the teacher might provide negative reinforcement (brief breaks) for completing small amounts of work or for asking appropriately for assistance. Finally, as a reductive component, problem behavior might be placed on extinction (i.e., no breaks from work) or might receive punishment in the form of more work or loss of break time. These antecedent, reinforcement, and reductive components are internally consistent because each is matched to the function of destructive behavior. When reinforcement as well as punishment components are included, the student is directly taught to engage in adaptive responses that are reinforced and learns that destructive behaviors produce punishment.

In this chapter, we first describe a function-based approach to treatment and some historical references to initial applications of this approach. We then discuss epidemiological studies that have summarized the results of function-based treatments. Next, we describe two series of longitudinal research projects funded by the National Institutes of Health—one series focusing on socially maintained destructive behavior (Wacker and Berg, 1992, Wacker, Berg, and Harding, 1996; Wacker, Berg, and Harding, 2000; Wacker, Berg, and Harding, 2004) and one series on automatically maintained destructive behavior (Berg, Ringdahl, Wacker, and Bosch, 2000; Berg, Wacker, Ringdahl, and Bosch, 2003)—to provide more specific exemplars of how we have used a function-based model to treat destructive behavior. Finally, we describe some directions for future research.

Function as the Basis for Treatment

Severe topographies of problem behavior, such as self-injury, aggression, stereotypy, and property destruction, have been observed in as many as one-third of individuals with developmental disabilities (Tassé, 2006). Approaches to treatment, including behavioral treatment, often have been based on trial and error. Historically, behavioral treatments included arbitrarily selected reinforcement, extinction, and punishment procedures in an attempt to "overwhelm" unknown, existing sources of reinforcement for these destructive behaviors. Thus, treatment succeeded when an arbitrarily selected contingency competed effectively against the unknown contingency that maintained the destructive behavior.

Early operant researchers, such as Lovaas and Simmons (1969), showed that even severe destructive behaviors could be maintained by specific social reinforcers (in this study, attention), but a method for either conceptualizing or identifying specific sources of reinforcement for specific behaviors was not available. As a result, behavioral researchers relied heavily on punishment contingencies because they were often the most effective way to reduce destructive behavior (Cataldo, 1989).

Carr (1977) provided the first conceptual model of operant contingencies maintaining destructive behavior. Based on previously published empirical studies, Carr hypothesized that there were three distinct operant functions for destructive behavior: (a) positive reinforcement in the form of attention or access to preferred items, (b) negative reinforcement in the form of escape or avoidance of nonpreferred tasks or activities, and (c) sensory or automatic reinforcement, which refers to reinforcement produced by the behavior itself. Early studies evaluating these sources of reinforcement showed that attention (Lovaas and Simmons, 1969), tangible (Day, Rea, Schussler, Larsen, and Johnson, 1988), escape (Carr, Newsom, and Binkoff, 1980), and sensory stimuli (Lovaas, Newsom, and Hickman, 1987) functioned as reinforcers for destructive behavior in at least some cases.

Iwata, Dorsey, Slifer, Bauman, and Richman (1982/1994) developed the first operant methodology for identifying the specific functions of destructive behavior. This methodology, termed a functional analysis, permitted researchers, clinicians, and teachers to determine which specific sources of reinforcement were maintaining the destructive behavior of any given individual. Assessment was conducted by observing rates of destructive behavior within tightly controlled analogue conditions that tested for positive, negative, and automatic reinforcement. If rates in any of the test conditions were higher than in a control (free play) condition, then a function was identified. For the 9 participants in Iwata et al.'s 1982/1994 study, 6 showed higher levels of problem behavior during one or more of the test conditions than during the control condition. These results supported Carr's (1977) operant conceptual model and provided the first clinical assessment procedure that could be used to prescribe treatment for destructive behaviors.

The major clinical benefit of the functional analysis methodology described by Iwata et al. (1982/1994) is that it directly tests each operant hypothesis and reduces the need for inference. In the test for negative reinforcement, for example, the child is given a demand that continues until the child engages in destructive behavior. Destructive behavior produces brief (20- to 30-s) periods of negative reinforcement followed by the re-presentation of the demand. If higher rates of destructive behavior occur during the demand condition than during free play, negative reinforcement is a function of problem behavior. Even very brief (e.g., 90-min) versions of this procedure are often sufficient for identifying a function (Northup et al., 1991), making it a clinically useful procedure in most contexts. Other approaches to identifying function, such as those that are based on antecedents (e.g., Carr and Durand, 1985), are also useful for identifying function but require a greater degree of inference in interpreting the results because the response-reinforcer relation is not directly tested. For this reason, we most often use the methodology described by Iwata et al. (1982/1994).

In a clinical context, function refers to the reinforcers that maintain destructive behaviors. Identifying the function permits clinicians to determine the menu of treatment procedures that should be most effective in reducing destructive behavior. Of equal importance, identifying function eliminates treatments that may be ineffective or counter-therapeutic. As described previously, exclusionary time-out in which a child is removed from a task may be highly effective when teacher attention is reinforcing. However, time-out may be counter-therapeutic when the child's behavior is maintained by escape from task demands.

Identifying function increases the probability of effective treatment because we no longer have to hope that an arbitrarily selected contingency will compete against the unknown contingency maintaining destructive behavior. Instead, we can match the treatment to the function of destructive behavior (Iwata, Pace, Kalsher, Cowdery, and Cataldo,1990); that is, the identified reinforcer can be discontinued for destructive behavior and provided contingently for desired behavior.

One important outcome of matching treatment to function is that reinforcement- based approaches to treatment have increased in the literature. Pelios, Morren, Tesch, and Axelrod (1999) reviewed articles from five peer-reviewed journals to examine the overall effects of functional analysis procedures on selection of treatments for self-injurious and/or aggressive behaviors. Pelios et al. reviewed articles published between 1963 and 1997 and found an increase in the use of reinforcement-based procedures across years beginning in the late 1980s; however, the use of punishment-based procedures remained fairly stable. They further examined the treatment of self-injury and aggression using reinforcement- and punishment-based procedures with and without pre-treatment functional analyses. They found that in studies in which a functional analysis identified maintaining variables for self-injury and aggression, reinforcement-based treatments were used more frequently than punishment-based treatments. These results suggest that identification of the maintaining variables for problem behavior may allow better use of reinforcement-based treatments because of a better understanding of the function of the behavior.

Epidemiological Studies of Functional Approaches to Treatment

Iwata, Pace, Dorsey, and colleagues (1994) summarized the results from 152 functional analyses of individuals with developmental disabilities referred for assessment and treatment of self-injury during an 11-year period. The total length of assessments ranged from 2 to 16.5 hr (average = 6.5 hr). The assessments were conducted while clients were inpatients in a pediatric hospital or were living in a state residential facility. The sessions were conducted two to eight times per day, usually 5 days per week. The results indicated that at least one maintaining condition was identified in 95.4% of the cases. The effects of intervention were also evaluated, with results indicating that when appropriate interventions were applied to the self-injury (i.e., the intervention was matched to the function of the behavior), there was a reduction in behavior to below 10% of baseline in over 80% of the cases. Interventions included antecedent manipulations (mostly noncontingent reinforcement), differential reinforcement, and extinction.

Wacker et al. (1998) summarized the results of functional analyses and treatments for 28 children (ages 1 through 6 years) with developmental disabilities who displayed problem behaviors. The assessments and treatments were conducted by parents in their homes with training from the researchers. The problem behaviors included self-injury, aggression, stereotypy, and property destruction. Functional analyses identified the maintaining condition(s) of the problem behaviors for 86% of the children. Treatment consisted of functional communication training, which involved teaching a communication response (e.g., vocal response, picture exchange) that served the same function as the problem behavior. For example, a child was taught to request attention by using a word card rather than by head banging. Following initiation of treatment, problem behavior decreased an average of 87%. Wacker and colleagues also reported improvements in the children's appropriate behaviors, such as use of appropriate communication, with improvements averaging a 69% increase above baseline.

Kurtz et al. (2003) summarized the results of functional analyses for children under the age of 5 years who engaged in problem behaviors that included self-injury and aggression and in dangerous behaviors, such as touching electrical outlets. The children's cognitive levels ranged from profound mental retardation to no developmental delays. The children received intensive outpatient services for 2 to 3 hours per day, usually 2 to 3 days per week for 12 to 16 weeks. Sources of reinforcement for all problem behaviors were identified in 87.5% of cases. Of the 24 children who completed treatment, self-injury and other problem behaviors were reduced by 95% and 87%, respectively. The most frequently prescribed intervention was functional communication training.

Asmus et al. (2004) summarized the results for 138 clients who were admitted for up to 10 days to an inpatient unit for assessment and treatment of severe behaviors. The clients ranged in age from 1 to 49 years and varied in levels of functioning (e.g., from normal development to severe or profound mental retardation). Behaviors included self-injury, aggression, stereotypy, destruction, disruption, pica, elopement, and rumination. Functional analyses were conducted for an average of 4 hours for each participant, but ranged from 50 min to 11 hr. A maintaining condition for problem behavior was identified for 96% of the clients. Selected treatments were based on the results of the functional analyses and were implemented for an average of 4 hours (range = 10 min to 13 hr). Following the initiation of treatment, problem behavior was reduced for 97% of all clients, with 76% of the clients showing a reduction of 80% or more in problem behavior.

In summary, functional analyses identified the categories of reinforcement (negative, positive, or automatic) that maintained destructive or other problem behavior for the majority of the participants in each of the four studies reviewed (see Table 1.1). Treatments that were selected based on functional analysis outcomes for each participant resulted in mean reductions in destructive behavior of at least 90% for most participants. The findings from these summary studies provide a strong empirical base for function-based approaches to the treatment of destructive behavior. However, these are only the summary studies; a very large empirical literature on functional analysis has developed since its initial dissemination in 1982. An August 2006 search of the *Journal of Applied Behavior Analysis* using the keywords "functional analysis" produced 348 results. This finding suggests that the identification of function has been a very active goal of behavioral researchers.

In the next two sections, we describe how we have applied function-based models of treatment with two distinct subgroups. The first subgroup was composed of children, 6 years or younger, whose parents conducted all assessment and treatment procedures in their homes. The majority (90%) of these children showed social functions, meaning that their behavior was maintained by positive or negative reinforcement.

Table 1.1. Summary of Epidemiological Studies

Study	% of cases with identified function	% of cases with identified social function	% of cases with at least 90% reduction of target behavior
Iwata et al. (1982/1994)	95	69.7	80
Wacker et al. (1998)	89	86	62.5
Kurtz et al. (2003)	87	83	79
Asmus et al. (2004)	96	89	66

The second subgroup was composed of both children and adults who showed automatic functions. All assessment and treatment procedures were conducted in an outpatient clinic setting by both trained therapists and care providers.

IN-HOME ASSESSMENT AND TREATMENT OF DESTRUCTIVE BEHAVIOR MAINTAINED BY SOCIAL REINFORCEMENT

Our research team at The University of Iowa Center for Disabilities and Development has conducted a series of research projects funded by the National Institute of Child Health and Human Development of the National Institutes of Health (Wacker and Berg, 1992; Wacker, Berg, and Harding, 1996; Wacker, Berg, and Harding, 2000; Wacker, Berg, and Harding, 2004). These projects have focused on the in-home assessment and treatment of young children (6 years of age or younger) with developmental disabilities who displayed severe destructive behavior such as self-injury and aggression. Referrals for participation in these projects have come from outpatient clinics at the University of Iowa Hospitals and Clinics and early childhood intervention teams from the children's communities.

During these projects, research team members scheduled weekly to monthly visits to participants' homes for up to 3 years. The parents served as therapists during in-home assessment and intervention procedures with coaching from project investigators. Research investigators provided instruction to parents, prescriptive feedback on conducting treatment sessions, and evaluations of the child's progress via ongoing graphical representations of data collected from videotapes of the assessment and intervention sessions.

ASSESSMENT AND TREATMENT PROCEDURES

Across all projects, the children's assessment and treatment were conducted in three phases (see Table 1.2). During Phase 1, we conducted a descriptive assessment (e.g., A-B-C assessment; Bijou, Peterson, and Ault, 1968) to acquire information about situations that were associated with destructive behavior. In Phase 2, we conducted a functional analysis (Iwata et al., 1982/1994) to identify conditions that maintained destructive behavior. During

Phase 3, we implemented a functional communication training program (Carr and Durand, 1985). We also asked parents to complete a treatment acceptability survey, *Treatment Acceptability Rating Form-Revised* (Reimers and Wacker, 1988 [TARF-R]), at the beginning and end of treatment.

Table 1.2. Assessment and Treatment Phases for Social Function Projects

Phase	Procedure	Purpose
Phase 1	Descriptive assessment: Daily behavior record Interview Preference assessment	Identify events associated with destructive behavior, generate hypotheses, and identify preferred toys
Phase 2	Functional analysis	Identify conditions that maintained destructive behavior
Phase 3	Functional communication training	Teach child to perform appropriate communicative behavior as an alternative to destructive behavior

Daily behavior record. During the first phase in our assessment, parents completed a daily behavior record for 7 days. These records gave us an indication of the frequency of destructive behavior throughout the day (Touchette, MacDonald, and Langer, 1985), the situations associated with destructive behavior, a description of the type of behavior that was displayed, and parental response to the behavior (Bijou et al., 1968). Discussing each of these elements with the parents gave us an emerging picture of the children's response to events that were part of their daily routines as well as their parents' efforts to manage the behavior.

The final step in our descriptive assessment phase was to ask parents to list the toys that were available to the child and to rate these toys with respect to preference. Our objective was to identify toys that might serve as reinforcers for adaptive behavior and tasks that might serve as non-preferred activities during assessment and treatment. To increase our confidence that we had identified preferred toys for our functional analysis, we conducted a direct preference assessment (Windsor, Piché, and Locke, 1994). During these conditions, the child was allowed to play with a selection of toys identified as both preferred and non-preferred, and the parent provided non-contingent attention. We used a 6-s partial interval recording system to record the percentage of intervals that the child engaged with each toy during 5-min sessions. This allowed us to identify preferred and less preferred toys based on the amount of time that the child played with each toy.

The results of our descriptive assessments often provided information that was useful for generating initial hypotheses regarding relations between child behavior and environmental events. However, in some cases, the results of the descriptive assessments were unclear with respect to the function of the behavior (Lerman and Iwata, 1993). To be more prescriptive in our treatment recommendations, we conducted a more rigorous evaluation of behavioral function via a functional analysis (Iwata et al., 1982/1994).

Functional analysis. During Phase 2, we conducted a functional analysis to test hypotheses regarding specific consequences that potentially maintained destructive behavior. The functional analysis consisted of a series of brief (e.g., 5-min) conditions in which the child was provided with a specific reinforcer (attention, tangible, or escape from demands) contingent on displaying destructive behavior. For example, during an attention condition, the parent was directed to ignore the child unless he or she engaged in destructive behavior. If destructive behavior occurred, then the parent provided a small amount of attention (e.g., "Stop doing that"). During a demand condition, the child was asked to complete an age-appropriate but non-preferred task (e.g., picking up toys). If destructive behavior occurred, the task was removed and the child was allowed a brief (20- to 30-s) break (negative reinforcement).

Test conditions were alternated with a free play (control) condition. During the free play condition, the child had access to preferred toys, the parent provided non-contingent attention, and no demands were presented to the child. Thus, during the control condition, we attempted to eliminate social motivation to engage in destructive behavior.

The free play and test conditions were conducted within a multielement design to demonstrate experimental control. For example, if destructive behavior consistently occurred during a demand condition but never during a free play condition, this indicated that the child's destructive behavior was occasioned by the presentation of a specific demand and maintained by negative reinforcement (i.e., escape from demands). We conducted the functional analysis conditions until we observed a consistent pattern of behavior, meaning that higher levels of destructive behavior occurred in one or more test conditions relative to the free play condition.

Functional communication training (FCT). We have used FCT (Carr and Durand, 1985) as a primary treatment program for most of the children in our projects. During FCT, we teach the child an appropriate communicative response (mand) to replace destructive behavior as a way for the child to obtain reinforcement. There are a number of important considerations in developing an effective FCT program. First, the mand must produce the reinforcers identified as maintaining destructive behavior (Durand and Carr, 1985). Second, the mand must be efficient (i.e., easy for the child to perform).

If the mand is more effortful for the child than destructive behavior, it is less likely that the child will use the mand (Horner and Day, 1991). Caregivers must be prepared to provide reinforcement as consistently as possible when the child is first learning the mand. Finally, destructive behavior must be placed on extinction. Destructive behavior that continues to produce reinforcement may persist.

It is also important to consider the form of the mand based on the child's speech and language abilities. Some children have difficulty emitting vocal responses but are capable of using a manual sign, word/picture card, or electronic device to communicate. In our projects, we typically provide the child with a multi-modal approach to communication. For example, if a child is being trained to ask for attention by saying or signing, "Mom," we attach a photograph of the parent and the word "Mom" to a microswitch recording device that emits, "Mom, play please," when activated.

Thus, the child has multiple cues regarding "what" to say and, if vocalizing is difficult, the child can touch the photograph on the microswitch. Furthermore, the presence of the picture/word card and the microswitch may serve as a discriminative stimulus for the child that communication will produce attention.

CASE EXAMPLE

Tina was a participant in our most recent project (Wacker et al., 2004). She was 3 years 11 months old and was diagnosed with ASD and developmental delays. Her language was limited to a few spoken words. Destructive behavior included aggression (hitting, kicking), property destruction (throwing objects), and noncompliance. Investigators visited Tina's home on a weekly basis over a 2-year period. Tina's mother served as the therapist for all procedures with investigator coaching. All procedures were videotaped for data collection and analysis.

A functional analysis was conducted to compare free play, attention, demand, and tangible conditions. A 6-s partial-interval recording system was used to measure the occurrence of destructive behavior. Figure 1.1 shows the mean percentage of intervals of destructive behavior that occurred during each of the conditions. These results showed that Tina's destructive behavior was maintained by escape from demands (negative reinforcement) and access to tangibles (positive reinforcement).

During treatment, we compared baseline and FCT conditions within a reversal design. During baseline, Tina's mother asked her to stack colored blocks during a series of eight trials conducted within each 5-min session. There were no programmed consequences for compliance, and Tina was not provided with any cues to communicate.

During FCT, Tina was shown a "work" picture/word card and was directed to sit at a desk. She was asked to stack one colored block. If she engaged in destructive behavior, her mother provided hand-over-hand assistance to complete the task and then presented Tina with another block. If she complied, she was shown a microswitch recording device with a "play" picture/word card attached. Touching the card activated the recorded message, "Play, please." If Tina touched the switch, she was given a 1-min break to play with her toys, and her mother provided attention.

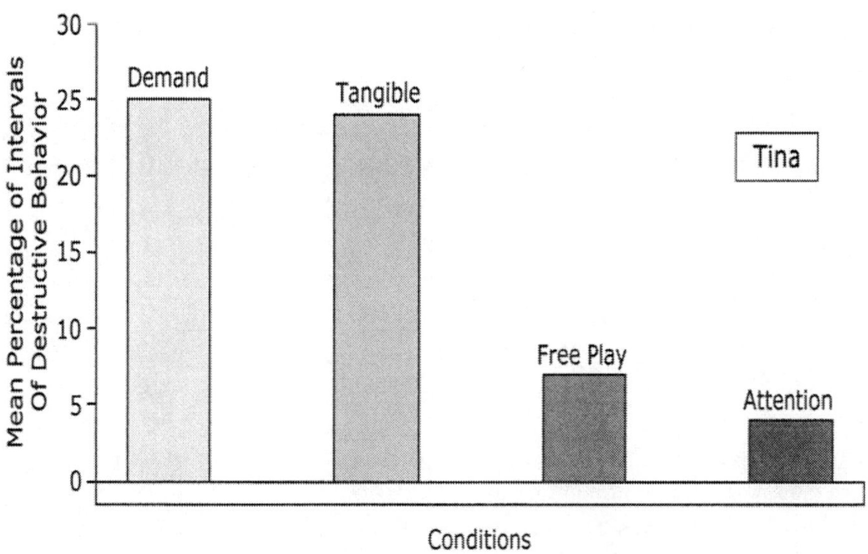

Figure 1.1. Mean percentage of intervals of destructive behavior during functional analysis conditions for Tina.

At the end of her break, she was again shown the "work" card and directed back to her desk for another trial. Initially, the objective was for Tina to complete two task requests during each 5-min session. Over time, her task requirements were increased to baseline levels (eight task requests).

A summary of the results of Tina's functional communication training program over a 12-month period is shown in Figure 1.2. These results compared mean percentages of destructive behavior during repeated baseline sessions with three consecutive FCT sessions that were conducted immediately after the baseline sessions. Data from these two conditions are shown at the beginning of treatment and at approximately 3-month intervals over a 1-year period. In each of these comparisons, destructive behavior is at a higher level during the baseline condition than during the following FCT condition. Thus, Tina's performance was better when the FCT program was implemented.

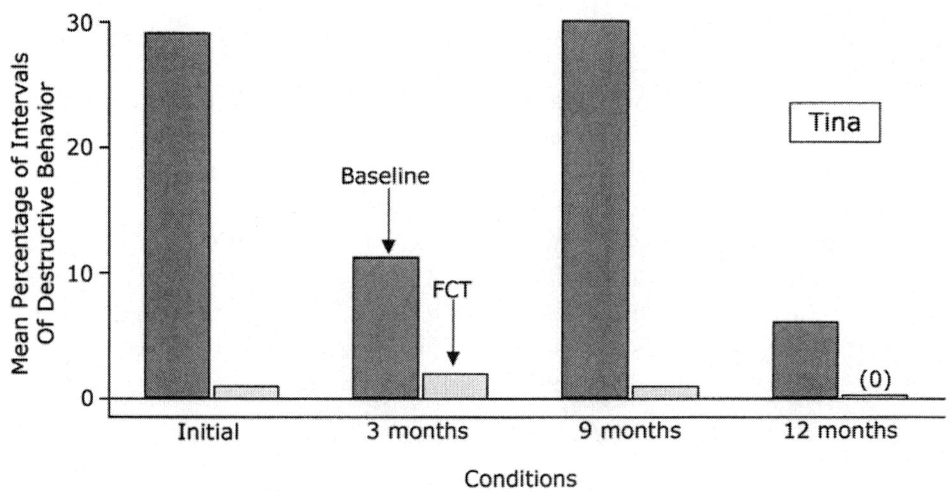

Figure 1.2. Mean percentage of intervals of destructive behavior during baseline and functional communication training conditions for Tina.

Assessment and Treatment Results for Children Diagnosed with ASD

To date we have enrolled 86 children in our research projects. Of these 86 children, 17 children (13 boys, 4 girls) were diagnosed with autism (9) or pervasive developmental disorder (8). The average age of this subgroup was 4 years 6 months (range = 2 years, 8 months to 6 years, 6 months), and estimated intellectual functioning ranged from mild delays to moderate mental retardation. All 17 children displayed destructive behavior such as self-injury, aggression, and property destruction, as well as other forms of problem behavior such as screaming, elopement, and noncompliance.

A functional analysis was conducted with all 17 children. Thirteen children displayed destructive behavior that was maintained by both positive and negative reinforcement, 2 children showed behavior that was maintained by positive reinforcement, 1 child showed destructive behavior maintained by negative reinforcement, and 1 child displayed an undifferentiated pattern of responding. Thus, 16 of the 17 children displayed destructive behavior that was maintained by social contingencies.

Although the children with ASD represented a distinct diagnostic subgroup, there were no major differences between these children and the other children in the research projects with respect to parent involvement, treatment outcomes, or parent ratings of treatment acceptability. Final treatment results were available for 72 children who showed an average decrease in destructive behavior of 90%.

Final treatment outcomes were available for 14 of the children diagnosed with ASD. Twelve of these children showed a 90% to 100% decrease in destructive behavior compared to baseline levels, 1 child showed an 87% decrease, and 1 child did not show improvement during treatment probes. The mean reduction in destructive behavior across all 14 children was 90%. Thus, the overall effects of FCT for the ASD group were similar to the overall group.

Parent satisfaction with the program was evaluated by asking parents to complete the *Treatment Acceptability Rating Form-Revised* (Reimers and Wacker, 1988 [TARF-R]). With regard to the question, "How acceptable do you find the treatment to be regarding your concerns about your child?," parents responded by indicating a number on a Likert scale of (1) *Not at all acceptable* to (7) *Very acceptable*. The average rating on this question across all participants was 6.37 (range = 4 to 7). For parents who had children diagnosed with ASD, the average rating on this question was 6.7 (range = 6 to 7). These results show that in addition to being effective, the assessment and treatment procedures were rated as being highly acceptable.

Clinic-Based Assessment and Treatment of Problem Behavior Maintained by Automatic Reinforcement

As demonstrated by the results reported in epidemiological studies (Asmus et al., 2004; Iwata et al., 1982/1994; Kurtz et al., 2003; Wacker et al., 1998), the combination of functional analyses of destructive behavior and function-based treatments has been an effective approach for reducing destructive behaviors and increasing adaptive responses. In the majority of cases, functional analyses identify social reinforcers (attention, escape from demands, or access to tangibles) that maintain destructive behaviors. In these cases, the results of the functional analysis are prescriptive for treatment because the response-reinforcer relationship maintaining destructive behavior has been identified, and treatments can be arranged to weaken that relationship and strengthen more adaptive responses. In some cases, however, the results of the functional analysis show that destructive responses occur primarily when the person is alone without leisure or work materials or occur in an undifferentiated pattern across all functional analysis test and control conditions. These two patterns of results are problematic in that specific response-reinforcer relationships are not identified, and no direction is provided for selecting a reinforcement-based treatment. In these cases, the function of destructive behavior is described as being automatic because it appears that engaging in the behavior results in its own reinforcement rather than a change in the environment (e.g., increasing the delivery of attention or decreasing the delivery of task demands).

Individuals whose functional analysis results fit these two patterns have been the focus of two research projects at the Center for Disabilities and Development at The University of Iowa (Berg, Ringdahl, Wacker, and Bosch, 2000; Berg, Wacker, Ringdahl, and Bosch, 2003). One purpose of this line of research has been to evaluate the effectiveness of additional assessment procedures in prescribing treatment approaches to reduce the occurrence of destructive behaviors maintained by automatic reinforcement. The evaluations of destructive behavior have been conducted in four phases: Phases 1 through 3 are assessment phases, and Phase 4 is the treatment phase (see Table 1.3).

The three assessment phases evaluate the occurrence of destructive responses across different reinforcement schedules. Phase 1 is a functional analysis of destructive behaviors and is conducted using the procedures described in Iwata et al. (1982/1994). The purpose of Phase 1 is to determine whether the contingent delivery of social reinforcers for destructive responses results in differentiated responding across assessment conditions. Only those participants whose functional analysis results fit the patterns identified for automatic reinforcement were enrolled in this project. Phase 2 involves a pairwise comparison (Iwata, Duncan, Zarcone, Lerman, and Shore, 1994) of destructive behavior in the absence of social contingencies across two functional analysis control conditions (play, in which the participant has noncontingent access to attention and preferred materials, and alone/ignore, in which no attention or materials are provided to the participant). The purpose of this phase is to evaluate the persistence of destructive responses in the presence and absence of alternative stimuli. Phase 3 is a concurrent operants assessment (Harding et al., 1999) in which access to social reinforcers is provided contingent on one response, and access to destructive behavior (automatic reinforcers) is provided contingent on an alternative response. In this phase, access to each type of reinforcer (social or automatic) is mutually exclusive. Destructive responses are blocked if the participant engages in the response associated with social reinforcers, and social reinforcers are withheld if the participant engages in the response associated with automatic reinforcers.

Table 1.3. Assessment and Treatment Phases for Automatic Function Projects

Phase	Procedure	Purpose
Phase 1	Functional analysis of destructive behavior	Identify the reinforcers that maintain destructive responding.
Phase 2	Pairwise comparison	Assess the occurrence of destructive responses in the absence of social contingencies both with (play) and without (alone) social stimuli.
Phase 3	Concurrent operants	Identify social reinforcers that the participant selects to the exclusion of automatic reinforcers.
Phase 4	Treatment	Evaluate the effectiveness of treatment procedures prescribed from the results of Phases 1 – 3 in reducing destructive behavior.

Results of the three-phase assessment procedure are used to assign each participant to one of three treatment approaches. The first category of treatment consists of providing noncontingent access (NCR) to alternative social reinforcers. (e.g., Ringdahl, Vollmer,

Marcus, and Roane, 1997; Shore, Iwata, DeLeon, Khang, and Smith, 1997; Vollmer, 1997). The hypotheses guiding selection of these treatments are that (a) dense schedules of social reinforcers will alleviate the establishing operations associated with automatic reinforcement, or (b) the social reinforcers will overwhelm the automatic reinforcers through reinforcer competition.

The second treatment approach is based on making access to social reinforcers contingent on the absence of destructive behaviors (differential reinforcement; e.g., Falcomata, Roane, Hovanetz, Kettering, and Keeney, 1997; Vollmer, 1994). These treatments are based on the hypothesis that some social reinforcers are of greater value to the individual than the automatic reinforcers maintaining destructive responding. It is expected that access to these social reinforcers contingent on the absence of the destructive response or contingent on engagement in a response that is incompatible with the destructive response will decrease destructive responding and increase the occurrence of the incompatible response.

The final treatment approach involves blocking the participant's access to the destructive responses, thereby blocking access to the automatic reinforcers maintaining the destructive responses (e.g., Fisher, Lindauer, Alterson, and Thompson, 1998; Rincover, Cook, Peoples, and Packard, 1979; Roscoe, Iwata, and Goh, 1998). This third approach to treatment is a default treatment and is prescribed only when we cannot identify social reinforcers that compete with destructive behavior during Assessment Phases 2 and 3. We hypothesize that blocking the participant's access to automatic reinforcers will weaken the response-reinforcer relationship maintaining destructive responding. We also hypothesize that the participants will increase their engagement with social reinforcers when access to automatic reinforcers is prevented.

The effectiveness of each prescribed treatment was evaluated on a monthly basis over a 6-month (Berg et al., 2000) or 12-month (Berg et al., 2003) period. Data were collected on the occurrence of destructive and adaptive responding during probes of the treatment sessions. In addition, data were collected during probes in which the treatment component hypothesized to reduce problem behavior was temporarily removed from the treatment package. Comparisons of the occurrence of destructive and adaptive responding in the presence and absence of the different treatment components provided information on the operant mechanisms responsible for reductions in destructive behavior.

To date, we have enrolled 32 participants across the two projects. Eleven of these participants were diagnosed with autism. The participants with autism ranged in age from 5 to 49 years, and all were diagnosed with mental retardation (moderate to profound). Of these participants, 11 engaged in self-injury, 8 engaged in property destruction, and 11 engaged in stereotypy that interfered with participation in daily activities (all participants engaged in more than one topography of destructive behavior). See Table 1.4 for a complete list of destructive behaviors for the 11 participants.

Functional analysis results showed that all participants engaged in destructive behavior across test and control conditions during the functional analysis, but 1 participant engaged in destructive behavior primarily during the alone conditions of the pairwise analysis and engaged in little to no destructive behavior during the play control condition. This participant received treatment based on noncontingent access to preferred leisure items. Nine participants received treatments based on differential reinforcement in which access to attention and/or preferred leisure items was contingent on the absence of destructive behavior, and 1 received a treatment that included response blocking of destructive responding and differential reinforcement (preferred leisure materials and attention).

Table 1.4. Percentage of Participants with Autism (N = 11) who Engaged in Specific Topographies of Destructive Behavior

Topography of behavior	Definition of behavior	% of participants
Self-injury	Any of the following behaviors displayed in a manner that could produce tissue damage:	100
Hit/slap head or body	Contact between a closed fist or open palm against any part of the head or body	73
Rub or scratch ear, face, or neck	Any part of the hand making contact with the face, neck, or ears in a back and forth movement that occurs more than two times before the hand is removed	55
Bite hands or arms	Contact between the teeth and hand or arm	55
Mouth or bite objects	Contact between the lips or teeth and non-edible materials	36
Bang head on surface	Contact between the head and a hard surface as a result of movement of the head	36
Hit surface with hands, arms, legs or feet	Contact between the hand, arm, leg, or foot against a hard surface as a result of movement of the body part	27
Drop to floor	Rapid movement from a sitting or standing position to lying on the floor	9
Eye gouge	Insertion of finger into the eye socket	9
Stereotypy	Any of the following behaviors displayed in a manner that interfered with daily activities:	100
Repetitive movements with object	Holding object in the hand and shaking the object, twirling the object, or dropping the object to the floor in a repetitive manner	91
Jump or bounce	Repetitive vertical movement of the body that results in momentary loss of contact between the floor and the person's feet or knees	36
Repetitive movements with hands	Repetitive, non-functional, rapid movements of the hands without making contact with other body parts or items	55
Rock body	Moving body back and forth in a repetitive manner while seated	27
Scream	Repeated loud vocalizations with or without tears	73
Property destruction	Any of the following behaviors:	64
Throw objects	Contact of the hand with an object that results in the object being moved away from the body rapidly and contacting another surface	45
Destroy items	Bending, tearing, or breaking item with the hands	36
Aggression	Contact of the hands, feet, or mouth with another person that has the potential to cause tissue damage to the other person. Aggressive behaviors did not fit the patterns associated with automatic reinforcement and were not targeted for intervention in this project.	64

Treatment has been completed with 10 of these 11 participants. A summary of the results for each treatment procedure is provided in Table 1.5.

Table 1.5. Treatments Prescribed Based on the Results of the Three-Phase assessment Model and Treatment in Automatic Function Projects

Treatment Procedure	Noncontingent access to preferred stimuli (NCR)	Differential access to preferred stimuli contingent on the absence of destructive behavior (DR)	Differential access to preferred stimuli plus physical blocking of destructive responses (RB + DR)
Number of participants assigned to treatment	1	8	2
Number of participants who have completed treatment	1	6	1
Mean % reduction in destructive behavior from Phase 1 and 2 alone conditions to final three treatment sessions for the participants who have completed treatment	97	89	96

The NCR treatment resulted in a 97% reduction in destructive behavior for the 1 participant who received this treatment. Treatments based on differential reinforcement (DR) resulted in a mean reduction in destructive behavior of 91% for the 8 participants who completed these treatments. One participant completed treatment that was based on response blocking plus differential reinforcement (RB+DR) and showed a 96% reduction in destructive behavior at the end of treatment. Overall, of the 10 participants who completed treatment, 80% showed a reduction in problem behavior of at least 90% for an overall reduction of 92%. These results are similar to those obtained for behavior maintained by social reinforcement described in the previous section and support the benefits of basing treatments on a prescriptive assessment.

Summary and Directions for Future Research

In this chapter, we provided two examples of our current longitudinal research that show the clinical benefits of basing treatment on the assessed functions of destructive behavior. Our goal in both projects was to arrange the environment so that the child's responding was biased toward appropriate topographies of responding to gain social reinforcers rather than toward destructive topographies of responding. Our results to date suggest that this approach to treatment is often effective and is applicable across functions, distinct topographies of destructive behavior, settings, and distinct subgroups (e.g., children and adults). Although these results are encouraging, further research is needed to better understand why these results have occurred and to promote generalization and maintenance.

Within each project, we used a multi-component package of procedures, and further research is needed to determine which components are active at different points in treatment. For example, in the first project on social functions, the treatment package consisted of (a) stimulus control (e.g., the presence of a picture), (b) differential reinforcement, (c) extinction, and (d) demand fading. Although this package was effective for most participants, it remains unclear if individual components were active (affected responding) at any given point in treatment or changed over the course of treatment, or if all were needed to achieve the results. An analysis of each component at different points in treatment might identify some of the conditions that are necessary for maintenance or that are related to the resurgence in destructive behavior that often occurs following successful treatment.

Relative to our project on automatic functions, the competition between social and automatic reinforcers appears to be a key component, but our understanding of why successful competition occurs for any given individual is still incomplete. Matching the sensory consequences obtained from alternative stimuli with those inferred to be obtained from destructive behavior has proven promising but continues to result in inconsistent findings (Ahearn, Clark, DeBar, and Florentino, 2005). Similarly, the dimensions of reinforcement (e.g., effort) that underlie the different effects of noncontingent and differential reinforcement schedules on destructive behavior warrant further study.

In general, we suggest that sufficient applications of function-based models of treatment have been disseminated in the literature to support this approach to treatment. Second generation studies need to focus on the behavioral mechanisms that underlie or disrupt these results at different points in treatment.

ACKNOWLEDGMENTS

This chapter was supported, in part, by Grant #R01 HD029402-15 and Grant #SR01 HD042813-04 from the National Institute of Child Health and Human Development of the National Institutes of Health. The opinions expressed do not necessarily reflect the position or policy of that agency. We express our appreciation to the families who participated in these projects, to Agnes DeRaad for her editing and preparation of the chapter, and John Lee for his graphics expertise. Correspondence should be addressed to David P. Wacker, Ph.D., Center for Disabilities and Development, 100 Hawkins Dr, Rm 251, Iowa City, IA 52241; david-wacker@uiowa.edu.

REFERENCES

Ahearn, W. K., Clark, K. M., DeBar, R., and Florentino, C. (2005). On the role of preference in response competition. *Journal of Applied Behavior Analysis, 38,* 247-250.

Asmus, J. M., Ringdahl, J. E., Sellers, J. A., Call, N. A., Andelman, M. S., and Wacker, D. P. (2004). Use of a short-term inpatient model to evaluate aberrant behavior: Outcomes data summaries from 1996 to 2001. *Journal of Applied Behavior Analysis, 37,* 283-304.

Berg, W. K., Ringdahl, J. E., Wacker, D. P., and Bosch, J. (2000). *Competing stimuli and automatic reinforcement.* Department of Human Services. National Institute of Child Health and Human Development.

Berg. W. K., Wacker, D. P., Ringdahl, J. E., and Bosch, J. (2003). *Competing stimuli and automatic reinforcement.* Department of Human Services. National Institute of Child Health and Human Development.

Bijou, S. W., Peterson, R. F., and Ault, M. H. (1968). A method to integrate descriptive and experimental field studies at the level of data and empirical concepts. *Journal of Applied Behavior Analysis*, 1, 175-191.

Carr, E. G. (1977). The motivation of self-injurious behavior: A review of some hypotheses. *Psychological Bulletin,* 84, 800-816.

Carr, E. G., and Durand, V. M. (1985). Reducing behavior problems through functional communication training. *Journal of Applied Behavior Analysis*, 18, 111-126.

Carr, E. G., Newsom, C. D., and Binkoff, J. A. (1980). Escape as a factor in the aggressive behavior of two retarded children. *Journal of Applied Behavior Analysis,* 13, 101-117.

Cataldo, M. F. (1989) Punishment and behavior reducing procedures on the destructive behavior of persons with developmental disabilities. In *National Institutes of Mental Health Consensus Development Conference* (NIH Publication No. 91-2410), 231-341.

Day, R. M., Rea, J. A., Schussler, N. G., Larsen, S. E., and Johnson, W. L. (1988). A functionally based approach to the treatment of self-injurious behavior. *Behavior Modification,* 12, 565-589.

Durand, V. M., and Carr, E. G. (1985). Self-injurious behavior; Motivating conditions and guidelines for treatment. *School Psychology Review,* 14, 171-176.

Falcomata, T. S., Roane H. S., Hovanetz, A. N., Kettering, T. L., and Keeney, K. M. (2004). An evaluation of response cost in the treatment of inappropriate vocalizations maintained by automatic reinforcement. *Journal of Applied Behavior Analysis,* 37, 83-87.

Fisher, W. W., Lindauer, S. E., Alterson, C. J., and Thompson, R. H. (1998). Assessment and treatment of destructive behavior maintained by stereotypic object manipulation. *Journal of Applied Behavior Analysis,* 31, 513-527.

Harding, J. W., Wacker, D. P., Berg, W. K., Cooper, L. J., Asmus, J. A., Mlela, K., et al. (1999). An analysis of choice making in the assessment of young children with severe behavior problems. *Journal of Applied Behavior Analysis,* 32, 63-82.

Horner, R. H., and Day, H. M. (1991). The effects of response efficiencies on functionally equivalent competing behaviors. *Journal of Applied Behavior Analysis*, 24, 719-732.

Iwata, B. A., Dorsey, M. F., Slifer, K. J., Bauman, K. E., and Richman, G. S. (1982/1994). Toward a functional analysis of self-injury. *Journal of Applied Behavior Analysis*, 27, 197-209. (Reprinted from *Analysis and Intervention in Developmental Disabilities*, 2, 3-20, 1982).

Iwata, B. A., Duncan, B. A., Zarcone, J. R., Lerman, D. C., and Shore, B. A. (1994) A sequential, test-control methodology for conducting functional analyses of self-injurious behavior. *Behavior Modification,* 18, 289-306.

Iwata B. A., Pace, G. M., Dorsey, M. F., Zarcone, J. R., Vollmer, T. R., Smith R.G., et al. (1994). The functions of self-injurious behavior: An experimental epidemiological analysis. *Journal of Applied Behavior Analysis,* 27, 215–240.

Iwata, B. A., Pace, G. M., Kalsher, M. J., Cowdery, G. E., and Cataldo, M. F. (1990). Experimental analysis and extinction of self-injurious behavior. *Journal of Applied Behavior Analysis,* 23, 11–27.

Iwata, B. A., Vollmer, T. R., Zarcone, J. R., and Rodgers, T. A. (1993). Treatment classification and selection based on behavioral function. In R. Van Houten and S. Axelrod (Eds.), *Behavior analysis and treatment* (pp. 101-125). New York: Plenum Press.

Kurtz, P. F., Chin, M. D., Huete, J. M., Tarbox, R. S. F., O'Connor, J. T., Paclawskyj, T. R., et al. (2003). Functional analysis and treatment of self-injurious behavior in young children: A summary of 30 cases. *Journal of Applied Behavior Analysis*, 6, 205-219.

Lerman, D. C., and Iwata, B. A. (1993). Descriptive and experimental analysis of variables maintaining self-injurious behavior. *Journal of Applied Behavior Analysis*, 26, 293-319.

Lovaas, O. I., Newsom, C., and Hickman, C. (1987). Self-stimulatory behavior and perceptual reinforcement. *Journal of Applied Behavior Analysis,* 20, 45-68.

Lovaas, O. I., and Simmons, J. Q. (1969). Manipulation of self-destruction in three retarded children. *Journal of Applied Behavioral Analysis*, 2, 143–157.

Northup, J., Wacker, D., Sasso, G., Steege, M., Cigrand, K., Cook, J., et al. (1991). A brief functional analysis of aggressive and alternative behavior in an outclinic setting. *Journal of Applied Behavior Analysis,* 24, 509-522.

Pelios, L., Morren, J., Tesch, D., and Axelrod, S. (1999). The impact of functional analysis methodology on treatment choice for self-injurious and aggressive behavior. *Journal of Applied Behavior Analysis*, 32, 185-195.

Reimers, T., and Wacker, D. (1988). Parents' ratings of the acceptability of behavioral treatment recommendations made in an outpatient clinic: A preliminary analysis of the influence of treatment effectiveness. *Behavioral Disorders*, 14, 7-15.

Rincover, A., Cook, R., Peoples, A., and Packard, D. (1979). Sensory extinction and sensory reinforcement principles for programming multiple adaptive behavior change. *Journal of Applied Behavior Analysis,* 12, 221-233.

Ringdahl, J. E., Vollmer, T. R., Marcus, B. A., and Roane, H. S. (1997). An analogue evaluation of environmental enrichment: The role of stimulus preference. *Journal of Applied Behavior Analysis,* 30, 203-216.

Roscoe, E. M., Iwata, B. A., and Goh, H. (1998). A comparison of noncontingent reinforcement and sensory extinction as treatments for self-injurious behavior. *Journal of Applied Behavior Analysis,* 31, 635-646.

Shore, B. A., Iwata, B. A., DeLeon, I. G., Kahng, S., and Smith, R. G. (1997). An analysis of reinforcer substitutability using object manipulation and self-injury as competing responses. *Journal of Applied Behavior Analysis,* 30, 21-40.

Tassé, M. J. (2006). Functional behavioural assessment in people with intellectual disabilities [mental retardation and developmental disorders]. *Current Opinion in Psychiatry*, 19, 475-480.

Touchette, P. E., MacDonald, R. F., and Langer, S. N. (1985). A scatter plot for identifying stimulus control of destructive behavior. *Journal of Applied Behavior Analysis*, 18, 343-351.

Vollmer T. R. (1994). The concept of automatic reinforcement: Implications for behavioral research in developmental disabilities. *Research in Developmental Disabilities,* 15, 187-207.

Wacker, D. P., and Berg, W. K. (1992). *Inducing reciprocal parent/child interactions.* Washington, DC: Department of Health and Human Services, National Institute of Child Health and Human Development.

Wacker, D. P., Berg, W. K., and Harding, J. W. (1996). *Promoting stimulus generalization with young children.* Washington, DC: Department of Health and Human Services, National Institute of Child Health and Human Development.

Wacker, D. P., Berg, W. K., and Harding, J. W. (2000). *Functional communication training augmented with choices*. Washington, DC: Department of Health and Human Services, National Institute of Child Health and Human Development.

Wacker, D. P., Berg, W. K., and Harding, J. W. (2004). *Maintenance effects of functional communication training.* Washington, DC: Department of Health and Human Services, National Institute of Child Health and Human Development.

Wacker, D. P., Berg, W. K., Harding, J. W., Derby, K. M., Asmus, J. M., and Healy, A. (1998). Evaluation and long-term treatment of aberrant behavior displayed by young children with disabilities. *Journal of Developmental and Behavioral Pediatrics,* 19, 260-266.

Windsor, J., Piché, L. M., and Locke, P. A. (1994). Preference testing: A comparison of two presentation methods. *Research in Developmental Disabilities*, 15, 439-455.

In: Behavioral Theories and Interventions for Autism
Editor: Phil Reed
ISBN 978-1-60741-165-9
© 2009 Nova Science Publishers, Inc.

Chapter 2

STIMULUS OVERSELECTIVITY IN DISCRIMINATION LEARNING

William V. Dube
University of Massachusetts Medical School – Shriver Center
Waltham, Massachusetts, USA

During the 1960's, O. I. Lovaas and his colleagues initiated a program of behavioral analysis and intervention with children who had been diagnosed with autism. One aspect of the children's behavior was described as follows: "Operationally, our data show that when autistic children are presented with multiple stimulus inputs, their behavior comes under the control of a range of input that is too restricted. This problem was referred to as 'stimulus overselectivity' (Lovaas, Schreibman, Koegel, and Rhem, 1971) because the children overselected a limited number of stimuli from those available in their environment" (Lovaas, Koegel, and Schreibman, 1979, p. 1237). Overselectivity seems consistent with characteristics of Autistic Spectrum Disorders (ASD) identified in the *Diagnostic and Statistical Manual of Mental Disorders* (APA, 2000): abnormally restricted patterns of interest, persistent preoccupation with parts of objects, and lack of variation in play. Perhaps less obviously, overselectivity may also be related to impairments in social interaction and communication; these will be considered later in this chapter.

The experimental methods used by Lovaas and colleagues to define the problem most often involved initial discrimination training with multi-element stimuli followed by testing with the individual elements to determine how many of those elements had gained stimulus control of behavior. For example, if initial training established stimulus ABC as positive and XYZ as negative, tests would present the various combinations of individual elements, A vs. Y, B vs. X, etc. When given such tests, typically developing children are highly likely to respond correctly to all combinations of elements, but children with developmental disabilities may respond to only a subset of elements (e.g., Wilhelm and Lovaas, 1976). It seems important to note that overselectivity was defined in relation to the typical range of controlling stimuli for a given subject population. Given a sufficiently large number of relevant features or elements, a rapid increase in task difficulty, or some concurrent and distracting activity, a failure to establish stimulus control by some subset of available stimuli could be predicted for any subject population, including intellectually normal adults (e.g.,

Dube, Balsamo, Fowler, Dickson, Lombard, and Tomanari, 2006; McHugh and Reed, 2007; Reed, 2006; Reed and Gibson, 2005). Limitations on the range or breadth of stimulus control constitute a learning problem when they are atypically restricted.

Overselectivity Problem Areas

One problem associated with overselectivity in special-education settings is sometimes referred to as prompt dependency. When supplemental cues are given to prompt new learning (e.g., as in modeling use of a selection-based communication device), the student may seem to attend only to the prompt (e.g., the teacher's pointing finger) and not to the training stimulus. Failures of stimulus control transfer from prompts and supplemental cues to teaching materials will result if stimulus control is restricted to the prompt. This problem may be especially evident with extra-stimulus prompts like pointing cues, where the prompting stimulus is physically separate from the target stimulus (e.g., Schreibman, Charlop, and Koegel, 1982).

More broadly, children with developmental disabilities may experience problems associated with stimulus overselectivity in social and communicative behavior. Social behavior could be affected if the student identifies other people on the basis of a limited number of cues. For example, Schreibman (1997) described cases in which children with ASD suddenly failed to recognize familiar people when there was a change in some personal feature that would not challenge identification for typically developing children, such as a change in eyeglasses or hairstyle.

Laboratory studies provide some supporting evidence for this with stimuli that depict people. Schreibman and Lovaas (1973) tested typically developing children and children with ASD in a discrimination task with realistic dolls as stimuli. On test trials, stimulus control by various features of the dolls was evaluated by switching those features between the two dolls. Typically developing children identified dolls by their heads, but children with ASD were just as likely to do so by idiosyncratic cues such as an item of clothing.

Dickson, Wang, Lombard, and Dube (2006b) found overselectivity in a matching-to-sample task with six digital images of adult faces. Participants were students at a residential special-education school. After verifying accurate discrimination of the six different images, test trials were presented in which one feature of the correct stimulus was added to one of the incorrect stimuli, for example, a hat that was present in the correct stimulus was also added to one of the incorrect stimuli. The results showed overselectivity in several participants with ASD, but an unexpected finding was a lack of control by specific features in these individuals, for example, stimulus control by a woman's eyeglasses on one trial, but her scarf on another trial. Only one participant showed overselectivity for a consistent feature (hats), and this individual was not diagnosed with ASD.

Deficits in the acquisition of language and communication skills may be related to overselectivity in discriminations of auditory (vocal speech) or visual (e.g., printed words) cues (e.g., Koegel, Schreibman, Britten, and Laitinen, 1979). For example, it may be discovered that the student who had apparently learned to recognize her printed name was actually responding to the initial letter only. The material to be presented in this chapter will include research findings that are directly relevant to overselectivity with visual multi-stimulus arrays such as printed words.

OVERSELECTIVITY IN DISCRIMINATION LEARNING

This chapter will address the problem of stimulus overselectivity within the context of discrimination learning, and with an emphasis on discrete-trials instruction for individuals with developmental disabilities such as ASD and mental retardation. Discrete-trials instruction usually consists of a series of trials on which the teacher presents stimuli and the student responds to those stimuli. Each response can be judged as correct or incorrect, and learning is often measured by an accuracy score. Ordinarily, some form of positive reinforcement follows correct responses, and there is a short (e.g., 2-5 s) pause between trials.

The focus on discrete-trials instruction is not intended to suggest that it is superior to other forms of instruction (cf. discussions of the relative merits of stimulus selection-based vs. topography-based communication systems; Sundberg and Sundberg, 1990; Vignes, 2007), nor that its sole use constitutes a sufficient instructional program. Rather, the discrete-trials approach is one useful component of a comprehensive special-education program. (In some ways discrete-trials instruction seems analogous to a jazz musician's practice routines for scales, arpeggios, and other patterns of notes. The mechanical exercises are not the music, but this type of practice provides a foundation to support musical improvisation.) As Sigafoos, O'Reilly, Schlosser, and Lancioni (2007) pointed out recently, the relation between discrete-trials and naturalistic training approaches need not be seen as a dichotomy but may be better cast as a continuum (see also Prizant and Wetherby, 1998). There are a number of approaches toward integrating the two styles of instruction. A good example of a parallel integration of the two approaches is seen in Kasari, Freeman, and Paparella (2006), a study that examined interventions to improve joint attention or symbolic play in preschool children with ASD. Each intervention session began with a brief period of discrete-trials training that focused on a specific behavior or skill. Then, the experimenter and child immediately moved on to a semi-structured play session during which the targeted skill was incorporated into naturally occurring opportunities. Thompson (2007) describes a more serial relation between discrete trials and naturalistic teaching. He observed that discrete-trial teaching is often useful early in therapy or instruction, especially with children who have severe intellectual disabilities and problems attending to instruction. Then, after some period of initial training, skills that were first taught by discrete-trial methods may be embedded in typical daily routines. Sundberg and Partington (1999) have proposed that discrete-trials and naturalistic training target different types of expressive language (e.g., discrete-trials for identifying objects, naturalistic training for requesting desired objects). Because of this, the relative emphasis on each type training procedure may shift back and forth during language instruction as teaching objectives change over time.

Because the response requirements for discrete trials procedures are not complex – perhaps simply pointing to a stimulus – they are practical for special-education students who have relatively severe learning difficulties. For example, teaching via discrete-trials procedures can contribute to overall educational goals by building and elaborating networks of stimulus-stimulus relations, independently of other forms of instruction designed to establish and refine response forms such as speech or writing.

Simple-discrimination tasks. The behavior established by *simple discrimination* learning tasks may be analyzed in terms of the three-term operant contingency: discriminative stimulus, response, reinforcing stimulus. Simultaneous simple-discrimination tasks involve a series of trials with a choice between two or more stimuli on each trial (successive simple-discrimination tasks, sometimes referred to as "go/no-go" tasks, are not considered here; e.g., Matthews, Shute, and Rees, 2001). One stimulus is always correct (S+), and the other(s) are always incorrect (S-). Because of the invariant S+ and S- stimulus functions, the simple-discrimination procedure has limited utility for delivering instruction in educational settings (e.g., identifying the appropriate symbols for public restrooms). Simple-discrimination training has also been useful as an early component in some programmed methods to teach matching-to-sample tasks (e.g., Dube, Iennaco, Rocco, Kledaras, and McIlvane, 1992; Dube and Serna, 1998; Saunders and Spradlin, 1989, 1990).

Matching-to-sample tasks. Perhaps the most common format for discrete-trials instruction is the matching-to-sample (MTS) procedure. MTS is a form of multiple-choice testing. On each trial, the student is presented with a sample stimulus (equivalent to the question) and an array of two or more comparison stimuli (the multiple choices). The sample may be an auditory or visual stimulus, and the comparison stimuli are usually visual. For example, on an auditory-visual MTS trial, the sample may be the word "Cat" spoken by the teacher, and the comparison array may be pictures of a cat (S+), dog (S-), and horse (S-). On the next trial, the sample may be "Dog," and thus the dog picture becomes S+ and the cat picture is S-. This is a *conditional discrimination* because the discriminative stimulus functions of the comparison stimuli change conditionally upon the sample for each trial. The behavior may be analyzed as an elaboration of the three-term contingency with the addition of stimuli (the samples) that signal the trial-to-trial changes in S+ and S- stimulus functions of the comparison stimuli. For a visual-visual MTS procedure, the sample is a visual stimulus that may remain displayed for the entire trial (*simultaneous* matching to sample) or removed before the comparisons are presented (*delayed* matching to sample; DMTS). For example, a visual-visual MTS trial may present a picture of three dots as the sample and the printed numerals 2, 3, and 4 as the comparison stimuli.

Relational stimulus control is required for accurate MTS performance because it involves stimulus-stimulus relations between sample and comparison stimuli. These include relations that have been termed *select* and *reject* (Carrigan and Sidman, 1992), or *sample/S+* and *sample/S-* (e.g., Dube and McIlvane, 1996), and these terms refer to relations between the sample and the correct and incorrect comparisons, respectively. Although sometimes taken for granted, sample/S- relations are necessary to account for all of the behavior that occurs within a matching-to-sample session. With three comparison stimuli, for example, the chances are only one in three that the first comparison the student observes is the correct one. Accurate MTS performance, therefore, includes both selecting correct comparisons and rejecting incorrect ones.

Stimulus overselectivity affects accuracy in the MTS context because of failures to reject incorrect comparison stimuli. This may happen when the specific feature that has gained stimulus control is shared by both correct and incorrect comparisons. For example, if discrimination of the letter "A" were restricted to the "/" feature, the student might fail to reject comparison stimulus "Z" because the controlling feature was present.

Naming tasks. Naming tasks are sometimes used to assess the outcomes of MTS training with auditory sample stimuli. As with simple discrimination, the behavior can be analyzed in terms of the three-term operant contingency, but in the case of naming tasks the response form varies from trial to trial. For example, in a picture-identification task the teacher may display a picture of a dog (discriminative stimulus) and the student's correct response is to say "Dog," followed by a reinforcer. On the next trial, the picture might be of a cat, and so forth. Other common stimuli for naming tasks like this are printed words, numerals, and quantities.

Examples of Stimulus Overselectivity in a Special-Education Setting

Two examples of stimulus overselectivity within discrete-trials tasks come from a residential special-education program for children and young adults. Teaching sessions included discrete-trials instruction, often with a computer and touch screen monitor used as an interactive teaching machine. Students earned poker-chip tokens for all correct responses and the tokens were exchanged after sessions for students' choices of reinforcer items or activities.

Sam was a 21-year-old man with moderate mental retardation (Peabody Picture Vocabulary Test - Revised mental age equivalent score [PPVT MAE], 5.75 years) and a seizure disorder. Sam was learning to read printed words aloud. New words were introduced via auditory-visual matching-to-sample trials in the context of an accumulating baseline that reviewed previously learned words. On these matching-to-sample trials, the computer would present a spoken-word name and Sam selected the corresponding printed word by touching it on the monitor screen. After he reliably touched the printed word that corresponded to the spoken sample, he was given a naming test. On naming test trials, the printed word was presented in the center of the computer screen and the teacher asked Sam, "What is it?"

Figure 2.1 shows accuracy scores for the naming tests. The first four words were EXIT, MEN, WALK, and PUSH, and teaching went smoothly; naming accuracy scores were always 100% correct. The fifth word was PULL. As soon as it was introduced, naming accuracy fell to approximately 50%, and almost every error was saying "Push" when PULL was presented. After several sessions, Sam also began to say "Pull" on approximately half of the trials on which PUSH was presented. In subsequent sessions, the teachers sometimes eliminated one or the other of the words, PUSH or PULL, but accuracy did not improve. Finally, after 15 sessions, both PUSH and PULL were eliminated from the baseline. Accuracy recovered immediately, and there were no problems as the new word SUN was introduced. Later, however, when the word MUG was introduced, accuracy once again fell due to errors reading "Men" for MUG. Apparently, stimulus control was overselective in that it was restricted to the initial letters of the words.

In Sam's case, the problem was readily apparent because it occurred within a teaching structure that introduced new words individually and within the context of previously learned words. A second classroom example illustrates that a more detailed analyses sometimes may be necessary to uncover learning problems related to overselectivity.

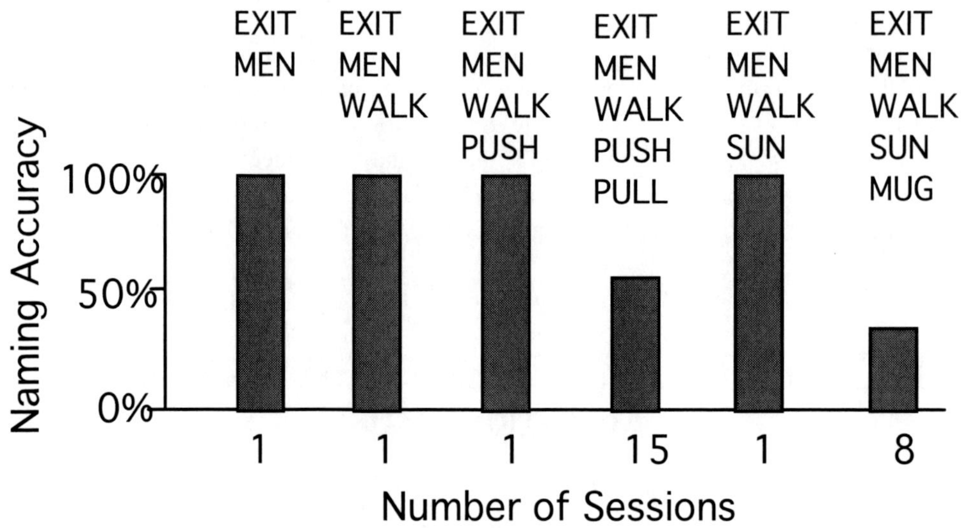

Figure 2.1. Sam's mean accuracy scores for naming printed words. The set of words presented in each test session is shown above the bars. Numbers beneath the bars show the number of sessions that contributed to each accuracy score.

Paul was a 15-year-old boy with Cerebral Palsy and moderate mental retardation (PPVT MAE 6.1 years; Gardner Expressive One-Word Picture Vocabulary Test MAE 3.4 years). The curriculum included instruction in identifying useful words by reading them aloud, and the words were presented in sets of six words. His teachers were about to begin a new set of words: POISON, EXIT, WOMEN, DANGER, POLICE, and WALK. New sets of words were first presented in an identity matching-to-sample format, in which the sample and correct comparison stimulus were identical. High accuracy on an identity-matching test was taken as evidence for discrimination among the words, a prerequisite for the instruction that was to follow. The words were presented in a two-choice identity-matching task, in all possible combinations, for five 36-trial sessions.

The leftmost portion of Figure 2.2, labeled "All trials," shows the overall accuracy score of 91% correct for the five sessions, a total of 180 trials. On the basis of this score alone, his teachers may have proceeded to the next phase of training. A closer analysis, however, with a separate accuracy score calculated for each sample stimulus, is shown in the center portion of the figure. Here, the scores for four of the words are still at least 90%, but the scores for trials on which POISON or POLICE were the samples were 83% and 73%, respectively. Finally, the right portion of the figure shows accuracy scores for only those trials on which both POISON and POLICE appeared together in the comparison array (and thus one or the other was the sample). This score, 54%, is at the "chance" level and it indicates that there was no discrimination between these two words. As with Sam's data above, it appears that Paul was matching the printed words on the basis of the first one or two letters only, an instance of stimulus overselectivity that was not as obvious as Sam's because of differences in the discrimination teaching and evaluation procedures.

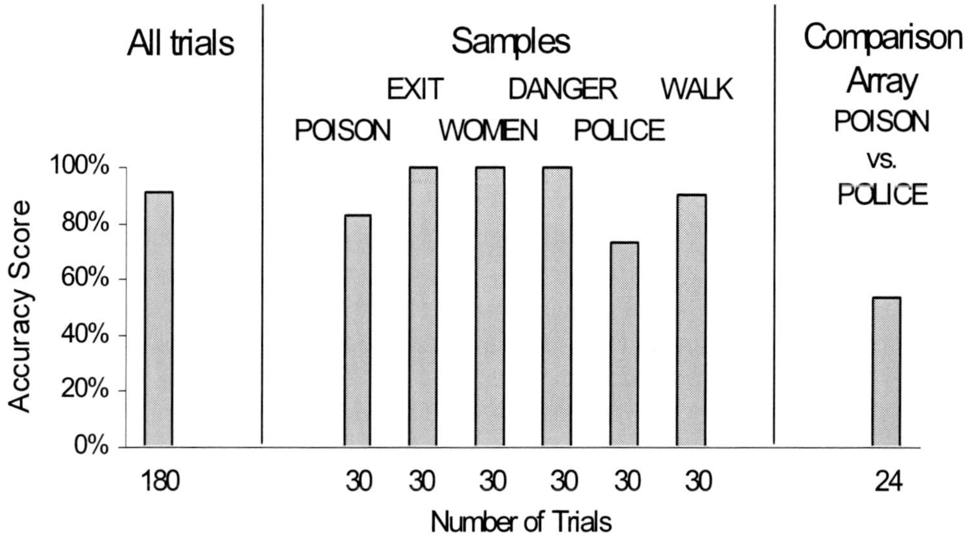

Figure 2.2. Paul's accuracy scores for identity matching to sample with a set of six printed words. Numbers beneath the bars show the number of trials that contributed to each accuracy score. The left portion shows global accuracy for all trials. The center portion shows accuracy broken down by sample stimulus; sample stimuli are shown above each bar. The right portion shows accuracy score for only those trials in which the comparison array was POISON and POLICE.

Experimental Procedures in Overselectivity Research

Simple discrimination. Simple-discrimination procedures were predominant in the initial experimental studies that defined the problem of stimulus overselectivity in children with ASD (reviewed in Lovaas et al., 1979). Since then, a substantial portion of the research literature in individuals with intellectual disabilities has been conducted with these procedures, and they continue to be used in contemporary research (e.g., Reed and Gibson, 2005). As noted above, in simple discrimination the positive and negative functions of experimental stimuli do not change from trial to trial and thus relational or conditional stimulus control is not required. In a typical experimental implementation, simple discriminative control is first established with multi-component stimuli, and then stimulus control by the components is tested separately. Component tests are usually conducted without differential reinforcement (i.e., in extinction) because (a) repeated test trials are necessary to obtain a meaningful accuracy score and (b) differential reinforcement on test trials may result in new learning within the test and thus contaminate the test results.

Matching-to-sample procedures. The use of matching-to-sample procedures in studies of overselectivity in individuals with developmental disabilities began to increase approximately 25 years ago (e.g., Mackie and Mackay, 1982; Schneider and Salzberg, 1982; Whiteley, Zaparniuk, and Asmundson, 1987). This followed work about a decade earlier in animal cognition laboratories (Maki and Leith, 1973; Maki and Leuin, 1972; Maki, Riley, and Leith, 1976) and it also has roots in analyses of breadth of attention using "demonstration-trial" discrimination procedures (described in Fisher and Zeaman, 1973). Typically, multielement or multidimensional sample stimuli are presented for some observation period, and then the sample is removed from view prior to presentation of an array of comparison stimuli.

Performance baselines are established with comparison stimuli that are identical to the sample (e.g., sample AB, and comparisons AB, CD, and EF). On tests for restricted stimulus control, only one sample element or dimension (or a subset of them) is represented in the comparison array. With sample AB, for example, high accuracy when comparison displays include A, C, and E, and chance accuracy when displays include B, D, and F (i.e., A is not present), indicate stimulus control restricted to sample element A.

Our laboratory at the Shriver Center has made extensive use of matching-to-sample procedures to study stimulus overselectivity as it occurs with arrays of discrete forms (e.g., Stromer, McIlvane, Dube, and Mackay, 1993). Prerequisites for testing include accurate discrimination of the stimulus set to be tested when the stimuli are presented individually, as verified by high accuracy on simultaneous and delayed identity matching to sample. The primary task is delayed matching to sample (DMTS) with multi-element sample stimuli. A two-sample version of the procedure is illustrated in Figure 2.3. Trials begin with the sample stimuli presented in the center of a computer touch screen. After the participant has observed the samples, he or she touches the sample display area, the samples disappear, and three single comparison stimuli are presented in three corners of the screen. One comparison matches one of the samples, the other two comparisons match neither sample, and one of the samples has no matching comparison. All stimuli appear in both the left and right sample positions equally often, and so the participant cannot predict which of the samples will subsequently appear as the correct comparison. Sessions usually consist of 36 trials. High accuracy scores (near 100%) indicate reliable control by both sample stimuli; regardless of which stimulus appears in the comparison array, the participant is able to match it. With two samples, typically developing individuals and many children with developmental disabilities have high accuracy scores (e.g., Dickson, Deutsch, Wang, and Dube, 2006a; Dickson et al., 2006b; Dube et al., 2006). Chance-level accuracy scores (near 33%) would result if there were no stimulus control by any sample stimuli, and scores in this range indicate that the participant could not be meaningfully tested with this procedure.

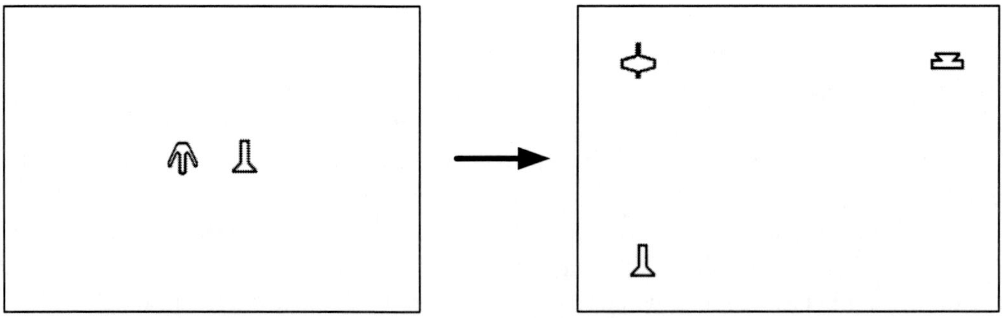

Figure 2.3. Stimulus displays for two-sample delayed matching to sample (DMTS) with arbitrary forms as stimuli. The left panel shows the two sample stimuli. The right panel shows the comparison display; the correct comparison is in the lower left corner.

Intermediate accuracy scores (near 67%) are consistent with overselectivity: If stimulus control were limited to only one sample stimulus per trial, then on an average of half the trials, that stimulus would appear in the comparison array and the participant would always be correct. On the remaining half of the trials, the stimulus with the potential to control a correct response would not appear as a comparison and the participant would be correct “by chance” on one-third of those trials. The overall accuracy score near 67% results from averaging, across the entire session, the 100% score for those trials with a comparison identical to a controlling sample and the 33% score for those trials with no stimulus control by a sample.

Relative merits of simple-discrimination and MTS procedures. When research subjects are developmentally limited, simple-discrimination procedures offer an advantage in that performance baselines are relatively easy to establish. For those subjects who do not learn readily, several generally successful programmed or "errorless learning" procedures (e.g., stimulus fading; reviewed by Lancioni and Smeets, 1986) are available to supplement simple-discrimination training.

Matching-to-sample procedures, however, seem to offer some useful advantages over simple-discrimination procedures. Because stimulus functions in simple discrimination are defined entirely by positive or negative relation to reinforcement, testing contingencies interact with the relations tested. Testing in extinction may not provide adequate measures of stimulus control, while testing with reinforcement may establish control that is not a result of the pre-test contingencies or create conditions where pretest conditions cannot be recovered. For example, in an early demonstration of selective stimulus control, pigeons acquired a simple discrimination in which a triangle on a red background was positive and a circle on a blue background was negative (Reynolds, 1961). Tests for control by the component colors and forms were conducted in extinction; some subjects responded with high rates to red and others with high rates to the triangle, and, in both cases, with equally low rates to the other three stimuli. The results were interpreted as showing selective stimulus control by the component stimulus producing high rates. Several years later Wilkie and Masson (1976) repeated Reynolds' experiment with similar results on extinction tests. Wilkie and Masson, however, then conducted tests where all responses were reinforced. On these tests, rates of responding increased faster to red than blue *and* faster to the triangle than circle. Apparently, stimulus control had been acquired by both elements of the positive compound although it was not measured on the extinction test. The reinforcement tests revealed this control but did so, of course, at the expense of creating a reinforcement history for negative stimuli and therefore irrevocably altering the baseline performance.

In contrast to simple-discrimination procedures, stimulus functions in matching to sample are defined by stimulus-stimulus relations between samples and comparisons. Relation to reinforcement is equated for all stimuli because all stimuli exhibit both positive and negative functions (i.e., are correct and incorrect) equally often. Matching to sample produces a stable baseline of stimulus control that can be maintained for extended periods. Further, matching to sample permits testing without altering the reinforcement contingencies for the baseline performance and so allows a wider range of testing options.

A Selective Summary of Research Findings

Subject characteristics. As might be expected with any test of discrimination learning, the severity and/or prevalence of overselectivity in individuals with developmental disabilities has been related to mental age equivalent scores on standardized tests (e.g., Schover and Newsom, 1976; Wilhelm and Lovaas, 1976). For example, a recent study by Dickson et al. (2006a) reported the results of matching-to-sample and stimulus overselectivity testing in 70 individuals attending residential special-education schools. The stimuli were *arbitrary forms*, so termed because they were likely to be unfamiliar to the participants; examples of the stimuli were shown in Figure 2.3. The testing procedure was the two-sample DMTS task described above. Before the test for overselectivity was given, participants received a set of preliminary tests to evaluate prerequisite performances such as accurate matching-to-sample with single sample stimuli. Twenty-one of the 70 participants failed the pre-tests and the mean PPVT MAE for these individuals was 3.70 years. Results were consistent with overselectivity for 35 participants and mean MAE for this group was 5.28 years. Finally, the results showed no overselectivity for 14 participants with mean MAE of 7.44 years. Thus, MAE scores were related to both matching-to-sample performance and stimulus overselectivity.

Overselectivity was assessed with a wider range of stimuli by Dickson et al. (2006b). The method was DMTS and the stimuli included form/color compounds (nine possible combinations of three colors and three forms), pairs of alphanumeric characters, and digital images of adult faces. The results showed overselective stimulus control with at least one set of stimuli for 18 of the 29 participants. Although a finding of overselectivity was more likely in individuals with lower PPVT MAE scores, it was found across a relatively wide range of PPVT MAE scores, from 1 to 8 years. Overselectivity was more prevalent in individuals with Autism Diagnostic Observation Scale (ADOS; Lord, Rutter, DiLavore, and Risi, 2001) scores that met the clinical criterion for autism, but it was also found in almost half of the participants with ADOS scores that did not meet the criterion for autism. This finding is consistent with a number of previous studies that have reported overselectivity in individuals with mental retardation but without autism (Allen and Fuqua, 1985; Dube and McIlvane, 1997; Huguenin, 2000, 2004; Litrownik, McInnis, Wetzel-Pritchard, and Filipelli, 1978; Meisel, 1981; Schneider and Salzberg, 1982; Stromer et al., 1993; Wilhelm and Lovaas, 1976).

Stimulus modality. Overselectivity has been demonstrated with auditory stimuli (e.g., Schreibman, Kohlenberg, and Britten, 1986), but the primary focus for most research and intervention has been on visual stimuli. Overselective responding has been documented with several types of multi-element visual stimuli, including those with elements of the same stimulus dimension (e.g., arrays of discrete forms; Koegel and Wilhelm, 1973) and multidimensional elements (differences in color, form, etc.; Kovattana and Kraemer, 1974). Overselectivity has also been shown in contexts that included accurate discrimination of all stimulus elements when presented individually (Dube, Kledaras, Iennaco, Stoddard, and McIlvane, 1990) and tests verifying discrimination of the individual stimuli when presented in multiple-stimulus arrays (Stromer et al., 1993).

Observing behavior. Ongoing research in our laboratory is investigating the relation between observing behavior and overselectivity. We are using an eye tracking apparatus to obtain direct measures of observing behavior during two-sample DMTS performances. The eye tracking imaging components include miniature cameras mounted on a lightweight and comfortable headband. Because these cameras move in concert with the participant's head, it is not necessary to restrict head movement in order to obtain eye tracking data, and thus we have been able to study observing behavior in individuals with developmental disabilities who might not tolerate prolonged restrictions on head movement, or for whom such restrictions may themselves interfere with discriminative performances (the training program is described in Dube et al., 1999).

Results to date with the two-sample DMTS procedure indicate that normal adults and individuals with mental retardation who are not overselective observe each sample stimulus at least one time on every trial, and often twice. In contrast, individuals with mental retardation who are overselective on the task often fail to observe one of the sample stimuli (Dube et al., 1999, 2003). Analyses of the relation between DMTS errors and observing behavior indicate that the errors are closely related to observing failures or extremely short observing durations. Ongoing research indicates that interventions that increase the number of observations per trial and the duration of each observation may produce an immediate increase in two-sample DMTS accuracy scores. Although this research is not complete as of this writing, the results thus far suggest that stimulus overselectivity may not necessarily indicate an attentional deficit *per se*, but may result at least in part from incomplete or poorly organized observing behavior.

Reinforcement variables. Dube and McIlvane (1997) reported that relative rates of reinforcement could influence the specific stimuli that gain stimulus control in overselective responding. Initial identity matching-to-sample training was conducted with a set of four stimuli. For two of the stimuli, correct matching responses produced a high rate of reinforcement; for the other two stimuli, correct responses produced a substantially lower reinforcer rate. When pairs of sample stimuli consisting of one high- and one low-rate stimulus were presented on subsequent DMTS test trials, the results showed overselective stimulus control by the high-rate stimulus. Following more training with the individual stimuli and reversed reinforcement schedules for all stimuli, the differences in stimulus control on two-sample tests also reversed. These results demonstrate experimental control by reinforcement contingencies of which of two sample stimuli controlled selections in the two-sample task.

RESEARCH ON REMEDIATION OF OVERSELECTIVITY

Reinforcement schedules. There were three early reports that overselectivity could be reduced by overtraining or repeated testing with intermittent reinforcement (Koegel et al., 1979; Schover and Newsom, 1976; Schreibman, Koegel, and Craig, 1977). There have been, however, no further reports of successful remediation by reducing the reinforcement schedule. Remington and Clarke (1993), for example, did not find a similar effect in a study teaching matching-to-sample skills to children with mental retardation in the context of augmentative and alternative communication training (see also Meisel, 1981). Dube and McIlvane (1997) found no amelioration of overselectivity in extensive two-sample DMTS training with intermittent reinforcement schedules. With continuous reinforcement, however, Huguenin (2000, 2004) has reported that extensive training with individual stimuli may reduce overselectivity when those stimuli are presented within multi-stimulus compounds.

Multiple cue training. Perhaps the most promising approach to remediation was documented in four studies of multiple-cue training. Participants were given extended practice with tasks where high accuracy required simultaneous discrimination of two or more stimuli. Three of these studies used simple-discrimination procedures and the correct response was, for example, to select on every trial the compound stimulus A+B, and to reject the incorrect alternatives A+C, and A alone (Allen and Fuqua, 1985; Koegel and Schreibman,

1977; Schreibman, Charlop, and Koegel, 1982). The fourth study employed a matching task with multiple verbal cues; for example, "[touch the] big red pencil," where the incorrect alternatives included a small red pencil, big blue pencil, etc. (Burke and Cerniglia, 1990; cf. training techniques described in Rosenblatt, Bloom, and Koegel, 1995; and Schreibman, 1997). In all four studies, the stimulus sets were such that responding based on only one cue would not be consistently reinforced. Results showed that children who were overselective on initial assessments improved at least to some extent with trial-and-error training on multiple-cue problems. These studies documented that differential reinforcement for responding based on multiple cues could broaden stimulus control.

REMEDIATION VIA DIFFERENTIAL OBSERVING RESPONSES

For discrete-trials instruction with matching-to-sample procedures, overselectivity with respect to sample stimuli can often be greatly reduced by incorporating *differential observing responses* (DOR). DOR contingencies require a specific response to each sample stimulus, and one that is different for each stimulus. DORs thus control observing behavior and verify discrimination of relevant stimulus features. For matching-to-sample procedures, the DOR may be contrasted with the more common non-differential observing response of simply touching the sample stimulus (i.e., non-differential because it is the same response for every sample stimulus). The DOR technique arose originally in the basic research laboratory (e.g., Cohen, Brady, and Lowry, 1981; Urcuioli and Callender, 1989) and it has been successfully applied to discrimination learning in developmentally disabled populations. For example, Constantine and Sidman (1975) found that DMTS accuracy with pictures improved in young men with severe mental retardation when they were required to name the sample pictures (cf. Geren, Stromer, and Mackay, 1997).

Gutowski, Geren, Stromer, and Mackay (1995) examined the effects of imposing a DOR requirement in two individuals with moderate mental retardation who responded overselectively in a two-sample DMTS task. The stimuli were pictures of common objects. When the participants were required to name the two stimuli aloud before making a comparison selection, accuracy scores improved. The same approach could be implemented with printed-word stimuli; a convenient differential observing response would be to have the student spell the word aloud. For example, given the printed-word stimulus JOHN, the student must observe each letter to produce the responses, "J, O, H, N," and the forms of the responses verify accurate discrimination of each letter.

For non-vocal students, or for students that do not know the names of the stimuli, naming is not an option. Dube and McIlvane (1999) adopted the logic of the multiple-cue procedures described earlier to test a nonverbal DOR that capitalized on generalized identity-matching repertoires. Participants were three individuals with mental retardation who had intermediate accuracy scores on the two-sample DMTS procedure. The DOR procedure prompted participants to make simultaneous identity-matching responses that required observation and discrimination of both sample stimuli. For example, if the sample were AB, then the simultaneous identity-matching DOR displayed the comparison stimuli AB, AC, and DB (the actual stimuli were arbitrary forms). When observing responses were prompted, participants' accuracy scores improved. In a return to the baseline condition, when differential observing responses were no longer prompted, accuracy returned to intermediate levels (a similar finding has been reported with non-disabled adults; Broomfield, McHugh, and Reed, 2008). The results thus showed that stimulus overselectivity could be greatly reduced by a behavioral intervention that controls observing behavior and verifies discrimination, but that exposure to such procedures alone may be insufficient for lasting benefits.

A study by Walpole, Roscoe, and Dube (2007) extended the use of identity-matching DORs to educational stimuli. A participant with ASD had high matching-to-sample accuracy scores with printed words that had no letters in common (e.g., cat, lid, bug) but poor accuracy with words that had two letters in common (e.g., cat, can, car). In the DOR intervention, she matched the distinguishing letters of the overlapping words (e.g., t, n, r) immediately prior to matching the whole words. Accuracy scores improved to high levels and accuracy remained high when DOR requirements were withdrawn.

Identity-matching DORs with whole words or sets of distinguishing letters for different word combinations, however, could become cumbersome for the teacher to arrange with increases in the number of letters in the words and the number of different words. A convenient option is to match the individual letters of a word, one by one. A similar approach was taken to teach spelling in Mackay and Sidman (1984, on tabletop using anagram letters like those of the game Scrabble) and Dube, McDonald, McIlvane, and Mackay (1991), via interactive computer software: An initial stage of the spelling program taught an identity-matching task; the procedure is illustrated in Figure 2.4. A printed word was displayed as a sample stimulus and the student selected identical individual letters, one by one, from a *choice pool* of individual letters. As each letter was selected, it was moved from the choice pool to a *construction area* adjacent to the sample. This task was termed *constructed-response matching to sample* (CRMTS) because the student constructed a word identical to the sample, rather than merely selecting it. In some situations, constructed-response matching could be used as a differential observing response for discrimination training with printed words, groups of coins in money skills training (e.g., Stoddard, Bradley, and McIlvane, 1987), or other tasks with similar requirements.

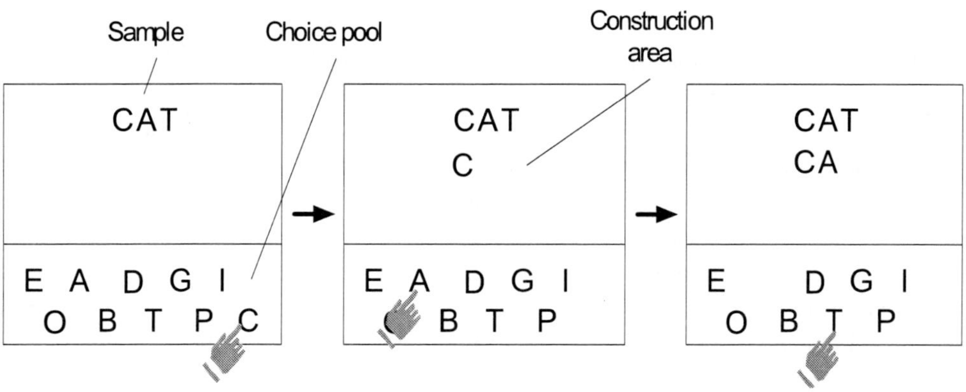

Figure 2.4. Stimulus displays for identity constructed-response matching to sample (CRMTS). The gray hands in the lower portion of the figure show three successive correct responses. In a tabletop implementation, the letters in the choice pool are on individual tiles and the student moves them from the choice pool to the construction area. In a computer-based implementation, the choice-pool letters move via on-screen animation when they are touched.

Mackay and Sidman (1984) and Dube et al. (1991) include descriptions of the identity-matching CRMTS training programs for tabletop and computer-based instruction, respectively. (Although obtaining and using specialized software for CRMTS in the classroom seems somewhat impractical at present, many of the training steps in Dube et al., 1999 could be adapted for tabletop use.) A prerequisite is accurate identity matching with the letters of the alphabet. CRMTS training begins with single-letter samples and only two or three letters in the choice pool. The task requirements are thus virtually the same as identity MTS, and the student familiar with identity matching should be able to select the matching letter. The transition to constructed-response matching requires four steps: (a) In a tabletop setting, the student is taught to move the letter from the choice pool to the appropriate spot in the construction area, rather than merely touching it. (b) The number of letters in the choice pool is gradually increased to an appropriate number, which is at least a few more than the number of letters in the longest word to be taught. (c) Two-letter samples are introduced and the student is taught to match the sample letters in order from left to right. (d) The number of sample letters is increased and accurate left-to-right matching is maintained. If generalized CRMTS can be established in the student, it can provide a convenient way to add a nonverbal differential observing response requirement to a MTS task with printed-word stimuli: After the printed word(s) are presented, the student could construct identical printed words to verify discrimination of every letter in the word(s). In tabletop instruction CRMTS can be implemented with anagram letters, as in Mackay and Sidman (1984). A student such as Sam, in the example shown in Figure 2.1, could be required to construct the word PUSH, identical to the sample, before naming it aloud.

A computer keyboard may sometimes be a convenient option for DORs with printed words; the student who types a word identical to one displayed by a teacher has verified discrimination and observation of all letters within the word. Our laboratory has examined the feasibility of this approach with three boys, Joe (15 years old), Ben (10), and Chuck (13); all had autism (ADOS Module-1 Communication-Social Interaction total scores of at least 12, which meets the diagnostic criterion for a classification of autism) and severe intellectual disabilities (all failed to achieve a PPVT MAE basal score of 1.75 years). All three had participated in Dickson et al. (2006b) and met the criteria for stimulus overselectivity on a two-sample DMTS assessment with alphanumeric stimuli. Although all had played computer games and had used a mouse before, none were able to type displayed words with a keyboard in preliminary testing. Reinforcer preference testing identified preferred edible items for each participant and presentation of these items followed trials with correct responses.

The baseline task was the computer-based two-sample DMTS task, described above, with letters as stimuli. We asked if overselective responding on two-sample DMTS could be improved if the students emitted a DOR for each sample stimulus by typing an identical two-letter "word," prior to selecting a comparison stimulus. As with other research described previously, the essential elements of the instructional program do not require a computer and they could be implemented for tabletop settings.

Participants were given preliminary training in CRMTS with methods similar to those described in Dube et al. (1991). The purpose of this training was to provide a history of reinforcement for observing relatively large arrays of letters in an identity-matching context. Sample stimuli were individual letters at first, and then pairs of letters. Sample letters remained displayed throughout the trials as participants selected matching letters from a choice pool that was gradually increased from 3 to 12 letters. Joe and Chuck each received 8 sessions of CRMTS training, and Ben received 25 sessions.

The DOR teaching methods and results are summarized in Table 2.1. First, the earlier overselectivity finding with letters of the alphabet was confirmed in computer-based testing with letters presented in random order: DMTS accuracy was above 90% with single letters (not shown in Table 2.1) and 62% to 71% with two-letter samples (Table 2.1, Step 1).

Table 2.1. Letterboard (LB) and keyboard (KB) training and results. Numbers in parentheses following accuracy scores indicate number of sessions. DMTS = Two-sample delayed matching-to-sample test. DOR = Differential observing response.

Step		Joe	Chuck	Ben
1	DMTS all letters	69% (3)	71% (3)	62% (3)
2	Match letters to LB	100% (4)	99% (4)	92% (5)
3	DMTS Set 1	75% (6)	72% (6)	66% (6)
4	DMTS Set 1, LB DOR required	97% (6)	85% (6)	97% (6)
5	DMTS Set 1	76% (6)	75% (6)	66% (6)
6	DMTS Set 1, LB DOR required	94% (6)	95% (6)	96% (6)
7	DMTS Set 1, LB DOR optional	79% (10)	93% (6)	67% (3)
	Percent trials LB used	3%	100%	6%
8	DMTS Set 1, LB DOR required	97% (3)		90% (3)
9	DMTS Set 2	75% (6)	71% (6)	70% (6)
10	DMTS Set 2, LB DOR required	94% (6)	97% (6)	83% (9)
11	DMTS Sets 1 and 2, LB DOR required	98% (2)	94% (2)	78% (6)
12	DMTS Sets 1, 2, or both, LB DOR required			86% (20)
13	DMTS Sets 1 and 2, KB DOR required	96% (5)	96% (4)	84% (7)
14	DMTS Sets 1 and 2, KB DOR optional	92% (20)	94% (2)	85% (12)
	Percent trials KB used	99%	98%	99%
15	DMTS all letters	74% (15)	71% (4)	75% (3)
16	DMTS Sets 1 and 2, KB DOR optional	78% (6)	81% (6)	81% (6)
	Percent trials KB used	6%	0%	99%
17	DMTS Sets 1 and 2, KB DOR required	98% (6)	94% (6)	86% (8)

We introduced a *letterboard* as an intermediate step between responding to the touchscreen on CRMTS trials and responding to a keyboard as part of a DOR procedure. The letterboards were white laminated cardboard with black capital letters (the same as the choice-pool letters displayed on the computer screen) but approximately the same size and spacing between letters as the computer keyboard to be used later in instruction. Letters on the letterboard were always displayed in the same relative positions as those on a keyboard. One letterboard displayed Stimulus Set 1: 12 letters, QWER, ASDF, ZXCV arranged in three slightly offset rows. Another letterboard showed Stimulus Set 2, which included the remaining 14 letters of the alphabet, also in three offset rows as on a keyboard. A third letterboard included all 26 letters.

In training Step 2, participants matched individual and pairs of letters from Set 1, displayed on the computer screen, to identical letters on the Set-1 letterboard. During the initial session, the experimenter provided prompts as needed for the first few trials, including instructions (e.g., "Touch the same letter here") and holding the letterboard over the lower portion of the computer screen in the same position as the choice pool on CRMTS trials.

Within the first 10 trials, instructions were discontinued and the letterboard was placed on the desktop in front of the monitor. If the participant did not respond to a sample stimulus within 5 seconds, he was prompted to "Use the letterboard." If the student made an error, the experimenter said "No," pointed out the correct letter, and prompted the participant to make the correct response. If an error occurred on the second letter of a two-letter sequence, the participant was prompted to begin the sequence again, until the participant made a correct two-response sequence. Accuracy scores were high for all participants.

Step 3 presented only the Set-1 stimuli in the two-sample DMTS task, and overselectivity was confirmed for all three participants by accuracy scores of 66% to 75%. Step 4 continued to present the two-sample DMTS task with Set-1 stimuli, but with the addition of a letterboard DOR requirement. The letterboard was placed on the desktop. After the sample stimulus appeared, the participant touched the letterboard letters that were identical to those of the sample. Failures to respond and letterboard errors were treated as described above, and any responses to the sample stimulus had no effect. After the letterboard DOR response was complete, the participant touched the sample stimulus, the sample disappeared, and the comparison stimuli were immediately presented; there was no intervening consequence for the letterboard responses. As soon as the letterboard DOR requirement was imposed, accuracy scores improved to very high levels for Joe and Ben (97%) and to 85% for Chuck (Table 2.1, Step 4). Steps 5 and 6 replicated Steps 3 and 4: Intermediate accuracy with no DOR, and immediately high accuracy with the DOR, this time for all three participants.

We then asked if the participants would continue to use the letterboard if it were not required. Sessions in Step 7 were the same as those in Step 6, except that (a) the experimenter did not prompt letterboard use and (b) if the sample stimulus were touched at any point in the trial, it disappeared and the comparisons were presented, regardless of whether the DOR had been emitted. As Table 2.1 (Step 7) shows, the results were clear. Joe and Ben used the letterboard on less than 10% of the trials and their accuracy scores declined to intermediate levels; Chuck continued to use the letterboard and maintained high accuracy. When Joe and Ben were again required to use the letterboard (Step 8), their high accuracy scores recovered.

Steps 9 through 11 replicated the DOR effect in Joe and Chuck with Stimulus Set 2, and then Sets 1 and 2 combined. Ben's accuracy declined to intermediate levels when both stimulus sets were first combined, and improved somewhat to an average of 86% (range 75% to 92% for individual sessions) over 20 additional training sessions (Table 2.1, Step 12).

Transfer of the DOR from the letterboard to a keyboard was tested in Step 13. The first three trials of the first session were conducted with the letterboard as usual. Then, between trials, the experimenter replaced the letterboard with a computer keyboard with all keys removed except the 26 letters of the alphabet. The keyboard was connected to a laptop computer (that recorded the DORs in a text document), but the laptop's display screen was not visible to the participant. The transfer for all three participants occurred without problems. When the keyboard was presented in the first session, participants were initially slower to respond and the number of DOR corrections approximately doubled, but DMTS accuracy scores remained high and no additional prompting was necessary by the second half of the session, nor in subsequent sessions. The letterboard training had provided all of the necessary behavioral prerequisites for keyboard use in the DOR context.

In Step 14, keyboard DORs were optional. All participants continued to make DORs and two-sample DMTS accuracy scores remained high. Step 15 was a return to baseline; the two-sample DMTS task was presented without the keyboard available, and accuracy was again intermediate for all participants. The history of making DORs and producing high accuracy scores had little effect when the stimuli that controlled the DOR behavior (letterboard or keyboard) were not present. When the keyboard was re-introduced for optional use in Step 16, only Ben used it and his accuracy rose to approximately its former level. Finally, with the DOR requirement reinstated in Step 17, all participants again achieved high accuracy scores.

As an additional check on the effectiveness of keyboard DORs, Ben and Joe were tested with stimuli that had immediate educational relevance. Because of poor expressive language, both of these participants used alternative communication methods that included notebooks with Mayer-Johnson communication symbols consisting of icons and accompanying printed words (Mayer-Johnson LLC, Solana Beach, CA, USA). Matching-to-sample tests were conducted with sets of such stimuli to determine whether there was stimulus control by both the icons and the printed words. Figure 2.5 shows Ben's stimuli: book, bagel, and gym; and Joe's stimuli: book, ball, and bowl. Sample stimuli consisted of one icon and one printed word. On half of the trials in the session, the comparison stimuli were the three icons (without printed words), one identical to the sample icon and two non-matching; high accuracy on these trials would show stimulus control by the icon portion of the sample. On the remaining trials in the session, the comparison stimuli were the three printed words (without icons), one identical to the sample word and two non-matching; high accuracy on these trials would show stimulus control by the printed-word portion of the sample. Comparison types alternated irregularly from trial to trial so that the participant could not predict which type of comparison would appear on any particular trial.

Testing began with a simultaneous matching task (MTS; the sample stimulus remained displayed throughout the trial). Joe's accuracy scores were high and Ben's were high on trials with icon comparisons, but Ben made errors on trials with printed-word comparisons. The initial condition (MTS) in the upper portion of Figure 2.6 shows Ben's accuracy scores on trials with printed-word comparisons only. Mean accuracy for MTS was 69%. The keyboard DOR procedure was introduced for the next six sessions (Figure 2.6, MTS w/ KB) and accuracy improved to a mean of 92%. When the keyboard was no longer required, accuracy remained high on simultaneous matching trials.

Both participants were then tested with standard delayed matching trials (i.e., with no DOR). As with the simultaneous matching test, there were very few errors on trials with icon comparisons, but accuracy scores were low for both participants on the trials with printed-word comparisons. Thus, the DMTS tests documented stimulus overselectivity, with stimulus control restricted to the icons.

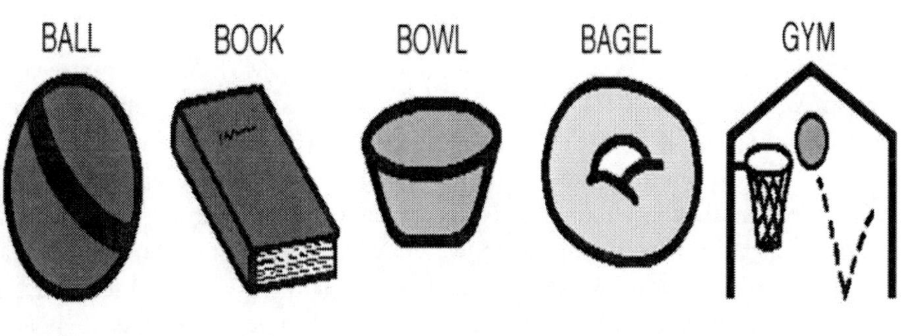

Figure 2.5. Mayer-Johnson symbols.

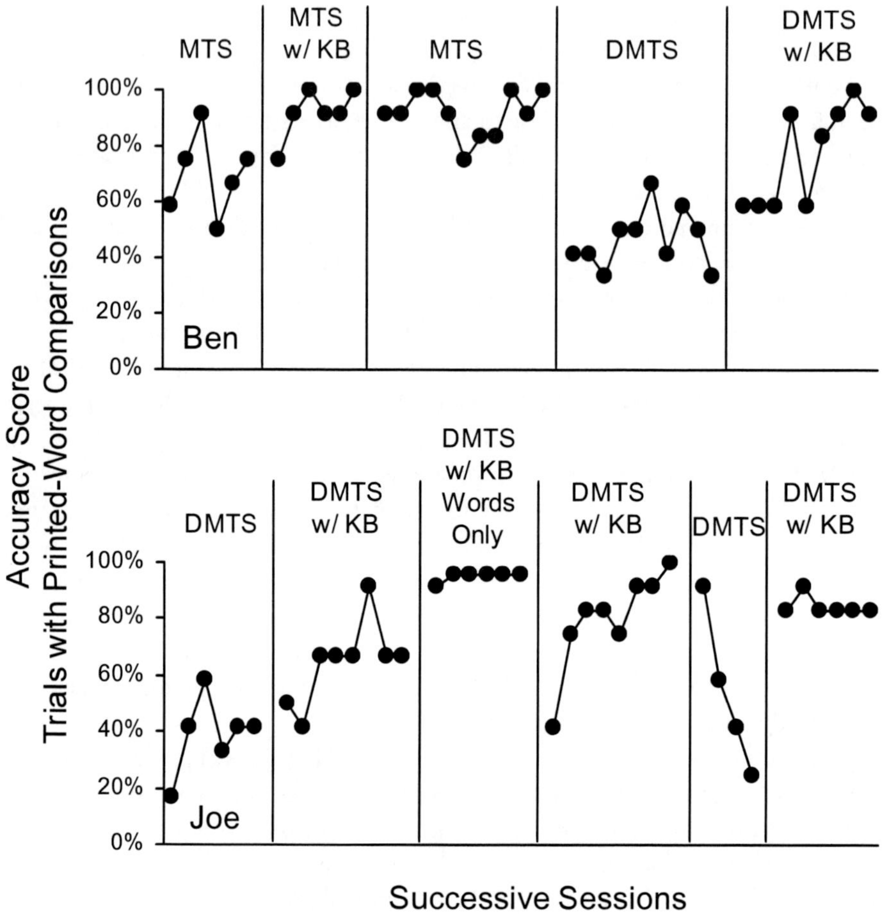

Figure 2.6. Matching-to-sample accuracy scores for Ben (upper portion) and Joe (lower portion). Sample stimuli were icons and printed words (see Figure 2.5) for all conditions except the bottom portion labeled, "DMTS w/ KB Words Only." The figure shows accuracy scores for only those trials with printed-word comparison stimuli (half the trials in each session). MTS indicates simultaneous matching, DMTS indicates delayed matching, and "w/ KB" indicates that the participant was required to make a differential observing response by typing the printed-word sample on a keyboard before the comparison stimuli were presented.

Figure 2.6 shows DMTS accuracy on trials with printed-word comparisons only; mean accuracy scores on these trials in the initial test condition were 47% for Ben (Figure 2.6, top panel, DMTS), and 39% for Joe (bottom panel, first condition).

When the keyboard DOR requirement was added, Ben's DMTS scores improved to high accuracy within nine sessions (94% for the last three sessions). At this point Ben transferred to another school and was not available for further testing. With the keyboard DOR, Joe's scores improved only to intermediate levels (mean 65%). He was then given six sessions in which all sample stimuli consisted of only the printed words, without the accompanying icons. Accuracy was high (Figure 2.6, DMTS w/ KB Words Only), and then improved to high levels when the icons were re-introduced. When the keyboard was removed for four sessions, performance rapidly deteriorated, but then recovered with a return to the keyboard DOR condition (see Figure 2.6).

In general, therefore, the results of our research in identity-matching DOR procedures indicate that they can be a very effective addition to discrete-trials teaching programs with printed-word stimuli. Accuracy scores almost always improved when DORs were required. Laptop computers are becoming increasingly available for special-education students. In situations where discrimination of all letters within printed words is important, it may be a generally useful skill if the student were able to construct identical words by typing them on a laptop. Our research also suggests that DOR requirements may have to be enforced by teachers in some situations. It was not uncommon for our participants to forego making DORs when they were optional, even with a recent history of improved accuracy with DORs. The reasons for this are unclear at present and remain a question for further research.

SUMMARY

Stimulus overselectivity refers to stimulus control by an atypically restricted range or number of stimuli or stimulus features. Overselectivity may present problems in discrimination learning for special-education students with intellectual disabilities. There is experimental evidence that overselectivity is related to insufficient observing behavior. Differential observing responses that verify observation and discrimination of all relevant stimuli may reduce overselectivity. Experience with differential observing responses alone, however, may not be sufficient to produce lasting effects; students may not engage in careful observing behavior unless it is required by the reinforcement contingencies. Thus, educational programming may be improved by adopting procedures with explicit or implicit observing response requirements.

ACKNOWLEDGMENTS

This research was supported by Grants HD25995 and HD37055 from the National Institute of Child Health and Human Development. The contents of this paper are solely the responsibility of the authors and do not necessarily represent the official views of NICHD.

I thank the staff and students of the New England Center for Children (Southborough, MA) and the Protestant Guild Learning Center (Waltham, MA) for their cooperation. Special thanks to Joanne Kledaras and Deborah Flusser for collecting the classroom data shown in Figures 2.1 and 2.2, to Kristin Lombard for programming many of the experimental sessions and performing preliminary data analyses, and to Bill McIlvane for advice on the research. Thanks are also due Kathy Clark, Jason Krienke, Sarah Luthern, Brooks Thompson, Sharon Wang, and many other research technicians of the Shriver Center who assisted with data collection.

Address any correspondence to William V. Dube, UMMS Shriver Center, 333 South Street, Shrewsbury, MA 01545, USA, or email to william.dube@umassmed.edu.

REFERENCES

Allen, K.D., and Fuqua, R.W. (1985). Eliminating selective stimulus control: A comparison of two procedures for teaching mentally retarded children to respond to compound stimuli. *Journal of Experimental Child Psychology,* 39, 55-71.

American Psychiatric Association (2000). *Diagnostic and Statistical Manual of Mental Disorders, Fourth Edition, Text Revision.* Arlington, VA: American Psychiatric Publishing, Inc.

Broomfield, L., McHugh, L., and Reed, P. (2008). The effect of observing response procedures on the reduction of over-selectivity in a match to sample task: Immediate but not long term benefits. *Research in Developmental Disabilities*, 29, 217-234.

Burke, J.C., and Cerniglia, L. (1990). Stimulus complexity and autistic children's responsivity: Assessing and training a pivotal behavior. *Journal of Autism and Developmental Disorders,* 20, 233-253.

Carrigan, P.F. Jr. and Sidman, M. (1992). Conditional discrimination and equivalence relations: A theoretical analysis of control by negative stimuli. *Journal of the Experimental Analysis of Behavior,* 58, 183-204.

Cohen, L.R., Brady, J., and Lowry, M. (1981). The role of differential responding in matching-to-sample and delayed matching performance. In M.L. Commons and J.A. Nevin (Eds.), *Quantitative analysis of behavior: Vol. 1. Discriminative properties of reinforcement schedules* (pp. 345-364). Cambridge, MA: Ballinger.

Constantine, B., and Sidman, M. (1975). The role of naming in delayed matching to sample. *American Journal of Mental Deficiency,* 79, 680-689.

Dickson, C.A., Deutsch, C.K., Wang, S.S., and Dube, W.V. (2006a). Matching-to sample assessment of stimulus overselectivity in students with intellectual disabilities. *American Journal on Mental Retardation,* 111, 447-453.

Dickson, C.A., Wang, S.S., Lombard, K.M., and Dube, W.V. (2006b). Overselective stimulus control in residential school students with intellectual disabilities. *Research in Developmental Disabilities,* 27, 618-631.

Dube, W.V., Balsamo, L.M., Fowler, T.R., Dickson, C.A., Lombard, K.M., and Tomanari, G.Y. (2006). Observing behavior topography in delayed matching to multiple samples. *The Psychological Record,* 56, 233-244.

Dube, W.V., Iennaco, F.M., Rocco, F.J., Kledaras, J.B. and McIlvane, W.J. (1992). Microcomputer-based programmed instruction in identity matching to sample for persons with severe disabilities. *Journal of Behavioral Education,* 2, 29-51.

Dube, W.V., Kledaras, J.B., Iennaco, F.M., Stoddard, L.T., and McIlvane, W.J. (1990). Observing complex visual stimuli: Effects of component pretraining. *Experimental Analysis of Human Behavior Bulletin,* 8, 7-11.

Dube, W.V., Lombard, K.M., Farren, K.M., Flusser, D.S., Balsamo, L.M., and Fowler, T.R. (1999). Eye tracking assessment of stimulus overselectivity in individuals with mental retardation. *Experimental Analysis of Human Behavior Bulletin,* 17, 8-14.

Dube, W.V., Lombard, K.M., Farren, K.M., Flusser, D.S., Balsamo, L.M., Fowler, T.R., and Tomanari, G.Y. (2003). Stimulus overselectivity and observing behavior in individuals with mental retardation. In S. Soraci and K. Murata-Soraci (Eds.), *Visual Information Processing* (pp. 109-123). Westport, CT: Praeger.

Dube, W.V., McDonald, S.J., McIlvane, W.J., and Mackay, H.A. (1991). Constructed response matching to sample and spelling instruction. *Journal of Applied Behavior Analysis,* 24, 305-317.

Dube, W.V. and McIlvane, W.J. (1996). Some implications of a stimulus control topography analysis for emergent stimulus classes. In T.R. Zentall and P.M. Smeets (Eds.), *Stimulus class formation in humans and animals* (pp. 197-218). Amsterdam, NL: Elsevier.

Dube, W.V., and McIlvane, W.J. (1997). Reinforcer frequency and restricted stimulus control. *Journal of the Experimental Analysis of Behavior,* 68, 303-316.

Dube, W.V. and McIlvane, W.J. (1999). Reduction of stimulus overselectivity with nonverbal differential observing responses. *Journal of Applied Behavior Analysis,* 32, 25-33.

Dube, W.V. and Serna, R.W. (1998). Reevaluation of a programmed method to teach generalized identity matching to sample. *Research in Developmental Disabilities,* 19, 347-379.

Fisher, M.A., and Zeaman, D. (1973). An attention-retention theory of retardate discrimination learning. In N.R. Ellis (Ed.), *International review of research in mental retardation, Vol. 6* (pp. 169-256). New York: Academic Press.

Geren, M.A., Stromer, R., and Mackay, H.A. (1997). Picture naming, matching to sample, and head injury: A stimulus control analysis. *Journal of Applied Behavior Analysis,* 30, 339-342.

Gutowski, S.J., Geren, M., Stromer, R., and Mackay, H.A. (1995). Restricted stimulus control in delayed matching to complex samples: A preliminary analysis of the role of naming. *Experimental Analysis of Human Behavior Bulletin,* 13, 18-24.

Huguenin, N.H. (2000). Reducing overselective attention to compound visual cues with extended training in adolescents with severe mental retardation. *Research in Developmental Disabilities,* 21, 93-113.

Huguenin, N.H. (2004). Assessing visual attention in young children and adolescents with severe mental retardation utilizing conditional-discrimination tasks and multiple testing procedures. *Research in Developmental Disabilities,* 25, 155-181.

Kasari, C., Freeman, S., and Paparella, T. (2006). Joint attention and symbolic play in young children with autism: A randomized controlled intervention study. *Journal of Child Psychology and Psychiatry,* 47, 611–620.

Koegel, R.L., and Schreibman, L. (1977). Teaching autistic children to respond to simultaneous multiple cues. *Journal of Experimental Child Psychology,* 24, 299-311.

Koegel, R.L., Schreibman, L., Britten, K., and Laitinen, R. (1979). The effects of schedule of reinforcement on stimulus overselectivity in autistic children. *Journal of Autism and Developmental Disabilities,* 9, 383-396.

Koegel, R.L., and Wilhelm, H. (1973). Selective responding to the components of multiple visual cues by autistic children. *Journal of Experimental Child Psychology,* 15, 442-453.

Kovattana, P.M., and Kraemer, H.C. (1974). Response to multiple visual cues of color, size, and form by autistic children. *Journal of Autism and Childhood Schizophrenia,* 4, 251-261.

Lancioni, G.E., and Smeets, P.M. (1986). Procedures and parameters of errorless discrimination training with developmentally impaired individuals. In N.R. Ellis and N.W. Bray (Eds.), *International Review of Research in Mental Retardation, Vol. 14*, (pp. 135-164). New York: Academic Press.

Litrownik, A.J., McInnis, E.T., Wetzel-Pritchard, A.M., and Filipelli, D.L. (1978). Restricted stimulus control and inferred attentional deficits in autistic and retarded children. *Journal of Abnormal Psychology,* 87, 554-562.

Lord, C., Rutter, M., DiLavore, P.C., and Risi, S. (2001). *Autism Diagnostic Observation Schedule*. Los Angeles, CA: Western Psychological Services.

Lovaas, O.I., Koegel, R.L., and Schreibman, L. (1979). Stimulus overselectivity in autism: A review of research. *Psychological Bulletin,* 86, 1236-1254.

Lovaas, O.I., Schreibman, L., Koegel, R.L., and Rehm, R. (1971). Selective responding by autistic children to multiple sensory input. *Journal of Abnormal Psychology,* 77, 211-222.

Mackay, H. A., and Sidman, M. (1984). Teaching new behavior via equivalence relations. In P.H. Brooks, R. Sperber, and C. MacCauley (Eds.), *Learning and cognition in the mentally retarded* (pp. 493-513). Hillsdale, NJ: Erlbaum.

Mackie, R., and Mackay, C.K. (1982). Attention vs. retention in discrimination learning of low-MA retarded adults and MA-matched retarded children. *American Journal of Mental Deficiency,* 86, 543-547.

Maki, W.S., and Leith, C.R. (1973). Shared attention in pigeons. *Journal of the Experimental Analysis of Behavior,* 19, 345-349.

Maki, W.S., and Leuin, T.C. (1972). Information processing by pigeons. *Science,* 176, 535-536.

Maki, W.S., Riley, D.A., and Leith, C.A. (1976). The role of test stimuli in matching to compound samples by pigeons. *Animal Learning and Behavior,* 4, 13-21.

Matthews B., Shute R., and Rees R. (2001). An analysis of stimulus overselectivity in adults with autism. *Journal of Intellectual and Developmental Disability,* 26, 161-176.

McHugh, L. and Reed, P. (2007). Age trends in stimulus overselectivity. *Journal of the Experimental Analysis of Behavior,* 88, 369-380.

Meisel, C.J. (1981). Stimulus overselectivity in mentally retarded adolescents: Effects of pretraining on cue identification. *American Journal of Mental Deficiency,* 86, 317-322.

Prizant, B. M. and Wetherby, A. M. (1998). Understanding the continuum of discrete trial traditional behavioral to social-pragmatic, developmental approaches in communication enhancement for young children with autism/PDD. *Seminars in Speech and Language*, 19, 329-353.

Reed, P. (2006). The effect of retention interval on stimulus over-selectivity using a matching-to-sample paradigm. *Journal of Autism and Developmental Disorders*, 36, 1115-1121.

Reed, P., and Gibson, E. (2005). The effect of concurrent task load on stimulus over-selectivity. *Journal of Autism and Developmental Disorders,* 35, 601-614.

Remington, B. and Clarke, S. (1993). Simultaneous communication and speech comprehension. Part I: Comparison of two methods of teaching expressive signing and speech comprehension skills. *Augmentative and Alternative Communication,* 9, 36-48.

Reynolds, G.S. (1961). Attention in the pigeon. *Journal of the Experimental Analysis of Behavior,* 4, 203-208.

Rosenblatt, J., Bloom, P., and Koegel, R.L. (1995). Overselective responding. In R.L. Koegel and L.K. Koegel (Eds.), *Teaching children with autism*. Baltimore: Brookes.

Saunders, K.J., and Spradlin, J.E. (1989). Conditional discrimination in mentally retarded adults: The effect of training the component simple discriminations. *Journal of the Experimental Analysis of Behavior,* 52, 1-12.

Saunders, K.J., and Spradlin, J.E. (1990). Conditional discrimination in mentally retarded adults: The development of generalized skills. *Journal of the Experimental Analysis of Behavior,* 54, 239-250.

Schneider H.C., and Salzberg, C.L. (1982). Stimulus overselectivity in a match-to sample paradigm by severely retarded youth. *Analysis and Intervention in Developmental Disabilities,* 2, 273-304.

Schover, L.R., and Newsom, C.D. (1976). Overselectivity, developmental level, and overtraining in autistic and normal children. *Journal of Abnormal Child Psychology,* 4, 289-298.

Schreibman, L. (1997). The study of stimulus control in autism. In D.M. Baer and E. M. Pinkston (Eds.), *Environment and behavior* (pp. 203-209). Boulder, CO: Westview.

Schreibman, L., Charlop, M.H., and Koegel, R.L. (1982). Teaching autistic children to use extra-stimulus prompts. *Journal of Experimental Child Psychology,* 33, 475-491.

Schreibman, L., Koegel, R.L., and Craig, M.S. (1977). Reducing stimulus overselectivity in autistic children. *Journal of Abnormal Child Psychology,* 5, 425-436.

Schreibman, L., Kohlenberg, B.S., and Britten, K.R. (1986). Differential responding to content and intonation components of a complex auditory stimulus by nonverbal and verbal autistic children. *Analysis and Intervention in Developmental Disabilities,* 6, 109-125.

Schreibman, L. and Lovaas, O.I. (1973). Overselective response to social stimuli by autistic children. *Journal of Abnormal Child Psychology,* 1, 152-168.

Sigafoos, J., O'Reilly, M.F., Schlosser, R.W., and Lancioni, G.E. (2007). Communication intervention. In P. Sturmey, and A. Fitzer (Eds.), *Autism spectrum disorders: Applied behavior analysis, evidence and practice* (pp. 131-185). Austin, TX: PRO-ED.

Stoddard, L.T., Bradley, D.P., and McIlvane, W.J. (1987). Stimulus control of emergent performances: Teaching money skills. In J.A. Mulick and R. Antonak (Eds.), *Transitions in mental retardation, Vol. 2* (pp. 115-149). Norwood, NJ: Ablex.

Stromer, R., McIlvane, W.J., Dube, W.V., and Mackay, H.A. (1993). Assessing control by elements of complex stimuli in delayed matching to sample. *Journal of the Experimental Analysis of Behavior,* 59, 83-102.

Sundberg, M.L., and Partington, J.W. (1999). The need for both discrete trial and natural environment language training for children with autism. In P.M. Ghezzi, W.L. Williams, and J.E. Carr (Eds.), *Autism: Behavior-analytic perspectives*, pp. 139-156. Reno, NV: Context Press.

Sundberg, C.T., and Sundberg, M.L. (1990). Comparing topography-based verbal behavior with stimulus selection-based verbal behavior. *Analysis of Verbal Behavior,* 8, 31-41.

Thompson, T. (2007). *Making sense of autism*. Baltimore, MD: Brookes.

Urcuioli, P.J. and Callender, J. (1989). Attentional enhancement in matching-to-sample: Facilitation in matching acquisition by sample-discrimination training. *Animal Learning and Behavior,* 17, 361-367.

Vignes, T. (2007). A comparison of topography-based and selection-based verbal behavior in typically developed children and developmentally disabled persons with autism. *Analysis of Verbal Behavior,* 23, 113-122.

Walpole, C.W., Roscoe, E.M., and Dube, W.V. (2007). Use of a differential observing response to expand restricted stimulus control. *Journal of Applied Behavior Analysis,* 40, 707-712.

Whiteley, J.H., Zaparniuk, J., and Asmundson, G.J.G. (1987). Mentally retarded adolescents' breadth of attention and short-term memory processes during matching to sample discriminations. *American Journal of Mental Deficiency,* 92, 207-212.

Wilhelm, H., and Lovaas, O.I. (1976). Stimulus overselectivity: A common feature in autism and mental retardation. *American Journal of Mental Deficiency*, 81, 26-31.

Wilkie, B.M., and Masson, M.E. (1976). Attention in pigeon: A reevaluation. *Journal of the Experimental Analysis of Behavior*, 26, 207-212.

In: Behavioral Theories and Interventions for Autism
Editor: Phil Reed
ISBN 978-1-60741-165-9
© 2009 Nova Science Publishers, Inc.

Chapter 3

RECIPROCAL IMITATION TRAINING: A NATURALISTIC BEHAVIORAL APPROACH TO TEACHING IMITATION TO YOUNG CHILDREN WITH AUTISTIC SPECTRUM DISORDERS

Brooke Ingersoll[1] and Laura Schreibman[2]
[1]Michigan State University, USA
[2]University of California, San Diego, USA

Autistic Spectrum Disorders (ASD) are characterized by pervasive deficits in social-communicative behaviors, including language, pretend play, and joint attention (APA, 2000). Children with ASD also have deficits in imitation (for reviews see Rogers and Williams, 2006; Smith and Bryson, 1994; Williams, Whiten, and Singh, 2004). In typical infants, imitation emerges early in development (Melzoff and Moore, 1977) and plays a role in the development of more advanced social-communication skills, such as language (e.g., Bates et al., 1988), play (Fiese, 1990; Uzgiris, 1990), and joint attention (Carpenter, Nagell, and Tomasello, 1998). Research with children with ASD suggests that imitation skills are associated with other social-communication skills, both concurrently (Curcio, 1978; Dawson and Adams, 1984; Stone, Ousley, and Littleford, 1997) and over time (Stone and Yoder, 2001). In fact, Carpenter and colleagues (2002) suggest that children with ASD may rely on imitation in the acquisition of language to a greater extent than typically developing children. Given the importance of imitation in the acquisition of other skills, it has been a central focus of intervention for young children with ASD.

Imitation serves two distinct functions in typical development: A learning function, through which infants acquire new skills and knowledge about the world, and a social function, through which infants engage in social and emotional exchanges with others (Uzgiris, 1981; 1990). Research is beginning to emerge that indicates children with ASD are particularly impaired in their ability to use imitation for social purposes (Hobson and Lee, 1999; Ingersoll, in press a; Rogers, Hepburn, Stackhouse, and Wehner, 2003; Whiten and Brown, 1998). For example, Ingersoll, Schreibman, and Tran (2003) found that children with ASD were more likely to imitate actions with objects when the action produced a non-social reinforcer (lights and sound) than when it did not. In contrast, typically developing children imitated equally well in both situations. Another study found that, unlike typically developing children who imitated equally well in both contexts, children with ASD were much less likely to imitate actions with objects when they were modeled in a spontaneous, interactive context than in a highly structured, elicited context (Ingersoll, in press b). Further, McDuffie and colleagues (2007) found that in young children with ASD, imitation in a spontaneous, interactive context was associated with social interaction skills, whereas imitation in structured, elicited context was associated with attention following.

These findings suggest that children with ASD may have particular difficulty imitating when the function of imitation is purely social and that the ability to imitate in spontaneous, interactive contexts is closely related to social ability, whereas the ability to imitate in structured contexts is not. Thus, targeting the *social* function of imitation may be particularly important, as it is more likely to be involved in social-communication development (the core deficits found in autism), than the learning function (Ingersoll, in press a). To do so, the field must utilize interventions that can teach imitation skills in a spontaneous, interactive context.

Structured Behavioral Approach

Early intervention programs for children with ASD typically use a structured behavioral approach for teaching imitation skills. Structured imitation training programs, which rely heavily on the use of discrete trials, stem from early imitation training research conducted in the 1960s (Baer, Peterson, and Sherman, 1967; Lovaas, Berberich, Perloff, and Schaeffer, 1966; Lovaas, Freitas, Nelson and Whalen, 1967; Metz, 1965) and vary little across intervention programs using this method today (e.g., Maurice, Green, and Luce, 1996). In this approach, the learning environment is highly structured and controlled by the therapist, usually with the child and therapist facing each other in child-sized chairs. Imitative behavior is broken into a series of discrete sub-skills, which are presented in multiple, successive trials. Specific sub-skills, such as individual non-verbal actions, are selected by the therapist from a variety of actions (meaningful and non-meaningful) that the child is not yet performing spontaneously. Acquisition is facilitated by the use of explicit prompting, starting with full physical prompts and fading to less intrusive prompts, and contingent reinforcement, usually a preferred food item or access to a preferred toy unrelated to the imitative act. Each action is taught individually in a set of trials (usually 10); however, several different actions may be targeted across different trial sets within a session. After mastery of an individual imitative action (e.g., 80% correct over three sets of 10 trials), random rotation of several mastered imitative actions is presented within a single set of trials. Eventually series of two or three actions are presented.

In this intervention, imitation is typically taught early on in treatment, as a means to facilitate the acquisition of higher level behaviors, such as verbal imitation, play, cognitive, and self-help skills. Thus, intervention programs targeting imitation using discrete trial training are concerned with teaching imitation as a cognitive skill on which to build other behaviors, rather than teaching the spontaneous use of imitation in a social context.

Structured behavioral techniques have demonstrated success in teaching children to imitate a variety of non-verbal actions and words. Metz (1965) demonstrated the development of body and object imitation in two children with ASD who had previously exhibited little to no imitative behavior. He used physical prompting and food reinforcers paired with verbal praise to teach behavioral responses that approximated the modeled action. He found that after intensive training, several imitative responses maintained in the absence of reinforcement. Baer et al. (1967) replicated this experiment using a more controlled reversal design with children with mental retardation. They found that as training progressed, new imitations were increasingly easy to teach. In addition, the children imitated probe trials of imitations that had never been reinforced during training. However, the imitative behavior extinguished during the reversal, demonstrating the control of reinforcement over the imitative behavior.

Lovaas and colleagues used a similar behavioral approach to teach verbal (Lovaas et al., 1966) and non-verbal (Lovaas et al., 1967) behavior in response to a verbal discriminative stimulus (S^D) to children with ASD. In both studies, the imitative behavior became increasingly easy to teach as it came under the control of the S^D. When reinforcement was delivered non-contingently, the imitative behavior deteriorated. Laying the groundwork for current, comprehensive early intervention programs using a traditional behavioral approach, Lovaas et al. (1977) used the newly acquired imitative behavior to teach a variety of more complex self-help and leisure behaviors.

Strengths of this approach include a basis on sound methodological research, impressive gains in children with otherwise poor prognoses (e.g., Lovaas, 1987), and accelerated skill acquisition (Miranda-Linne and Melin, 1992). However, several limitations have been noted. First, all training occurred in a highly structured environment and used artificial reinforcers. Although generalization across actions was found in all of the studies, none examined the generalization of these skills to non-treatment settings or therapists or the spontaneous use of imitation during play. Subsequent studies have shown that the highly structured teaching environment (Lovaas, 1977) and use of artificial reinforcers (Koegel, O'Dell, and Koegel, 1987) can prevent generalization to the natural environment (Spradlin and Siegel, 1982). Second, with the exception of one study (Metz, 1965), the imitative behavior was brought under the control of a specific verbal discriminative stimulus ("Do this" or "Say"). Research has shown that when a target behavior is brought under tight stimulus control, it can compromise the spontaneous use of the behavior (Carr, 1981). Third, the maintenance of the imitative behavior was dependent upon the continued reinforcement of at least some imitative responses, suggesting that the imitative behavior did not acquire its own reinforcing properties. And fourth, imitative behavior was targeted as an isolated skill rather than in the context of other co-occurring social-communicative behaviors and thus did not represent natural adult-child interactions (Schreibman, Kaneko, and Koegel, 1991). Therefore, this approach may actually hinder the development of spontaneous, self-initiated social and communication skills in the natural environment (Koegel and Koegel, 1995).

In short, the structured behavioral approach likely targets the *learning* function of imitation; it fails to incorporate the social-communicative process that typically occurs with the social use of imitation. While imitation in this form may be a useful tool for teaching other behaviors such as self-help skills, it may not serve as a building block for more advanced social-communication behaviors.

DEVELOPMENTAL APPROACH

Preliminary work has suggested that imitation can be taught using a more developmental, child-centered approach and might lead to changes in other social-communication skills. For example, Nadel and Peze (1992) targeted the use of reciprocal imitation in one 10-year-old, non-verbal child with ASD over the course of a year. The therapist alternated between imitating the child (contingent imitation) and modeling simple and motivating actions with toys. If the child failed to imitate the therapist, she would return to imitating the child. This child increased his use of imitation and role switching, but in a fixed pattern: the child would spontaneously switch from being imitated by the adult therapist to modeling an action for the adult to imitate, but would not switch from being imitated to imitating the adult. Additional findings suggested that, over time, the child relied less on imitating the actions of the therapist and used more complementary actions. Although the result from this report is intriguing, it did not employ a methodological design; thus change in imitative behavior cannot be attributed to the intervention per se.

Klinger and Dawson (1992) used a multiple baseline design to examine the effect of a developmental approach on the use of early social-communicative behavior in two five-year-old boys with ASD. One child was verbal, the other non-verbal. This approach included two levels of intervention strategies (Level One: contingent imitation and placement of objects near the therapist's eyes; Level Two: contingent imitation, modeling of familiar and novel actions, and environmental arrangement). The non-verbal child received Level One strategies aimed at increasing early social contingency, eye contact, and imitation while the verbal child received Level Two strategies aimed at increasing communication and joint attention skills. Both children showed increases in their social-communicative behavior, with the non-verbal child increasing his imitation of both familiar and unfamiliar body actions and actions with objects on the Uzgiris-Hunt Imitation Scale (Uzgiris and Hunt, 1975). Unfortunately, neither the non-verbal child's spontaneous use of imitation skills in the unstructured play environment nor his use of other targeted social-communicative skills were reported. This study offers additional preliminary support for the use of developmental strategies in the promotion of imitation skills. However, the inclusion of only one child per level limits the findings of this study considerably.

The previous studies, although promising, are limited by the lack of methodological control. To address this issue, Hwang and Hughes (2000) attempted to partially replicate Klinger and Dawson's (1992) intervention strategy using a multiple-baseline design with three preverbal preschool-aged children with ASD. This study used contingent imitation, naturally occurring reinforcement, expectant looks, and environmental arrangement. During baseline, classroom teachers played with the children as they typically did. During the treatment, an additional therapist implemented the social interactive training. Generalization probes with classroom teachers instructed to play with the children as they typically would were conducted in a separate room sporadically throughout treatment. All three children showed an increase in their frequency of eye contact, joint attention, and motor imitation concurrent with the onset of treatment. These increases and the acceptability of the treatment were found to be socially valid by naïve raters. The children also exhibited generalization, although minimal, to an untrained setting and teacher. Due to the length of the intervention (seven months), the treatment was never removed; therefore, maintenance of the acquired behaviors was not assessed.

These findings offer support for the ability of a developmental, child-centered approach to increase imitation behavior. However, the authors targeted the imitation of only familiar actions that were already in the children's repertoire. Therefore, while they were able to increase the spontaneous use of imitative behavior, they did not demonstrate that their technique could teach imitation of actions *outside* of the children's repertoire. In addition, the authors reported that increases in targeted behaviors occurred at a slower rate than anticipated, suggesting the acquisition of imitation behaviors using this method may be very time intensive.

There is empirical evidence that a commonly used developmental strategy, contingent imitation, is an effective treatment technique. Contingent imitation, in which the therapist imitates the actions and verbalizations of the child either concurrently or just after the child, has been shown to increase the use of eye contact (Tiegerman and Primavera, 1984), social responsiveness (Escalona, Field, Nadel, and Lundy, 2002); positive affect (Harris, Handleman, and Fong, 1987), coordinated joint attention (Lewy and Dawson, 1992), number of play schemes (Dawson and Galpert, 1990; Tiegerman and Primavera, 1981) and verbalizations (Gazdag and Warren, 2000) in young children with ASD or mental retardation. However, with all of the studies, the increase in child behavior did not maintain after the removal of treatment, suggesting that the therapeutic effects of contingent imitation may be limited.

The developmental approach is child-centered and conducted in the natural environment; therefore it theoretically addresses the problems with generalization and spontaneity found in the traditional behavioral method. In addition, it targets multiple, co-occurring social-communicative behaviors concurrently. However, outcomes from these studies suggest several limitations to a purely developmental approach. First, the rate of acquisition of the targeted behaviors was quite slow, ranging from 4 months (Klinger and Dawson, 1992) to 1 year (Nadel and Peze, 1992). It is likely that the exclusive reliance on child initiations to begin a teaching episode can prevent an adequate number of learning opportunities (Warren, Yoder, Gazdag, and Kim, 1993), resulting in slower acquisition. Second, the only controlled study (Hwang and Hughes, 2000) did not show evidence of the acquisition of imitation of novel behaviors. Without the use of explicit prompts or contingent reinforcement, certain skills which are not presently within the child's repertoire may be very difficult to teach (Quill, 1995). Third, evidence of the generalization and maintenance of the targeted behaviors over time and outside of the therapeutic environment is very limited. It is quite possible that the developmental strategies promote the use of early social-communicative behaviors that are already in the child's repertoire rather than teaching new behaviors. It is also possible that these behaviors may not maintain in the absence of the intervention.

NATURALISTIC BEHAVIORAL APPROACH

Naturalistic behavioral treatments, such as incidental teaching (Hart and Risley, 1968), milieu teaching (Alpert and Kaiser, 1992), and pivotal response training (PRT; Koegel et al., 1987; Koegel, Schreibman, Good, Cerniglia, Murphy, and Koegel, 1989), incorporate elements of the behavioral approach known to facilitate behavioral acquisition (i.e., multiple trials, explicit prompting and shaping, contingent reinforcement for correct responding) with techniques drawn from the developmental literature known to facilitate early social-communicative behavior in typical children (i.e., contingent imitation, following the child's lead, linguistic mapping; Warren et al., 1993). The naturalistic behavioral approach has been shown to provide increased generalization (Charlop-Christy and Carpenter, 2000; Spradlin and Siegel, 1982) through the use of naturally occurring teaching episodes and a direct response-reinforcer relationship (Kaiser, Yoder, and Keetz, 1992), increased spontaneity (Schwartz, Anderson, and Halle, 1989) by following the child's lead (Kaiser et al., 1992), and represents more natural adult-child interactions (Schreibman et al., 1991) because teaching is embedded in ongoing play interactions between the therapist and the child (Kaiser et al., 1992). In addition, naturalistic interventions increase the number of teaching opportunities by directly eliciting child response with a combination of environmental arrangement and behavioral techniques including explicit prompting (Kaiser et al., 1992; Warren et al., 1993).

There is an extensive literature to support the effectiveness of naturalistic behavioral teaching strategies for teaching language (see Kaiser et al., 1992, for review and Delprato, 2001). More recently, these procedures have been modified to teach other social-communication skills, including symbolic (Stahmer, 1995) and socio-dramatic play skills (Thorp, Stahmer, and Schreibman, 1995), peer interaction (Pierce and Schreibman, 1995), and joint attention skills (Whalen and Schreibman, 2003). This research has led to more diverse and effective intervention options for children with ASD that are now becoming more commonly used in the intervention community.

Reciprocal Imitation Training

Based the preliminary evidence that imitation can be targeted using more child-directed strategies and the success that naturalistic behavioral interventions have had in teaching other spontaneous, social-communication skills, we developed *Reciprocal Imitation Training* (RIT). This intervention addresses the shortcomings of the structured behavioral and developmental approaches. To address the limited generalization and spontaneity reported with the structured behavioral approach, RIT teaches imitation in the natural environment, using child-selected materials, multiple exemplars, varied S^Ds, and natural reinforcers. RIT also targets the social over the learning function of imitation by using interactive strategies (linguistic mapping, contingent imitation) and teaching imitation within the context of co-occurring social-communication skills. To address the issue of slow acquisition associated with the developmental approach (Quill, 1995), RIT uses direct prompting and reinforcement to teach imitation skills.

Our research has demonstrated that RIT is effective for teaching both object (Ingersoll and Schreibman, 2006) and gesture (Ingersoll, Lewis, and Kroman, in press) imitation that generalizes and maintains over time. This intervention is promising because it leads to changes in other social-communicative skills including language, pretend play, joint attention (Ingersoll and Schreibman, 2006) and spontaneous gesture use (Ingersoll et al., in press). Below, we provide a detailed description of the intervention along with specific points of departure from the structured behavioral approach.

Although RIT can be implemented during a variety of activities that do not use toys, such as the bath, or outside play, toys are an important part of teaching imitation skills. Toys are selected based on the child's preference. Toys that can be used in many different ways (such as balls, Slinkys, cups and containers, and doll/action figures are better than toys that have only one or two functions (such as mechanical toys). Also, toys that are interesting but not overly absorbing are better than very absorbing toys because the child is more likely to pay attention to the adult if he or she is not overly focused on the toys. In order to facilitate imitation, duplicate sets of developmentally appropriate toys are used in each session. By having several different sets of toys available (we use five sets for each 20 minute session), the child can select the toys that he or she is most motivated by. In order to encourage generalized imitation, toys are rotated each session, so that the child has access to a wide variety of materials over the course of intervention.

The goal of RIT is to teach imitation skills within on-going social interactions with a play partner (see Table 3.1). The focus is on the reciprocal aspect of imitation; thus, both the child and the adult take turns imitating each other. The adult begins the interaction by imitating the child's actions with toys, gestures, body movements, and vocalizations during play. The adult should be in the child's line of sight and should imitate the child's behavior in a playful, animated manner. For example, if the child were rolling a car back and forth, the adult would roll a second car back and forth in the child's line of sight. Research has shown that that contingent imitation of the child enhances social responsiveness and coordinated joint attention (Escalona et al., 2002; Ingersoll and Schreibman, 2006; Lewy and Dawson, 1992; Tiegerman and Primavera, 1984), which helps the child attend to the adult during modeling, increasing the likelihood of an imitative response. Although the adult is encouraged to imitate all of the child's behavior, both meaningful and non-meaningful, the adult should avoid imitating dangerous or destructive behaviors, since previous research has indicated that imitating a child's behavior may lead to increases in the behavior that is being imitated (Harris et al., 1987).

During contingent imitation, the adult describes the actions the adult and child are performing using simplified, repetitive language. This narration increases the correspondence between the child and the adult's behavior. For example, if the child were rolling a car back and forth, the adult would model, "Roll. Roll the car. The car is rolling. Roll the car." while imitating the child's behavior. This form of indirect language stimulation has been shown to increase spontaneous and imitative language in young children with ASD (Ingersoll, Dvortcsak, Whalen, and Sikora, 2005, Ingersoll and Schreibman, 2006).

In our original study (Ingersoll and Schreibman, 2006) contingent imitation of the child and linguistic mapping were used exclusively during the first two weeks of treatment prior to teaching the child to imitate the adult. In subsequent studies (Ingersoll et al., in press), imitation training has been introduced at the same time as contingent imitation and linguistic mapping. If training parents to implement the intervention, it might be best to begin with a short period of contingent imitation and linguistic mapping alone in order for the parents to become highly skilled in following their child's lead prior to teaching the child to imitate (Ingersoll and Gergans, 2007); however, when implemented by trained therapists, imitation training can begin immediately.

When teaching imitation the adult models a variety of interesting actions rather than teaching the imitation of a specific action to criterion.

Table 3.1. Goals, techniques and rationale for Reciprocal Imitation Training (RIT)

Goal	Teaching Component	Rationale
Increase child responsivity	*Contingent imitation* – The partner imitates the child's actions with toys, gestures/body movements, and vocalizations at the same time as the child	Increases eye contact and coordinated joint attention. Prepares child to imitate partner and teaches reciprocity.
Increase imitative language	*Linguistic mapping* – The partner describes what the child is attending to and/or doing using simplified language (e.g., "Dog is walking") or sound effects.	Provides appropriate language models. Increases imitative and spontaneous language.
Teach imitation	The partner implements the imitation training procedure once a minute on average during play. Once the child has successfully imitated the partner, the partner returns to imitating child and using linguistic mapping.	Teaches reciprocal turn-taking, allows child to take turns leading and following play partner. Enhances social components of imitation.
	Model – The partner models an action paired with a verbal marker that describes the action up to three times. The partner begins modeling familiar actions with the object the child is engaged with. As the child becomes more imitative, the partner begins to intersperse novel actions. The partner models a descriptive gesture that is functionally related to the child's play. Descriptive gestures include conventional, affective, object, attribute, and action gestures.	Verbal marker provides cue to imitate but, since it is consistently varied, it does not lead to prompt dependence. Beginning with familiar actions and following the child's lead enhances motivation and encourages spontaneous imitation. Gradually introducing novel actions builds play skills. Gestures are modeled within context to encourage spontaneous gesture use of meaningful gestures.
	Prompting – The partner uses physical guidance to encourage the child to imitate the modeled action if the child does not spontaneous imitate after the third model.	Provides child with information on what to do, assists with motor planning, and encourages future imitation via negative reinforcement.
	Contingent Reinforcement – The partner praises the child after imitating and allows the child continued access to the toys.	Encourages future imitation via positive social reinforcement (praise) and tangible reinforcement (continued access to materials).

Note: This table was reprinted with permission from Ingersoll, B. (in press). The social role of imitation in autism: Implications for the treatment of imitation deficits. Infants & Young Children.

For example, if the child is playing with a car, the adult might model a variety of actions related to car play, such as putting a man in the car, crashing the car into the wall, rolling the car down a ramp, or spinning the wheels of the car. Actions are chosen in the moment based on the child's interest and play. This strategy differs from the structured method, in which specific actions are chosen for each toy and taught one at a time to criterion (see Table 3.2).

Table 3.2. Comparison of Structured Imitation Training and RIT

Teaching Strategy	Discrete Trial Training	Reciprocal Imitation Training
Instructor	Therapist	Therapist/Caregiver
Setting	1:1, restricted	1:1, unrestricted
Materials	Adult selected; 1 or 2 sets of each toy.	Child selected; 2 sets of each toy.
Instructor's response to child's behavior	n/a	Contingent imitation of the child; Linguistic mapping of child's play
Discriminative Stimulus (S^D)	Specific and unvaried; (*"Do this"* or *"Do what I do"*)	General and varied; verbal description of action
Modeled Actions	All novel; pre-selected; Actions targeted one at a time to criterion.	Familiar, then novel; related to child's play/attentional focus; Multiple actions targeted concurrently.
Gestures	Arbitrary and meaningful; presented out of context	Meaningful; presented in context
Prompt strategies	Standard to criterion (full physical, partial physical, gesture, verbal); systematically faded	Physical guidance after 3rd model; no fading
Reinforcement Properties	Artificial-Social praise and access to preferred food or non-target play materials	Natural-Social praise and continued access to target play materials
Reinforcement Contingencies	Only for successive approximations	Loose shaping, reinforce attempts
Order of Training	Body/gesture before object	Object before gesture

By targeting a variety of actions at once, it is possible to keep the child interested in the activity and achieve generalized responding with limited intervention (Stokes and Baer, 1977). In addition, all attempts made by the child to imitate are reinforced with praise, even when they only approximate the adult's model. This strategy is used to increase motivation (Koegel et al., 1987) and to teach the child that our goal is for the child's behavior to match our behavior, rather than the accurate production of a specific action.

Early in treatment the adult models actions that are familiar and directly related to the child's current play. Thus, if the child typically plays with a car by rolling it back and forth or spinning its wheels, the adult might model rolling it back and forth while the child is spinning the wheels. Initially, familiar actions that are self-stimulatory, such as spinning the wheels of a car, might be modeled unless they are disruptive. By starting with familiar actions, we use the child's natural motivation for completing the action to teach imitation skills with the goal that imitation becomes intrinsically motivating and, therefore, more likely to maintain in the natural environment. This strategy differs significantly from the structured method, in which actions are chosen a priori from a list of actions that the child is not yet performing spontaneously.

As noted earlier research indicates that behavior that is brought under tight stimulus control often lacks spontaneity (Carr, 1981). Thus, in order to increase spontaneous responding, the modeled action is paired with a distinct, verbal marker, such as a sound effect or description of the action, rather than a specific S^D such as, "Do this", which is often used in the structured approach. The verbal marker is used to draw the child's attention to the action; however, it is consistently varied to prevent the child from becoming prompt dependent. For example, in placing a person in the car, the adult might say "Vroom, vroom" or "The boy is driving." Although the verbal marker provides a description of the action, specific verbal directions or commands (e.g., "Push the car") are avoided.

The action and verbal marker should be modeled up to three times. If the child fails to imitate on his or her own after three opportunities, the adult uses physical guidance to assist the child in completing the action. This guidance is provided for several reasons. First, it helps the child learn that he or she is expected to imitate the model. Second, it provides the child with a motor plan to complete new actions, which may be especially helpful for children who have motor planning difficulties. Third, it can be seen as a form of negative reinforcement, in that children can learn to avoid physical manipulation by completing the act spontaneously.

Once the child imitates the action, either spontaneously or with physical guidance, the adult provides contingent social praise and returns to imitating the child's behavior. Social reinforcement is more likely to mimic the reinforcers available during natural adult-child imitative interactions and thus, is more likely to promote the use of imitation outside of the treatment environment. In addition, by modeling interesting actions, the hope is that imitation itself becomes reinforcing. This strategy differs from the structured approach which typically provides artificial reinforcement (e.g., preferred snack item is used to reinforce object imitation).

Over time, the goal is to increase the complexity and flexibility of the child's imitation. Once the child begins to imitate familiar actions, novel actions can be introduced, such as placing a person in the car or filling the car with gas. Over time, self-stimulatory actions are replaced with more appropriate actions. In addition, once the child is able to consistently imitate actions modeled with the same object the child is engaged with, the adult can begin to present actions with a different toy. It is important to intermix familiar actions and actions with the same toy even while expanding the child's imitation, in order to keep motivation high (Koegel et al., 1987).

This intervention was originally designed to teach object imitation (Ingersoll and Schreibman, 2006), but has been modified to target gesture imitation as well (Ingersoll, Lewis and Kroman, in press). When teaching gesture imitation, conventional (e.g., waving as a greeting; palms up to indicate "where did it go?"), affective (e.g., clapping to indicate "good job"; hands on hips to indicate "mad"), and descriptive (e.g., arms out to indicate "big"; point in air to indicate "up") gestures are specifically targeted. In this training rather than modeling an action with an object, the adult models a gesture related to the child's play paired with a related verbal descriptor. Thus, if the child is rolling a car back and forth, the adult might model a sweeping hand motion ("Car is fast") or a circular hand motion ("Wheels are spinning").

Because object imitation is easier (DeMyer et al., 1972) and more intrinsically motivating, the adult typically targets object imitation before focusing on gesture imitation. However, object and gesture imitation can be targeted concurrently, depending on the child's ability. When teaching both object and gesture imitation, it is possible to present both types of trials within a session (Ingersoll and Gergans, 2007). However, it is often easier for the adult to focus on only one target at a time; thus in our current work, we alternate sessions.

RESEARCH ON RECIPROCAL IMITATION TRAINING

Several studies have been conducted on the effectiveness of this approach (see Figure 3.1). The first study used a multiple baseline design across five young children with ASD to examine the effectiveness of RIT for teaching object imitation (Ingersoll and Schreibman, 2006). The children ranged in age from 29 to 45 months (Mean CA=36.6 mos.). At intake all children exhibited significant developmental delay (Mean MA=19.1 mos.) and two of the children were non-verbal (Mean LA=16 mos.). The children received three, one-hour object imitation training sessions per week of RIT for 10 weeks. To assess generalization of skills to novel environments, probes were conducted at the end of treatment and at a one-month follow-up. During baseline, the children exhibited low rates of spontaneous imitation. After the onset of treatment, they showed substantial gains in their use of object imitation. Four of the five child participants maintained these gains after the removal of treatment and generalized their ability to imitate actions with objects to novel play materials, a therapist, and a setting. Follow-up data obtained after one month indicated that all children maintained higher than baseline rates of object imitation. Changes in object imitation were also evident on the Motor Imitation Scale (Stone et al., 1997), a structured imitation assessment, and during a naturalistic, structured observation with the therapist and the caregiver.

An additional important finding was that the children made gains in other non-targeted, social-communicative behaviors. All of the children increased their imitative language and four children used more coordinated joint attention and pretend play. For most of the children, increases in the non-targeted, social-communicative behaviors were maintained after treatment was withdrawn and at a one-month follow-up. Perhaps more exciting was the finding that using a 7-point Likert-type scale naïve observers blind to participants' treatment status rated the participants as exhibiting significantly more appropriate social-communication skills and appearing more typically-developing at post-treatment than pre-treatment This finding suggests that this treatment led to socially valid changes for the participants.

A second study targeted the imitation of meaningful gestures (Ingersoll, Lewis, and Kroman, in press). This study used a multiple baseline design across five young children with ASD who had difficulty with the imitation and spontaneous use of gestures. These children were slightly older (Mean CA=41.1 mos.) and had slightly higher mental ages (Mean MA=24.4 mos.) than the children in the object imitation study and all had at least single words (Mean LA=23.4 mos.) at intake. The children received two, one-hour sessions per week of RIT targeting gesture imitation for 10 weeks. To assess generalization of skills, generalization probes were conducted once a week throughout treatment and at a one-month follow-up. During baseline, the children exhibited few to no episodes of gesture imitation or spontaneous gesture use. With the onset of treatment, all children showed an increase in their imitation of gestures. The imitation skills generalized to novel environments and maintained at a one-month follow-up.

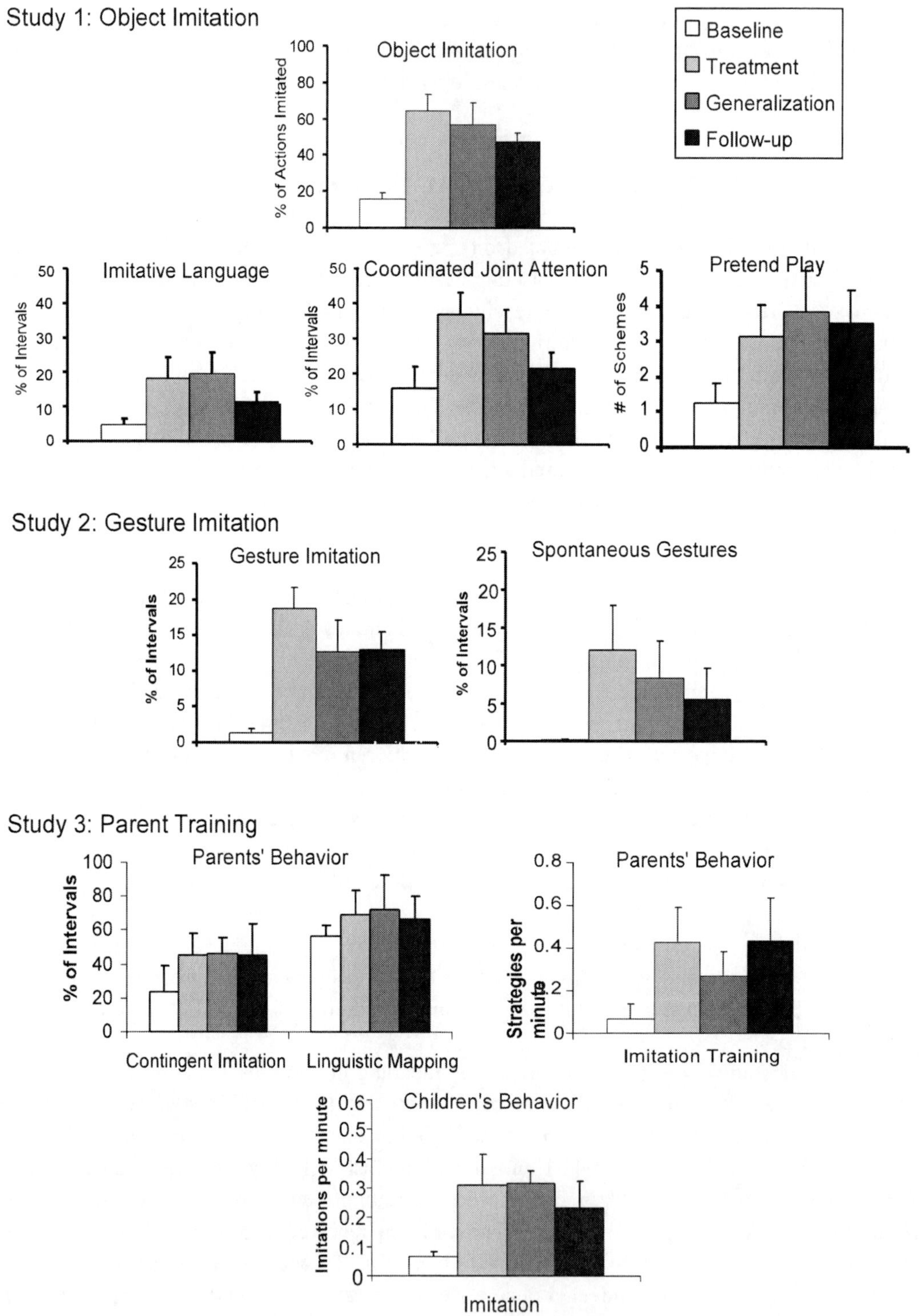

Figure 3.1. Summary data from Reciprocal Imitation Training studies. Original data analyses were conducted using visual analysis of single subject, multiple-baseline designs. Data were averaged across participants for presentation purposes. Error bars represent standard error.

Looking at spontaneous use of gestures, three of the children exhibited substantial gains while the other two exhibited small, but consistent gains. In addition, naïve observers blind to treatment status rated the children as using more appropriate social communication during treatment than at baseline. These findings suggest that RIT is effective for teaching gesture use and may have more global effects on social communication.

In a third study, three mothers were taught to implement RIT techniques with their child. Training sessions occurred twice a week for 10 weeks in a clinic setting (Ingersoll and Gergans, 2007). The children ranged in age from 31 to 42 months (Mean CA=36.7 mos.; Mean MA=17.3 mos.) and two of the children were non-verbal at intake (Mean LA=11 mos.). Within a multiple-baseline design, the mothers of the two non-verbal children were taught to use RIT to teach object imitation and the mother of the verbal child was taught to use RIT to target both object and gesture imitation. Generalization was assessed in the families' homes at the end of treatment and during a one-month follow-up. Results indicated that the parents learned to use the intervention strategies and their children improved their imitation skills. Importantly, the children's and parents' skills both generalized to the home and maintained over time. Parents rated the intervention as effective for improving a variety of social communication skills in their child, simple and easy to use, as well as enjoyable for them and their child. These findings suggest that RIT is appropriate as a parent training intervention.

ONGOING WORK

Our previous research suggests that RIT holds promise as an effective method for teaching imitation skills to young children with ASD. This approach leads to generalized imitation skills and concurrent changes in other important social-communication skills. We are conducting additional research to examine the efficacy of this intervention. Our current research will allow us to replicate and extend our previous findings of treatment efficacy using standardized assessments and a randomized control trial. We will compare young children with ASD receiving 12 weeks of RIT (3 hours per week) targeting object and gesture imitation to a control group receiving treatment-as-usual. We expect to find that the children who receive RIT will show more improvement in imitation, as well as other social-communication skills. We will also examine whether changes in generalized social-communication skills during treatment can be attributed specifically to the treatment's effect on imitation skills or are a generalized effect of the intervention. We expect to find that, in the RIT group, changes in imitation skills will mediate changes in other social-communication skills. We are also interested in determining what child characteristics at pre-treatment (language age, imitation skills, social reciprocity, cognitive ability and autism severity) predict response to RIT. Hopefully, these results will allow us to determine a priori which children are most likely to benefit from RIT.

FUTURE RESEARCH

If the research on RIT continues to support its efficacy, another important question would be whether RIT leads to better outcomes than other currently available imitation interventions, more specifically structured. We would predict that children with ASD would learn imitation skills at a similar rate using the two approaches; however, children learning imitation via RIT would be more likely to use imitation in the natural environment and would also experience additional gains in other social-communication skills. It would also be important to examine whether different child characteristics predict whether children would respond better to one type of imitation intervention than another. For example, we might predict that children with initially low levels of object interaction might benefit more from a structured behavioral approach, while children with moderate levels of object interaction might benefit more from RIT. Clearly additional research is needed to answer these questions.

To this point, we have examined the effectiveness of RIT exclusively with young children with ASD. Our reasons for limiting our research to this population has been theoretical more than clinical; we have been interested in examining the hypothesis that teaching imitation skills early in development may lead to broader changes in social communication (Rogers, 1999). Thus, it is unknown whether older children would also benefit from RIT. We would predict that RIT would be an appropriate intervention for older children with limited language, imitation, and play skills. However, older, more able children may benefit more from learning additional peer interaction skills, since as children age, reciprocal imitation becomes significantly less common and children are much more likely to engage in complimentary actions (Eckerman and Didow, 1996). However, it is also possible, that RIT could be adapted for older, more able children to target more subtle forms of imitation, particularly in the area of gestures.

Given the simplicity of the treatment techniques, it is likely this intervention would be suitable as a peer-mediated strategy. Peers or siblings could be taught to use RIT strategies with children with ASD. In fact, given the significance of reciprocal imitation during peer play, it may be more important to teach young children with ASD to imitate their peers rather than adults. A variety of research has focused on teaching children with ASD and other developmental disabilities to imitate specific peer behaviors (e.g., Apolloni, Cooke, and Cooke, 1977; Tryon and Keane, 1986). The majority of these interventions involve the adult training the child peer to model specific actions while the adult prompts the target child to imitate. A similar approach that incorporates training peers to imitate the child with ASD (i.e., reciprocal imitation) may increase social interaction as well as imitation. In some preliminary work, we found that typically developing children as young as two and a half could be taught to contingently imitate the behavior of a peer with ASD. In addition we found that the use of contingent imitation corresponded to increases in the toddler with ASD's use of coordinated joint attention (Ingersoll and Stahmer, 2002).

Another important question is whether RIT can be easily incorporated into existing early intervention (EI) and early childhood special education (ECSE) programs, many of which are group-based. Research suggests that this approach may be adapted for use in group settings. Using a small group intervention Garfinkle and Swartz (2002), taught four-year-old children with ASD to imitate their typically developing peers. Each child in the group took turns being the "leader" during which time he or she modeled preferred actions with toys. The other children in the group were then prompted by an adult to imitate the leader's behavior using a duplicate set of toys and the adult provided praise for successful imitation. Generalization sessions conducted during free play indicated that the intervention resulted in increases in social interactions between the children with ASD and the typical peers. This study suggests that peer interventions incorporating contingent imitation and prompts for imitation may be effectively used in preschool classrooms. Future research is necessary to examine the best ways to teach intervention providers to use RIT and how RIT can be best incorporated into existing EI/ECSE curricula.

In conclusion, children with ASD exhibit significant deficits in imitation skills that disrupt the development of more advanced cognitive and social-communication skills. Structured behavioral treatment options are limited in their ability to teach flexible, generalized imitation skills that maintain in the natural environment. *Reciprocal Imitation Training*, a naturalistic behavioral intervention, shows promise for teaching generalized imitation skills and promoting the use of more advanced social communication. Future research further evaluating this intervention's effectiveness will likely lead to more effective interventions for children with ASD who do not imitate.

ACKNOWLEDGMENTS

Preparation of this chapter was supported by a grant from the Cure Autism Now Foundation (Ingersoll, P.I.) and by U.S.P.H.S. research grant MH39434 from the National Institute of Mental Health (Schreibman, P.I.).

REFERENCES

Alpert, C.L., and Kaiser, A.P. (1992). Training parents as milieu language teachers. *Journal of Early Intervention,* 16, 31-52.

American Psychiatric Association (2000). Diagnostic and statistical manual of mental disorders-Text revision.

Apolloni, T., Cooke, S.A., and Cooke, T.P. (1977). Establishing a normal peer as a behavioral model for developmentally delayed toddlers. *Perceptual and Motor Skills,* 44, 231-241.

Baer, D.M., Peterson, R.F., and Sherman, J.A. (1967). The Development of Imitation by Reinforcing Behavioral Similarity To A Model. *Journal of the Experimental Analysis of Behavior,* 10, 405-416.

Bates, E., Bretherton, I., Snyder, L., Beeghly, M., Shore, C., McNew, S., Carlson, V., Williamson, C., and Garrison, A. (1988). *From first words to grammar: Individual differences and dissociable mechanisms*. New York: Cambridge University Press.

Carpenter, M., Pennington, B.E., and Rogers, S.J. (2002). Interrelations among social-cognitive skills in young children with autism. *Journal of Autism and Developmental Disorders,* 32, 91-106.

Carr, E.G. (1981). Sign language. In O.I. Lovaas, A. Ackerman, D. Alexander, P. Firestone, M. Perkins, and A.L. Egel (Eds.). *The me book: Teaching manual for parents and teachers of developmentally disabled children* (pp. 153-161). Baltimore: University Park Press.

Charlop-Christy, M.H. and Carpenter, M. (2000). Modified incidental teaching sessions: A procedure for parents to increase spontaneous speech in their children with autism. *Journal of Positive Behavior Interventions,* 2, 98-112.

Curcio, F. (1978). Sensorimotor functioning and communication in mute autistic children. *Journal of Autism and Childhood Schizophrenia,* 8, 281-292.

Dawson, G., and Adams, A. (1984). Imitation and social responsiveness in autistic children. *Journal of Abnormal Child Psychology,* 12, 209-226.

Dawson, G., and Galpert, L. (1990). Mothers' use of imitative play for the facilitation of social responsiveness and toy play in young autistic children. *Development and Psychopathology,* 2, 151-62.

Delprato, D.J. (2001). Comparisons of discrete-trial and normalized behavioral intervention for young children with autism. *Journal of Autism and Developmental Disorders*, 31, 315-325.

DeMyer, M., Alpern, G., Barton, S., DeMyer, W., Churchill, D., Hingtgen, J., Bryson, C., Pontius, W., and Kimberlin, C. (1972). Imitation in autistic, early schizophrenic, and non-psychotic subnormal children. *Journal of Autism and Childhood Schizophrenia,* 2, 264-287.

Eckerman, C., and Didow, S. (1996). Nonverbal imitation and toddlers' mastery of verbal means of achieving coordinated action. *Developmental Psychology,* 32, 141-152.

Escalona, A., Field, T., Nadel, J., and Lundy, B. (2002). Brief report: Imitation effects on children with autism. *Journal of Autism and Developmental Disorders,* 32, 141-144.

Fiese, B. (1990). Playful relationships: A contextual analysis of mother-toddler interaction and symbolic play. *Child Development,* 61, 1648-1656.

Gazdag, G. and Warren, S.F. (2000). Effects of adult contingent imitation on development of young children's vocal imitation. *Journal of Early Intervention,* 23, 24-35.

Garfinkle, A.N. and Schwartz, I.S. (2002). Peer imitation: Increasing social interactions in children with autism and other developmental disabilities in inclusive preschool classrooms. *Topics in Early Childhood Special Education,* 22, 26-38.

Harris, S.L., Handleman, J.S., and Fong, P.L. (1987). Imitation of self-stimulation: Impact on the autistic child's behavior and affect. *Child and Family Behavior Therapy,* 9, 1-21.

Hart, B.M, and Risley, T.R. (1968). Establishing Use of Descriptive Adjectives in the Spontaneous Speech of Disadvantaged Preschool Children. *Journal of Applied Behavior Analysis,* 1, 109-120.

Hobson, R.P., and Lee, A. (1999). Imitation and identification in autism. *Journal of Child Psychology and Psychiatry,* 40, 649-659.

Hwang, B., and Hughes, C. (2000). Increasing early social-communicative skills of preverbal preschool children with autism through social interactive training. *Journal of the Association for Persons with Severe Handicaps,* 25, 18-28.

Ingersoll, B. (in press a). The social role of imitation in autism: Implications for the treatment of imitation deficits. *Infants and Young Children.*

Ingersoll, B. (in press b). The effect of context on imitation skills in children with autism. *Research in Autism Spectrum Disorders.*

Ingersoll, B., Dvortcsak, A., Whalen, C., and Sikora, D. (2005). The effect of a developmental, social pragmatic language intervention on expressive language skills in young children with autism spectrum disorders. *Focus on Autism and other Developmental Disabilities,* 20, 213-222.

Ingersoll, B. and Gergans, S. (2007). The effect of a parent-implemented naturalistic imitation intervention on spontaneous imitation skills in young children with autism. *Research in Developmental Disabilities,* 28, 163-175.

Ingersoll, B., Lewis, E., and Kroman, E. (in press). Teaching the imitation and spontaneous use of descriptive gestures to young children with autism using a naturalistic behavioral intervention. *Journal of Autism and Developmental Disorders.*

Ingersoll, B. and Schreibman, L. (2006). Teaching reciprocal imitation skills to young children with autism using a naturalistic behavioral approach: Effects on language, pretend play, and joint attention. *Journal of Autism and Developmental Disorders, 36,* 487-505.

Ingersoll, B., Schreibman, L., and Tran, Q. (2003). The effect of sensory feedback on immediate object imitation in children with autism. *Journal of Autism and Developmental Disorders, 33,* 673-683.

Ingersoll, B. and Stahmer, A. (2002, May). Teaching peer interaction skills in toddlers with autism: Effects of contingent imitation training. In A. Stahmer (Chair), *The role of typical toddlers in the early social development of children with autism.* Symposium conducted at the annual meeting of the Association for Behavior Analysis, Toronto, Canada.

Kaiser, A.P., Yoder, P.J., and Keetz, A. (1992). Evaluating mileu teaching. In S.F. Warren and J. Rcichlc (Eds.), *Causes and Effects in Communication and Language Intervention* (pp. 9-48). Baltimore, MD: Paul Brooks Publishing Co.

Klinger, L.G., and Dawson, G. (1992). Facilitating early social and communicative development in children with autism. In S. F. Warren and J. E. Reichle (Eds.), *Causes and effects in communication and language intervention.* (pp. 157-186). Baltimore, MD, US: Paul H. Brookes Publishing.

Koegel, R.L. and Koegel, L.K. (Eds.). (1995). *Teaching children with autism: Strategies for initiating positive interactions and improving learning opportunities.* Baltimore: Paul H. Brooks Publishing Co.

Koegel, R.L., O'Dell, M.C., and Koegel, L.K. (1987). A natural language teaching paradigm for nonverbal autistic children. *Journal of Autismand Developmental Disorders,* 17, 187-200.

Koegel, R.L., Schreibman, L., Good, A., Cerniglia, L., Murphy, C., and Koegel, L. (1989). *How to teach pivotal behaviors to children with autism: A training manual.* Santa Barbara: University of California.

Lewy, A.L. and Dawson, G. (1992). Social stimulation and joint attention in young autistic children. *Journal of Abnormal Child Psychology,* 20, 555-566.

Lovaas, O.I. (1977). *The autistic child: Language development through behavior modification.* New York, Irvington.

Lovaas, O.I. (1987). Behavioral treatment and normal educational and intellectual functioning in young autistic children. *Journal of Consulting and Clinical Psychology,* 55, 3-9.

Lovaas, O.I., Berberich, J.P., Perloff, B.F., and Schaeffer, B. (1966). Acquisition of imitative speech by schizophrenic children. *Science,* 151, 705-707.

Lovaas, O.I., Freitas, K., Nelson, and Whalen, C. (1967). The establishment of imitation and its use for the development of complex behavior in schizophrenic children. *Behaviour Research and Therapy,* 5, 171-182.

Maurice, C., Green, G., and Luce, S.C. (Eds.). (1996). *Behavioral intervention for young children with autism: A manual for parents and professionals.* Austin, TX, US: PRO-ED, Inc.

McDuffie, A., Turner, L., Stone, W., Yoder, P., Wolery, M. and Ulman, T. (2007). Developmental correlates of different types of motor imitation in young children with autism spectrum disorders. *Journal of Autism and Developmental Disorders, 37,* 401-412.

Meltzoff, A.N., and Moore, M.K. (1977). Imitation of facial and manual gestures by human neonates. *Science,* 198, 75-78.

Metz, J. R. (1965). Conditioning Generalized Imitation in Autistic Children. *Journal of Experimental Child Psychology,* 4, 389-399.

Miranda-Linne, F., and Melin, L. (1992). Acquisition, generalization, and spontaneous use of color adjectives: A comparison of incidental teaching and traditional discrete-trial procedures for children with autism. *Research in Developmental Disabilities,* 13, 191-210.

Nadel, J and Peze, A. (1993). What makes immediate imitation communicative in toddlers and autistic children. In J. Nadel and L. Camaioni (Eds.), *New perspectives in early communicative development* (pp. 139-156). New York : Routledge.

Pierce, K. and Schreibman, L. (1995). Increasing complex social behaviors in children with autism: Effects of peer-implemented pivotal response training. *Journal of Applied Behavior Analysis*, 28, 285-295.

Quill, K.A. (2000). *Do-watch-listen-say: Social and communication intervention for children with autism.* Baltimore: Paul H. Brooks Publishing Co.

Rogers, S.J. (1999). An examination of the imitation deficit in autism. In J. Nadel and G. Butterworth (Eds.), *Imitation in infancy* (pp. 254-279). Cambridge: Cambridge University Press.

Rogers, S. J. and Bennetto, L. (2000). Intersubjectivity in autism: The roles of imitation and executive function. In A. Wetherby and B. Prizant (Eds.), Autism spectrum disorders: A transactional developmental perspective (pp. 79-107). Baltimore, MD: Paul H. Brookes.

Rogers, S.J., Hepburn, S., Stackhouse, T., and Wehner, E. (2003). Imitation performance in toddlers with autism and those with other developmental disorders. *Journal of Child Psychology and Psychiatry,* 44, 763-781.

Rogers, S. J. and Williams. J. (Eds.). (2006). *Imitation and the development of the social mind: Lessons from typical development and autism.* New York: Guilford.

Schreibman, L., Kaneko, W.M., and Koegel, R.L. (1991). Positive affect of parents of autistic children: A comparison across two teaching techniques. *Behavior Therapy,* 22, 479-490.

Schwartz, I.S., Anderson, S.R., and Halle, J.W. (1989). Training teachers to use naturalistic time delay: Effects on teacher behavior and on the language use of students. *Journal of the Association for Persons with Severe Handicaps*, 14, 48-57.

Smith, I., and Bryson S. (1994). Imitation and action in autism: A critical review. *Psychological Bulletin,* 116, 259-73.

Spradlin, J.E. and Siegel, G.M. (1982). Language training in natural and clinical environments. *Journal of Speech and Hearing Disorders,* 47, 2-6.

Stahmer, A.C. (1995). Teaching symbolic play skills to children with autism using pivotal response training. *Journal of Autismand Developmental Disorders,* 25, 123-141.

Stokes, T.F. and Baer, D.M. (1977). An implicit technology of generalization. *Journal of Applied Behavior Analysis,* 10, 349-367.

Stone, W., Ousley, O., and Littleford, C. (1997). Motor imitation in young children with autism: What's the object? *Journal of Abnormal Child Psychology,* 25, 475-485.

Stone, W.L., and Yoder, P.J. (2001). Predicting spoken language level in children with autism spectrum disorders. *Autism,* 5, 341-361.

Thorp, D.M., Stahmer, A.C., and Schreibman, L. (1995). Effects of sociodramatic play training on children with autism. *Journal of Autism and Developmental Disorders, 25*, 265-282.

Tiegerman, E., and Primavera, L. (1981). Object manipulation: An interactional strategy with autistic children. *Journal of Autism and Developmental Disorders,* 11, 427-438.

Tiegerman, E., and Primavera, L. (1984). Imitating the autistic child: Facilitating communicative gaze behavior. *Journal of Autism and Developmental Disorders,* 14, 27-38.

Tryon, A.., and Keane, S.P. (1986). Promoting imitative play through generalized observational learning in autistic-like children. *Journal of Abnormal Child Psychology,* 14, 532-549.

Uzgiris, I. (1981). Two functions of imitation in infancy. *International Journal of Behavioral Development*, 4, 1-12.

Uzgiris, I. (1990). The social context of infant imitation. In M. Lewis and S. Feinman (Eds.), *Social influences and socialization in infancy* (pp. 215-51). New York: Plenum Press.

Uzgiris, I. and Hunt, J. (1975). *Assessment in infancy.* Urbana, IL: University of Illinois Press.

Warren, S.F., Yoder, P.J., Gazdag, G.E., and Kim, K. (1993). Facilitating prelinguistic communication skills in young children with developmental delay. *Journal of Speech and Hearing Research,* 36, 83-97.

Whalen, C. and Schreibman, L. (2003). Joint attention training for children with autism using behavior modification procedures. *Journal of Child Psychiatry and Psychology,* 44, 456-468.

Whiten, A., and Brown, J. (1998). Imitation and the reading of other minds: Perspectives from the study of autism, normal children, and non-human primates. In S. Braten (Ed.) *Intersubjective communication and emotion in early ontogeny* (pp. 260-80). New York: Cambridge University Press.

Williams, J.H.G., Whiten, A., and Singh, T. (2004). A systematic review of action imitation in autistic spectrum disorder. *Journal of Autism and Developmental Disorders,* 34, 285-299.

In: Behavioral Theories and Interventions for Autism ISBN 978-1-60741-165-9
Editor: Phil Reed © 2009 Nova Science Publishers, Inc.

Chapter 4

RELATIONAL FRAME THEORY INTERVENTIONS FOR PERSPECTIVE-TAKING DEFICITS IN AUTISTIC SPECTRUM DISORDERS

Louise McHugh*
Swansea University, UK

The inability to understand the meaning of social signals and mental states is a feature of children with Autistic Spectrum Disorder (ASD; Chin and Bernard-Opitz, 2000; Sigman and Ruskin, 1999). Underlying their communication difficulties, many autistic children also show profound deficits in the ability to take the perspective of another. These communication deficits make successful social interaction less likely. The criteria in the Diagnostic and Statistical Manual (DSM) for the diagnosis of ASD centre around 'qualitative impairment in social interaction' and 'qualitative impairments in communication'. Given the strong link between ASD, social interactions and language, understanding the processes underlying the development of these repertoires is essential.

The current chapter describes some of the precursors to the development of perspective taking, followed by relevant concepts from the cognitive literature on the development of perspective-taking, also referred to as Theory of Mind (ToM). Following on from this section is an account of behavioral approaches to the development of social interactions, with particular reference to a behavior analytic account of the development of human language and cognition, Relational Frame Theory (RFT; Hayes, Barnes-Holmes and Roche, 2001).

PRECURSORS TO PERSPECTIVE TAKING

Joint attention between an infant and caregiver has been empirically modeled as a precursor to the development of social interactions such as taking the perspective of another. Research indicates that at around 12 to 15 month's infants' interactions with others undergo a significant change. In a longitudinal study by Bakeman and Adamson (1984) a dichotomous

* Correspondence should be addressed to Louise McHugh, Department of Psychology, Swansea University, Singleton Park, Swansea, SA2 8PP, U.K.

category was coined to refer to distinct parent-infant engagements. These categories are "passive joint attention engagement" (i.e., passive infant-mother interaction) and "coordinated joint engagement" (i.e., where the infant actively participates in the interaction). While the former interactions occur from birth the latter do not emerge until 12 to 15 months of age.

One possible explanation for the development of coordinated joint attention is the organic emergence of the infants' understanding of the specific action plans of other persons, the knowledge of which they subsequently use in their activities with others. Evidence for this interpretation was provided by Ross and Lollis (1987), who observed that when an adult stops participating in a shared activity with an infant, infants who are fourteen months and older, will not only prompt the adult to reengage, but will even perform the adult's turn for them in order to reengage the adult. Carpenter, Tomasello, and Striano (2005) constructed scenarios in which an adult, for example, held out a basket in which the child should place a toy. When the child engaged in the task the adult then placed the basket in front of the child and held the toy themselves. Some 12-month-olds, and even more 18-month-olds, then took their turn by holding out the basket for the adult and, importantly, looked to the adult in anticipation of them placing a toy in it. Thus, after an initial encounter in one role of an interaction, infants often derive the other role. This has been referred to as reversal imitation (Ratner and Bruner, 1977).

In these interactions, infants are engaging in joint attention, (Tomasello and Haberl, 2003; Liszkowski, Carpenter, Henning, Striano, and Tomasello, 2004). Indeed, there is a shift in the manner in which infants look at others over the course of their first twelve months, a shift that coincides with emergent abilities in social interactions (e.g., Rochat and Striano, 1999). While early gaze patterns in social interactions are generally dyadic, with the infants' attentional focus remaining exclusively on one social partner, from twelve months onwards infants gazing behavior becomes increasingly coordinated between people and objects.

A wealth of research has been conducted in the area of referential looking in infants due to the theoretical link between this behavior and the development of a wider class of social cognitive abilities. Specifically, this referential looking is linked to an early understanding that people have intentions directed to the external environment. This emergent understanding of the intentions of others is a basic development fundamental to theories of mind that emerge in young children by three years of age (Wellman, 1993). The development of referential looking underlies many important social behavioral repertoires, such as, looking at others during joint play (Bakeman and Adamson, 1984), following people's gaze in relation to external events and situations (Corkum and Moore, 1998), and checking others emotional perspective to provide cues in novel situations (Sorce, Emde, Campos, and Klinnert, 1985).

Recently, behavioral researchers have taken an interest in the emergence of joint attention in infant mother interactions (Dube, MacDonald, Mansfield, Holcomb and Ahearn, 2004). According to Dube et al (2004) stimuli that an adult attends to become conditioned reinforcers after a learning history in which the stimuli have become predictors that the adult will respond to the event and also that the adult's response will result in reinforcement for the infant. These conditioned reinforcers (i.e., the adult-attending stimuli) function as links in a behavioral chain. Specifically, they function as conditioned reinforcers for where to look and as discriminative stimuli for an increased probability of reinforcers linked to the adult's behavior. From this perspective there are two reasons why an infant may engage in joint attention: 1) because of their relevant history of event-related consequences; 2). because of a reinforcement history (either positive or negative) that includes both event-related consequences and adult mediated consequences. For example, in the case of negative reinforcement one potential class of reinforcers that may maintain the initiation of joint attention is negative reinforcement, that is, the termination of an aversive event. If the child's past experience has been that the adult's behavior is a reliable guide to the level of threat in a given situation, then one consequence of joint attention may be to predict from the adult's behavior that the situation is safe.

Behavioral researchers have also conducted research on the development of social referencing, in which the child observes the emotional expressions of others to appraise events and guide action. Behaviorally, social referencing is viewed as an example of social knowledge. With experience, the child learns that if the mother is smiling when a stranger approaches, reinforcement is likely. Thus, the facial expression of the mother becomes a setting event that establishes the function of the stranger as being discriminative for positive or negative reinforcement. Although one view of social referencing has suggested that it is an innate 'pre-wired' ability (Campos and Barrett, 1984) behavioral research has provided an alternative emphasizing that social referencing can result from contingency-based learning.

For example, Gewirtz and Pelaez-Nogueras (1992) conducted two experiments in order to determine whether infants could learn to respond to maternal "expressive" cues in ambiguous situations. In the first experiment, the mother was trained to present emotionally neutral (i.e, meaningless) cues to the infant (e.g., the mother holding her palms against the sides of her face). Twenty infants (age range 9 to 12 months) participated in daily sessions with their mothers across 8 to 13 weeks. Each trial involved placing, a covered, ambiguous object in front of the infant while the mother gave a neutral cue when the child looked at her. After the mothers cue the object was uncovered and moved within reach of the infant. If the child reached for the object, one of the two consequences was delivered (positive Sd: a brief musical baby melody, or negative Sd: harsh door buzzer) based on the cue given by the mother. The findings indicated that the infants learned to use their mother's (originally meaningless) cue as a discriminative stimulus for reaching when the cue was paired with a positive consequence.

The second experiment replicated experiment one using maternal facial emotional expressions as the cues, in order to determine whether facial expressions could also function as conditioned cues for infant referencing (Pelaez-Nogueras,1992). The findings replicated those of the first experiment, indicating that maternal facial-emotional expressions can be trained as cues for infant social referencing. These experiments provide an operant account of the development of social referencing. That is, the child learns through operant conditioning that the mother's facial expression reliably predicts specific consequences.

While different theories have accounted for the development of joint attention and social referencing all accounts agree that the ability of infants to engage in these behaviors presupposes a rudimentary insight into the minds of others. The fact that infants seek and interpret others' focus of attention and corresponding emotional perspective is a precursor to understanding that people have emotions, intentions, and perspectives that differ from their own and thus the development of social interactions (Bretherton, 1991; Striano and Rochat, 1999; Tomasello, 1995; Wellman, 1993).

THEORIES OF THE DEVELOPMENT OF SOCIAL INTERACTIONS

The development of social interactions has attracted considerable attention from mainstream psychologists based on its link to Autistic Spectrum Disorder (Baron-Cohen, 1995). Many different approaches to the development of human social interactions have emerged, some researchers have suggested that the development of social interaction emerges through pre-wired organic processes while others view the development of these abilities as 'experience driven' or learnt. A wide body of empirical work has been conducted in order to determine how children come to develop an understanding of other peoples' perspective, beliefs and desires (sometimes referred to as a theory of mind).

(i) Hobson. One widely known approach is that of Hobson (2007) who tracks the evolution of the human mind back to early infancy and views its development as by-product of a series of interactions between the infant and caregiver. Hobson links the development of human cognition to the work of Trevarthen (1978), who viewed the development of understanding other minds intersubjectively (i.e., between two or more subjects). Trevarthen viewed intersubjective interaction as a distinct developmental phase which prepared the pre-lingual infant's developing brain with the prerequisites necessary for symbolic thought.

Hobson tested this prediction by extending a research program that employed populations who were unable to engage in intersubjective relationships (for either genetic or environmental reasons), such as those diagnosed with ASD, Down's syndrome, congenital blindness and extreme social deprivation. Findings from this work suggested that an innate emotional connection is critical for an infant to start the process of intersubjective learning. The experience of having an emotion elicited by another human being, and eliciting emotional responses in others, appeared to be critical to the development of a sense of self, understanding the perspective of another and understanding symbol referents, as evidenced by deficits in these areas in the populations who lacked intersubjective relationships. According to Hobson (2007) it is the dissociation between ASD children's ability to perceive and understand actions, and impaired abilities to perceive and understand subjective/emotional states, that contributes to their social-communication deficits.

(ii) Theory of Mind Approach. Theory of Mind can be loosely defined as "the appreciation of the representational nature of mind and its relation to behavior" (Suddendorf and Fletcher-Flinn, 2002, p. 1). Specifically, Baron-Cohen et al., (2000) suggested that an individual may be described as portraying a well-developed theory of mind when s/he demonstrates "the ability to infer or attribute to oneself and others the full range of mental states (i.e. beliefs, desires, intentions, imagination, emotions, etc.) that cause action" (p. 3). From this perspective, therefore, a well-developed theory of mind requires the attribution of *both* information and emotion.

Theory of mind researchers have suggested that children must demonstrate a number of key distinctions with regard to their knowledge or information about objects or events in the environment before this information can be fully attributed to the self and others. Much of the ToM research in this area has involved comparative studies between ASD children and their normally developing counterparts.

A number of researchers have reported differences in the abilities of these two groups with regard to the *mental-physical distinction* (Wellman and Estes, 1986). In studies of this kind, for example, a child may be asked to listen to a story in which one character experiences a psychological event (e.g. thinking about a dog) while another character experiences a physical event (e.g. holding an actual dog). The child will then be asked, for example, "Who will be able to stroke the dog?" Wellman and Estes observed that normally-developing children aged between three and four years old could easily distinguish between mental and physical events by attributing the correct action to the appropriate character, whereas ASD children could not (see also Baron-Cohen, 1989a). In a similar study, the same researchers (1986) also observed differences between normally-developing and ASD children with regard to the attribution of physical and mental functions to the brain. Specifically, the normally-developing children attributed both physical (e.g. staying alive) and mental (e.g. dreaming, wanting, thinking) functions to the brain, whereas ASD children attributed only the former but not the latter. Similarly, by four years of age, normally-developing children can choose words from a word list that coincide with what the mind can do (e.g. "think", "imagine", "dream", "pretend", "hope" and "wish"). For these children, these words are easily distinguished from other kinds of non-mental verbs like "run", "eat", or "jump". In contrast, children diagnosed with ASD have much more difficulty in making judgments and attributions of this kind (Baron-Cohen et al., 1994).

Researchers have also observed differences between normally-developing and ASD children with regard to the *appearance-reality distinction* (Flavell, Green and Flavell, 1986), another important feature in understanding informational states. These researchers demonstrated that normally-developing children can correctly categorize objects that appear to have dual identities, whereas ASD children cannot. When presented with a candle in the shape of an apple, for example, normally-developing children correctly identified the object as a candle whereas ASD children identified it as either an apple or candle, but they could not discriminate the object's dual identity. These findings not only suggest important differences between the capabilities of normally-developing and ASD children with regard to understanding informational states, but also highlight what appear to be fundamental features of cognitive development at the level of basic process.

In the language of ToM, there are five levels in the development of the attribution of information or mental states to the self and others that range from simple visual perspective-taking to predicting actions on the basis of false belief (Howlin, Baron-Cohen and Hadwin, 1999). Level 1 of this model consisted of *simple visual perspective-taking*. Individuals at this level of ability are said to act on the principle that different people can have different views of the same situation. For example, with a two-sided card placed between two individuals, one person can see only one side while the other person can see the other side. Level 2 involves *complex visual perspective-taking*, and is based on the principle that people can see things differently. For example, if a picture is placed between two individuals sitting opposite one another, the picture will appear upside down for one individual and the right way up for the other. In the language of ToM these first two levels are collectively referred to as *first-order false belief* because they involve the simple attribution of a mental state to another person. Many of the relevant studies on this level of cognitive ability have been concerned with developmental differences between normally-developing and ASD children. The findings have generally indicated that the latter population show notable deficits in first- order false belief, while the former do not (Baron-Cohen, Leslie and Frith 1985; Leekam, and Perner 1991; Perner, Frith, Leslie, and Leekham, 1989; Reed, and Peterson, 1990; Swettenham, 1996; Sweetenham, Baron-Cohen, Gomez, and Walsh, 1996).

According to ToM, Levels 3-5 in the development of informational states may be collectively referred to as second-order-false-belief because they involve the more complex understanding that a person can have mental states about another person's mental states (Baron-Cohen, 2001). Levels 3 and 4, in particular, are concerned with the attribution of false belief and the prediction of another person's actions on this basis. At Level 3, individuals are said to understand that *'seeing leads to knowing'*, based on the principle that people only know things that they have seen (Taylor, 1988). Although this cognitive ability is of obvious significance to the development of socially appropriate communication, it also precludes an understanding of deception. That is, an individual who cannot keep track of what another person may or may not know is unlikely to be able to determine whether the other person is being truthful or dishonest. Pratt and Bryant (1990), for example, presented three-year-old children with a story about two characters, one of whom looks in a box, while the other simply touches the box. The children were then asked: "Who knows what's in the box?" All of the children from this age group correctly determined that only the character who had seen inside the box would know what was inside and that the character who did not see would not know.

Level 4 of this model of informational states involves the principle that actions can be predicted on the basis of true belief (Howlin et al., 1999). Consider a traditional training task involving toys, in which two similar scenes are portrayed. In one scene, a car is placed beside a boat, and in the other scene, an identical car is placed beside a plane. A child is then provided with the following true belief story: "This morning, you saw the car next to the boat but you did not see the car next to the plane". The child is then asked, "Where do you think the car is? Why do you think it is near the boat? Where will you go to get the car? Why will you go to the boat?" The correct conclusions from this scenario involve the knowledge that one will only know what one has seen, and will act on this basis. Although Levels 3 and 4 of understanding informational states appear to cover the attribution of true belief to the self and others, these abilities are also believed to be important prerequisites to the attribution of false belief.

Level 5 of this model involves the principle that you can predict actions on the basis of false belief and can become aware that previous beliefs may have been false (Howlin et al., 1999). Cognitive researchers have emphasized the representational capabilities that are required for the representation of events and states (Bennett, 1978). In instances in which representations or beliefs are discriminated as incorrect or false (e.g. events may have occurred without a person's knowledge) the individual can alter the belief about these events. Moreover, the individual can recognise that prior to acquiring the new information he/she was behaving on the basis of a false belief. In this way, cognitive theorists have suggested that the representational capacity of the mind with regard to these events has a reflexive quality in which the mind is aware of its own representations even when these have been updated (Wimmer et al., 1983).

One such task the "Sally Anne task" (see Wimmer and Perner, 1983) compared typically developing children, children diagnosed with ASD, and children with Down syndrome (Baron-Cohen, Leslie, and Frith, 1985). The task begins with Sally placing a marble in a basket and then leaving the scene, at which time Anne enters the scene, removes the marble from the basket, and places it in a box. Sally returns to the scene, and participants are asked where Sally would look for the marble. Findings indicated that children with diagnosed with ASD showed poor performance on the task, whereas typically-developing children and children with Down syndrome could easily answer the experimenter's questions about Sally's perspective. Dawson and Fernald (1987) found that the performance of children diagnosed with ASD on a perspective-taking task was positively correlated with the children's social competence, as measured by two standardized scales. In other words, those children who performed worse on the task were clinically evaluated as being less socially competent.

Leekam and Perner (1991) compared the performance of ASD children and their normally developing counterparts on typical Sally Anne tasks and control tasks that involve responding to the contents of a photograph that was taken before the unexpected transfer. Findings from studies involving false-belief tasks indicate that young children can respond correctly to the photograph task (non-false belief) before they can respond to the unexpected transfer task, suggesting that false belief is a cognitive skill that appears at a particular point in normal development (Leekam and Perner, 1991; Leslie and Thaiss, 1992).

(iii) Relational Complexity Theory. An alternative approach to perspective taking views its development in terms of the level of relational complexity involved (Andrews, Halford, Bunch, Bowden and Jones, 2003). According to relational complexity theory (RC), the core predictor of performance on ToM tasks is the number of variables that are to be related (Halford, Wilson, and Phillips, 1998). For example, a commonly employed false belief task, involving the unexpected transfer of an object involves relating three variables: the person's environmental cue (object location), the setting condition (movement seen/not seen), and the person's representation (represented object location). Andrews et al (2003) demonstrated that performance on non-ToM tasks that involved relating three variables was predictive of positive outcomes on false belief tasks. This suggests that it may be level of relational complexity, and not ToM understanding *per se*, which is causing typical theory of mind test outcomes.

The emergence of the relational complexity theory approach to perspective taking/ false belief understanding and other phenomena is exciting as this approach appears to be able to shed new light on these phenomena. Viewing perspective taking and other types of cognitive performance as relational in nature also presents us with a number of broad and interesting questions which RC theory has not as yet addressed. For example, RC theorists suggest that the development of children's relational skills is 'experience driven'. This suggests the questions of how and under what circumstances children learn to relate and whether we might improve their linguistic and / or cognitive ability by providing them with training that specifically targets their relational ability?

LANGUAGE AND UNDERSTANDING OTHER MINDS

A number of researchers have linked linguistic ability and the ability to take the perspective of another/theory of mind (Arbib, 2005; Cutting and Dunn, 1999; Hughes and Dunn, 1997). One issue that is pertinent in the literature is whether perspective taking is a modular ability or whether linguistic prerequisites are necessary for its development (deVilliers, 2003). Indeed a number of studies have found significant correlations between standardized language measures and preschooler performance on typical theory of mind tasks (e.g, Cutting and Dunn, 1999; Hughes and Dunn, 1997).

Arbib (2005) has proposed the Mirror System Hypothesis (MSH) in order to account for understanding other minds. According to this approach the MSH links the brain mechanisms for language to the mirror system for execution and observation of manual actions. Arbib tracks the neural and functional basis of language skills evolutionarily and predicts stages in development that lead from abilities that exist in monkeys and apes. According to the Mirror System Hypothesis the mirror system for grasping (manual actions) can be considered the 'missing link', in evolutionary terms, between language able humans and their non-language able ancestors (Rizzolatti and Arbib, 1998). From this viewpoint this mirror system for grasping fundamentally underlies the ability to imitate. Imitation is widely documented to provide the basis for the emergence of interactive communication or shared intentionality as described previously (Trevarthen , 1984; 1994; Gopnik, Meltzoff and Kuhl, 1999). Indeed, the emergence of delayed imitation is one of the first linguistic moves away from echolalia and can be viewed as the first move towards using symbolic referents (Meltzoff and Prinz, 2002; Hauser, Chomsky and Fitch).

In line with the MSH approach, de Villiers, de Villiers, Schick and Hoffmeister (2000) have suggested that language is a prerequisite for ToM. In order to determine how language skills relate to the development of a ToM these researchers recruited groups of signing and non-signing children who were deaf. The findings indicated that the children who were deaf with deaf parents performed similarly to hearing children, however, the children with hearing parents were significantly delayed in development of a ToM. The findings also indicated a direct relationship between the language skills and ToM skills in the children who were deaf.

According to Diesendruck et al. (2004) understanding other minds is essential to the development of word learning supporting the debate on the coevolution of theory of mind and language capacities. Such predictions are based on the research base that children rely on cues about speakers' intents, rather than cues relevant to the other mechanisms, for understanding the referents of words and for interpretation of word meanings. According to Diesendruck et al. (2004) word learning without theory of mind is useless. Specifically, the research evidence suggests that there are differences between words learnt via a theory of mind mechanism and words learnt without a theory of mind mechanism. It has been empirically demonstrated that organisms without a ToM can acquire words (Pepperberg and Wilcox, 2000; Savage-Rumbaugh, Murphy, Sevcik, Brakke, Williams, and Rumbaugh, 1993), and various animal species have indicated, understanding, and production of word-like symbols. However, exactly the nature of the language abilities demonstrated in these studies is debatable (Diesendruck et al., 2004). And the generality of the use of words as symbolic word referents does not emerge in these studies, nor do these trained animals take into account a listener's state of knowledge in their communicative interactions, thus their use of word-like symbols merely functions to express what they perceive directly.

The ability to learn words without a ToM is not solely observed in nonhuman animals. Empirical work conducted with children as young as 14-months of age have successfully learnt word-to-object pairings (Werker, Cohen, Lloyd, Casasola, and Stager, 1998). In addition to this, research conducted with children diagnosed with ASD has demonstrated word learning without ToM. While these children are capable of developing a relatively extensive vocabulary, they have deficits in the area of ToM. An example, of the futility of such word learning was demonstrated with children with ASD where the trained children demonstrated difficulty associating a novel label to an object, when the label's referent was not the object they were attending to but rather an object the speaker was attending to (Baron-

Cohen, Baldwin, and Crowson, 1997) thus, lacking an understanding of a speakers' referential intents (Clark, 1990; Diesendruck and Markson, 2001).

TRAINING THEORY OF MIND

The ToM literature has recently moved towards attempts to train perspective taking in populations where these repertoires appear to be deficient (e.g., Slaughter and Gopnik, 1996; Fisher and Happé 2005). In one such study, Fisher and Happé (2005) tested and trained theory of mind in ten children diagnosed with ASD. Individual training sessions were administered with corrective feedback on all training trials. The participants were tested before training, after training and at a two-month follow-up. Significant improvements were seen in performance on theory of mind tasks as compared to a 'no training' control group, indicating that accelerated performances on Theory of Mind tasks can be achieved.

Hale and Tager-Flusberg (2003) investigated the role of language and corrective feedback on ToM tasks in the development of theory of mind. Preschool children were assigned to one of three groups, that is, linguistic training, theory of mind task training with corrective feedback or, a control group. The results indicated that the linguistic training group improved on both linguistic and ToM tasks. The ToM group demonstrated improved performance on theory of mind scores but not on linguistic tasks. The control group indicated no improvement on ToM tasks. The researchers suggested that their findings provided evidence that the acquisition of certain linguistic skills facilitated the development of understanding other minds.

Although the theoretical and empirical interest in ToM has been considerable, and there is growing empirical evidence of the applicability of the concepts in remediation packages for populations in whom these skills appear deficient (Fisher and Happé 2005), from a behavioral perspective, questions remain over the basic and functional processes that comprise perspective-taking and the most focused means of establishing these. For example, the success in ToM training studies in accelerating the acquisition of ToM understanding implies that its development is 'experience driven', but the details of this critical experience, or learning history, remain unclear.

BEHAVIORAL ACCOUNT OF UNDERSTANDING OTHER MINDS

While the shift in ToM research toward training is valuable, from the behavioral perspective, there is still a void in the literature in terms of understanding functionally the underlying behavioral processes involved. Understanding the history of reinforcement involved in the development of taking the perspective of another, and thus social interactions more generally, would facilitate the development of training procedures that target directly functional units involved in perspective-taking and may ameliorate the training procedures that have been employed by ToM and behavioral researchers.

Behavior analytic research on social deficits in ASD has typically focused on offering descriptions of how to teach basic social behavior (Leaf and McEachin, 1999; Lovaas, 2003; Maurice, Green and Luce, 1996; Maurice, Green and Fox, 2001). Areas targeted by behavior analysts, that ameliorated social skills include, social awareness (Leaf and McEachin, 1999), social communication (Thiemann and Goldstein, 2001), social interactions (Petursdottir, McComas, McMaster and Horner, 2007), spontaneous verbal responses (Jones, Feeley and Takacs, 2007) and social initiation (Nikopoulos and Keenan, 2004). The methodologies employed in all these studies were grounded in basic behavioral principles, such as, the use of modeling, prompts, selecting target skills, video feedback, discrete-trial instruction, error correction, peer initiated responding, self-management, social interaction probes, individualized reinforcers, and individualized performance criterion levels.

To a large extent social skills training has proven effective with individuals with ASD (Kavale, Mathur, and Mostert, 2004; Marriage, Gordon, and Brand, 1995; Sukhodolsky, Golub, Stone, and Orban, 2005) and one of the most widely used intervention packages for behavioral analytic social skills training is referred to as behavioral skills training (BST; Miltenberger, 2004). BST programs provide concrete instructions, modelling techniques and corrective feedback that directly target social skills (Miltenberger, 2004). However, one issue that has emerged across all the behavior analytic social skills training literature is the lack of generalization of the trained skills (Sheridan, Hungelmann, and Maughan, 1999). One possible reason for this lack of generalisation is that the skills taught fail to address the core of the ASD deficit in social interactions, that is, a lack of the ability to take the perspective of another.

The Theory of Mind literature, outlined above, has indicated the importance of understanding the beliefs, thoughts and perspective of another in terms of the development of social repertoires. In line with this assumption, one study employed ABA procedures in order to directly remediate perspective-taking deficits in the area of ASD (LeBlanc, Coates, Daneshvar, Charlop-Christy, Morris, and Lancaster, 2003). These researchers implemented an intensive behavioral intervention involving video modelling and positive reinforcement. The intervention employed typical ToM tasks such as the Sally Anne task. However, even after the intervention the ASD children's performance on generalization perspective-taking tasks was weak. While targeting perspective-taking skills directly was an important issue addressed in LeBlanc et al's study understanding the behavioral processes involved in perspective-taking and targeting those processes directly was not attempted by these researchers.

In terms of underlying processes linked to perspective-taking, as outlined in the section above, one area highlighted in the ToM literature is language development. ToM researchers, have suggested that the development of language might be critical to understanding other minds, and thus, social interaction. The development of *language* has attracted interest from behavioral psychologists, and this interest has been characterized most notably by Skinner's *Verbal Behavior* (1957). In this account, Skinner attempted to answer the nativist criticisms (e.g. of language generativity) by appealing to a relatively limited number of verbal operants (e.g. mands, tacts and intraverbals) governed by the same basic principles (i.e. operant contingencies) that appeared to govern non-verbal behavior.

Skinner's Verbal Behavior

While a behavior analytic account of precursors to a theory of mind such as joint attention and social referencing can be understood in terms of conditioned reinforcers, the development of complex cognitive abilities such as understanding other minds necessitates a behavioral account of language. The development of *language* in behavioral psychology has been characterized most notably by Skinner's *Verbal Behavior* (1957). In this account, Skinner attempted to answer the nativist criticisms (e.g. of language generativity) by appealing to a relatively limited number of verbal operants (e.g. mands, tacts and intraverbals) governed by the same basic principles (i.e. operant contingencies) that appeared to govern non-verbal behavior. In spite of widely publicized criticisms from Chomsky and the generating of relatively limited empirical research, Skinner's account remained the hallmark of the behavioral perspective on human language. Although behavior analytic interventions have been used to increase speech production and comprehension (e.g., Hart and Risley, 1980: Koegel and Koegel, 1995; Krantz, Zalenski, Hall, Fenske, and McClannahan 1981; Lovaas, 1981), little or no behavior analytic research has been conducted with VB to teach tacting of private events or more complex forms of understanding other minds (Maurice, Green and Foxx, 2001; McHugh and Reed, 2008). One possible reason for the relative void of such examples might be that the contingencies establishing verbal behavior for private events are often unclear and defective, which leads to a questioning of the scientific value of research on the form of emotional responses (see Skinner, 1945; 1957, p. 131). Recent developments, however, within the field of behavior analysis have suggested that this situation has begun to change considerably.

Relational Frame Theory is a functional analytic approach that accounts for the development of language and higher cognition in terms of learned generalized patterns of relational responding referred to as arbitrary relational responding (ARR). The simplest example of an arbitrary relation is the relation of co-ordination between words and their referents which children begin to learn at around the age of two. Continued exposure to the socio-verbal environment produces increasingly complex patterns of ARR including more extensive relations of co-ordination as well as relational patterns other than co-ordination including distinction, opposition, comparison and so forth (Reilly,Whelan and Barnes-Holmes, 2005). According to RFT, perspective-taking is based on a particular pattern of relational responding referred to as deictic relational responding.

Equivalence and Relational Frame Theory

A number of species, capable of complex forms of learning, can be taught to respond to relations among stimuli. For example, Harmon, Strong, and Pasnak (1982) taught adult rhesus monkeys to select the taller of two stimuli, and, in subsequent testing, they chose a taller novel stimulus, rather than the previously reinforced smaller stimulus, thus, demonstrating that the critical responses were made on the basis of the relative, rather than the absolute, properties of the stimuli. This form of relational responding is referred to as physical, or non-arbitrary, relational responding, because the relational responses are made on the basis of the physical, or formal, relations amongst stimuli.

According to Relational Frame Theory (RFT; Hayes, Barnes-Holmes and Roche, 2001) there is an additional, form of relational responding. In this form of relational responding, referred to as arbitrarily applicable relational responding (AARR), responding is not controlled solely by the physical or non-arbitrary relations between the stimuli, but by arbitrary contextual cues; that it, is has a hierarchical structure. RFT proposes that AARR is acquired on the basis of a unique history of reinforcement, often provided by the human verbal community. This would, of course, confer significant advantages to humans in learning this type of relationship, but does not exclude the possibility that non-humans with appropriate training would also acquire it.

The earliest and simplest form of AARR that is learnt, is responding to the symmetrical relations between words and objects. For example, a child may be taught to orient towards a particular object in the presence of a novel word in the context of an interaction, such as the following: 'Where is Teddy?', [Child looks at Teddy], 'Good boy!'.

This interaction may be represented as follows: Hear Name A - Orient towards Object B. The child may also be taught to produce the name or an approximation of the name in the presence of the object: [Teddy shown to Child] 'Who is this?' [Child: 'Teddy'], 'Good boy!' (See Object B – Produce Name A). Initially, the child must be explicitly taught each such symmetrical relation (i.e., A-B; B-A). However, according to RFT, after a child has received a sufficient number of exemplars of bi-directional training in this relational response, eventually generalization occurs, so that contextual cues, such as, 'is', or the object-naming context itself, become sufficient to instantiate derived symmetrical relational responding with novel word-object combinations. In other words, at this point in time, the child need be taught in only one direction (i.e., either 'name-object', or 'object-name') and can then derive in the other direction (i.e., 'object-name', or 'name-object', respectively).

Thus, the earliest and most basic form of AARR is also the earliest and most basic form of language (i.e., reference). From an RFT perspective, AARR and language are believed to be synonymous, and, thus, the continued development of AARR corresponds with the continued development of language and verbal skills, (e.g., Barnes, McCullagh, and Keenan, 1990)

There are a number of forms of AARR in addition to the relations of co-ordination. These include relations of 'opposition' (Dymond and Barnes, 1997; Roche and Barnes, 1996; 1997; Steele and Hayes, 1991), 'distinction' (Roche and Barnes, 1996), 'comparison' and 'perspective' (McHugh, Barnes-Holmes, and Barnes-Holmes, 2004). All examples of this phenomenon possess the following three characteristics:

(i) *Mutual entailment*, which refers to the fundamental bi-directionality of relational responding. In a specified context, if stimulus A is related to stimulus B in a characteristic way, for example, A is more than B, it is entailed that, in that context, stimulus B will be related to stimulus A in another characteristic way, continuing with this example, B is less than A. In this context, if A is more than B, then it can be derived that, in that context, B is less than A.

(ii) *Combinatorial entailment*, which refers to a derived stimulus relation where two or more stimulus relations mutually combine. In a specified context, if stimulus A is related to stimulus B in a characteristic way, and stimulus B is also related to stimulus C in a characteristic way, a derived stimulus relation can be entailed between stimulus A and stimulus C in that context. For example, if A is less than B, and B is less than C, then it can be derived that A is less than C. This combinatorially entailed relation between stimulus A and stimulus C, however, may not always be specified. For example, if A is less than B, and B is more than C, it can be derived that A and C are, in some way, related, but this relationship cannot be specified.

(iii) *Transformation of stimulus functions*, which refers to the transformation of psychologically relevant functions of a stimulus in accordance with the underlying derived relation in a given context. If stimulus A is related to stimulus B in a given context, psychologically relevant functions of stimulus A may be transformed to stimulus B, in accordance with that relation. This phenomenon is what gives relational responding its psychological significance. It allows functions of an event to be determined not only by an individual's direct history with that event, but also by how that event participates in derived relations with other events (Wilson and Blackledge, 2000). For example, if stimulus A is in an equivalence and/or co-ordination relation with the neutral stimulus B, and stimulus A acquires fear eliciting functions, these functions may be transferred to stimulus B, so that this previously neutral stimulus B may now elicit fear. Similarly, stimulus functions can also be transformed in accordance with other forms of arbitrarily applicable relations. For example, if stimulus A is in an opposition class with the neutral stimulus B, and stimulus A acquires aversive functions, these functions may be transformed to stimulus B, so that this previously neutral stimulus B may now acquire reinforcing functions. It should be noted that when a relation is one of equivalence, or sameness, or co-ordination, the term 'transfer' is used, because the psychological function that is derived, is the same as the original function, whereas, if the relation is other than equivalence (e.g., opposition, distinction), then the term 'transformation' is used, because the function that is derived is not the same as the original function (e.g., in the example of transformation via opposition relations just given, the aversive function is transformed into a reinforcing function).

Transformation of stimulus functions is particularly important in the RFT approach to language, in that this phenomenon can account for how language can change the psychological functions of an event. It also accounts for how words can acquire the meaning of their referents, allowing the psychological functions of referents and events to be mediated, or re-lived, through the individual's thoughts.

Thus, a significant quantity of empirical research has already been carried out in relation to this phenomenon. Transformation of a number of different varieties of psychological function has already been empirically demonstrated.

These include transformation of conditioned reinforcing functions (Hayes, Brownstein, Devany, Kohlenberg, and Shelby, 1987; Hayes, Kohlenberg, and Hayes, 1991), discriminative functions (Hayes et al., 1987), elicited conditioned emotional responses (Dougher, Auguston, Markham, Greenway, and Wulfert, 1994), ordinal functions (Green, Sigurdardottir, and Saunders, 1991), extinction functions (Dougher, et al., 1994), and self-discrimination functions (Dymond and Barnes, 1994). Transformation of function has also been empirically demonstrated in accordance with a number of different arbitrarily applicable relational patterns including opposition (Roche and Barnes, 1997; Roche, Barnes-Holmes, Smeets, Barnes-Holmes, and McGeady, 2000; Whelan and Barnes-Holmes, 2004), and comparison (e.g., more than/less than, see e.g., Dymond and Barnes, 1995).

PERSPECTIVE-TAKING AS DERIVED RELATIONAL RESPONDING

From the RFT perspective one family of relational frames that appear to be critical for the development of perspective-taking skills are deictic relational frames. Deictic relational frames specify a relation in terms of the perspective of the speaker (McHugh, et al., 2004). The three frames that appear to be most important in this regard are the frames of I and YOU, HERE and THERE and NOW and THEN.

Unlike other relational frames, these do not appear to have formal or non-arbitrary counterparts and cannot be traced to formal dimensions in the environment. In the language of RFT, it is the relationship between the individual and other events that serves as the constant variable upon which these frames are based.Responding to, and asking, many questions contained within our common verbal interactions with others (e.g. "What am *I* doing *now*?" or "What are *you* doing *there*?") appear to be critical in establishing these perspective-taking frames. Each time questions such as these are asked or answered, the physical environment is different. What remains constant across these and many similar questions, however, are the relational properties of I versus You, Here versus There and Now versus Then. Furthermore, according to RFT, these properties themselves are abstracted through learning to talk about one's own perspective in relation to the perspective of others. *I,* for instance, is always from this perspective *here*, but not from the perspective of another person *there*. Abstraction of an individual's perspective on the world, and that of others, requires a combination of a sufficiently well developed relational repertoire and an extensive history of exemplars that take advantage of that repertoire.

According to RFT, the three perspective-taking frames described above can generate a range of relational networks, including: I-HERE-NOW; YOU-HERE-NOW; I-HERE-THEN; YOU-HERE-THEN; I-THERE-NOW; YOU-THERE-NOW; I-THERE-THEN; and YOU-THERE-THEN. Many phrases common to our daily discourse are derived from these eight relational networks. Consider, for example, the phrases; "I am here now, but you were here then"; "You were there then, but I am here now"; and "You and I are both here now, but I was here then". Of course, when used in actual dialogue, these phrases would often include or substitute words co-ordinated with particular individuals, places and times. For illustrative purposes, consider the following example: "It is four o'clock and I am at work [HERE and NOW], but Fiona [YOU] is still at home" [THERE and NOW]. What appears to makes perspective-taking frames particularly complex and useful is that they cannot be defined in terms of particular words. That is, words such as, "I", "you", "here", "there", "now", and "then" (used to describe the perspective of the self and others) are merely examples of the relational cues that control the perspective-taking frames, and a range of other words and contextual features may serve the same function. As is the case for all relational frames, what is important is the generalised relational activity, not the actual words themselves.

According to RFT, the establishment of the deictic perspective-taking frames will likely be critical to the development of perspective-taking as traditionally defined.

From this perspective, the theory would argue that there should be some correlation between competence in deictic relational responding and more traditional tasks of perspective-taking. Furthermore, RFT would also argue that targeting the deictic frames directly should lead to improved performances on perspective-taking tasks.

Perspective-Taking as Derived Relational Responding: Empirical Evidence

Empirical support for the RFT account of perspective-taking is growing. One of the earliest studies in this area developed (McHugh, Barnes-Holmes, O'Hora, and Barnes-Holmes, 2004) a protocol that targeted the three perspective-taking frames of I-YOU, HERE-THERE, and NOW-THEN, in conjunction with three levels of relational complexity, referred to as: simple relations; reversed relations; and double reversed relations. To illustrate the distinction between these varying levels of complexity explicit examples are provided below (see Appendix 5.1 for the tasks employed in McHugh et al., 2004).

Consider a simple I-YOU perspective-taking task in which participants were presented with the following question: "If I (Experimenter) have a white brick and YOU (Participant) have a red brick: What do I have? What do YOU have?" Responding correctly to this trial (i.e., "You/Experimenter have a white brick and I/Participants have a red brick") requires that the participants respond in accordance with the I-YOU deictic relational frame, under the contextual control of the if-then relational frame (see Figure 4.1). In effect, the if-then frame determines the functions (i.e., the white and red bricks) that become attached to the I and YOU related events in the deictic frame. The perspective-taking protocol also included simple HERE-THERE perspective-taking trials. In a simple HERE-THERE trial the Participants may have been instructed as follows: "I am standing here at the yellow door, and you are standing there at the brown door. Where are you standing? Where am I standing?" A correct response on this trial requires that the participants respond in accordance with the I-YOU and HERE-THERE frames, under the contextual control of if-then. The third simple relational task involved simple NOW-THEN relations. These trial-types differed from the other simple relations in that they did not involve responding to I and YOU simultaneously. Consider the following example: "Yesterday I was shopping, today I am washing the car. What was I doing then? What am I doing now?" Once again, a correct response requires that the participants respond in accordance with the I-YOU and NOW-THEN frames, under the contextual control of if-then.

A more complex level of derived relational responding is required for reversed relations (see Figure 4.2 for an alternative example employing colored chairs). The protocol included reversed I-YOU, reversed HERE-THERE, and reversed NOW-THEN trials. Consider the following example of a reversed I-YOU trial: "If I have a pen and you have a cup, and if I was you and you were me: What would you have? What would I have?" A correct response to this trial involves a transformation of functions in accordance with a deictic relation between I and YOU. That is, the mutually entailed relation between I and YOU transfers "pen" from I to YOU and "cup" from YOU to I. Reversed HERE-THERE and NOW-THEN relations followed the same format in which transformations of functions occurred via mutually entailed relations.

An example of a reversed HERE-THERE task goes as follows; I am standing here at the yellow door and you are standing there at the brown door. If here was there and there was here. Where would I be standing? Where would you be standing? A correct response to this trial involves a transformation of functions in accordance with a deictic relation between HERE and THERE. That is, the mutually entailed relation between HERE and THERE transfers "yellow door" from HERE to THERE and "brown door" from THERE to HERE.

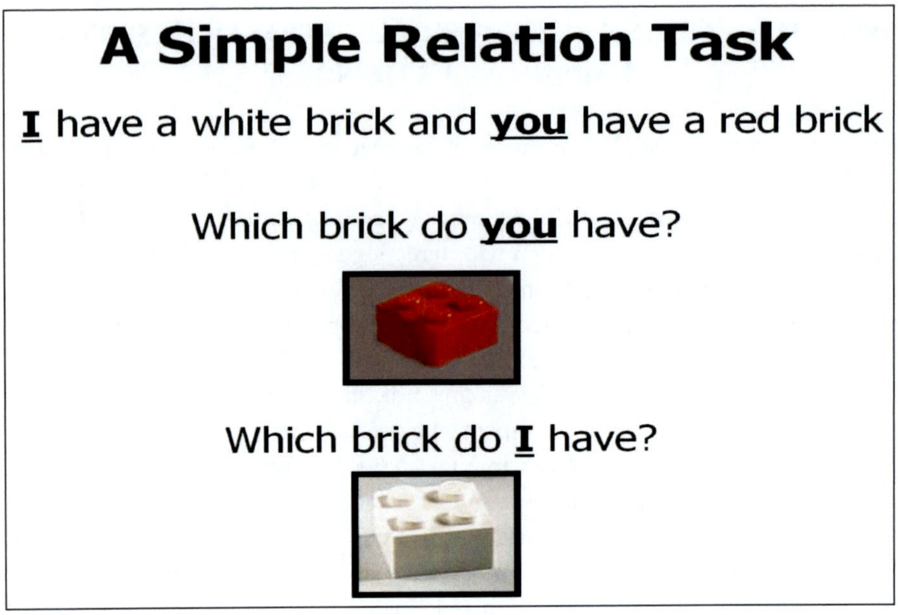

Figure 4.1. An example of a simple relation task.

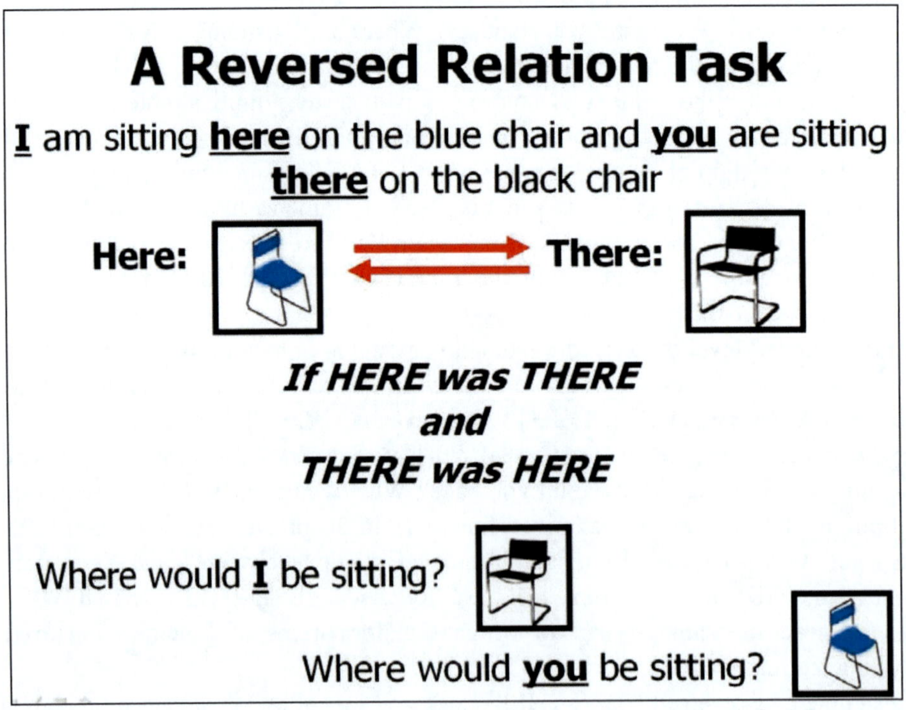

Figure 4.2. An example of a reversed task.

The protocol also contained exposures to trials involving NOW-THEN Reversals. A participant may be instructed, for example, “Yesterday you were watching television, today you are reading. If now was then and then was now. What would you be doing then? What would you be doing now?" The correct response in this case as with the I-YOU and the HERE-THERE reversed tasks is the reverse of the original locations. Reversed NOW-THEN relations followed the same format in which transformations of functions occurred via mutually entailed relations.

The most complex level of relational complexity was referred to as a double reversed relation, in which two relations were reversed simultaneously (see Figure 4.3). Consider the following double reversed trial referred to as an I-YOU/HERE-THERE double reversal: "I am sitting on the blue chair and you are sitting there on the black chair. If I was you and you were me, and if here was there and there was here: Where would you be sitting? Where would I be sitting?" In this trial, the I-YOU reversal followed by the HERE-THERE reversal involves two mutually entailed relations between I and YOU and HERE and THERE, thus reversing the initially reversed relation. In simple terms, the participants deriving these relations ends up sitting on the chair where they originally started.

The second form of double reversed trials followed the same format except that these trials were based on HERE-THERE and NOW-THEN rather than I-YOU and HERE-THERE. For example: "Yesterday I was standing there at the brown door, today I am standing here at the yellow door. If here was there and there was here, and if now was then and then was now: Where would you be standing now? Where would I be standing then?" Once again, in simple terms, the participants deriving these relations would respond by stating that they end up at the door where they started.

The findings from this study revealed differences between participants' responses on the various frames, and on the three levels of relational complexity. Specifically, the results for relation type revealed that participants emitted more errors on the HERE-THERE and NOW-THEN relations when each was compared with the I-YOU relations.

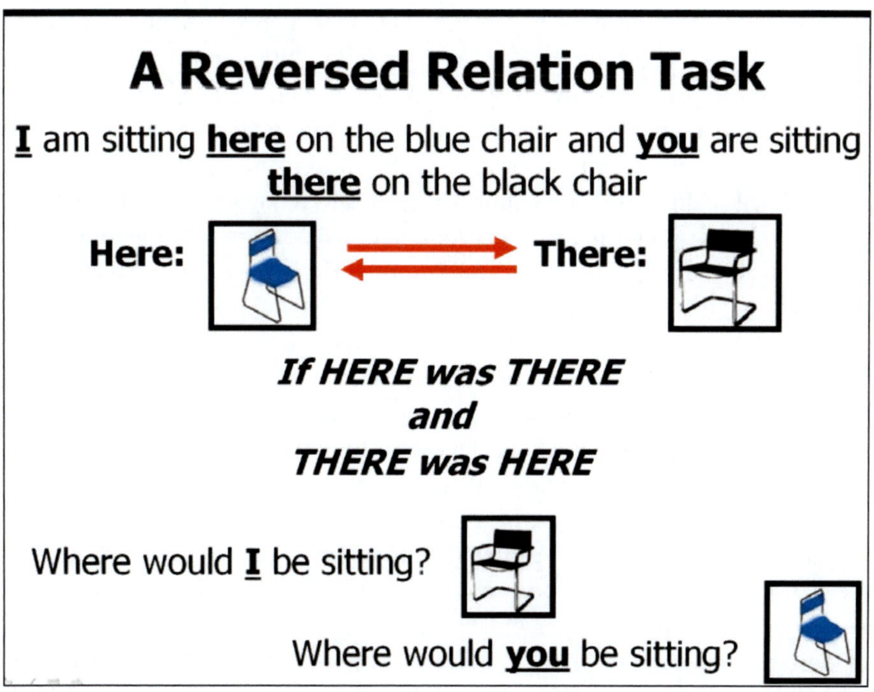

Figure 4.3. An example of a double reversed task

The results for relational complexity revealed that participants made significantly more errors on reversed and double reversed relations than on simple relations. Overall, these findings indicated that, even in adults, perspective-taking appears to consist of functionally distinct relational components.

In a subsequent study (McHugh et al., 2004) the same relational protocol was employed in an attempt to conduct a developmental profile of these perspective-taking skills with individuals of different age groups. The findings from this study indicated a clear developmental trend in the ability to perform the relational perspective-taking tasks from early childhood to adulthood. Children (aged 3-5 years) produced more errors than all of the older age groups (ranging from 6-30 years). Furthermore, these differences are broadly consistent with the mainstream cognitive literature, which has reported that performances on simple ToM tasks generally develop across the ages of four and five years old, and are usually well established by age six (Taylor, 1988).

It was suggested that the younger participants' poorer responding was due to the length of the statements contained within the tasks. McHugh et al. (2004) introduced a control study. To ensure that word length did not effect responding foils of the same word length which did not involve complex relational responding, were presented to the two younger groups of participants, that is, the 3-5 and the 6-8 year olds. An example of a foiled reversal trial is as follows "I'm sitting here on the blue chair and you are sitting there on the black chair. If here was here and there was there: Where would I be sitting? Where would you be sitting?" Responding to this trial does not involve the level of relational responding involved in responding to a typical HERE-THERE reversal as there is no transformation of functions between mutually entailed relations required (i.e., the participant and experimenter remain in the same positions in which they began).

An example of a double reversed foil trial goes as follows: "Yesterday I was sitting there on the black chair today I'm sitting here on the blue chair. If here was there and there was here and now was then and then was now: Where would I be sitting now? Where was I sitting then?" The 3-5 year old participants who were exposed to the foils produced less errors than children of the same age exposed to the original trials. The largest difference emerged for reversed relations. No significant difference emerged for the simple trial-types which replicates the original findings because simple trial-types were identical across both protocols. As with the 3-5 year old group the 6-8 year olds produced less errors than children of the same age exposed to the original trials. The largest difference between these groups was recorded on the double reversed relations. This supports the conclusion that the errors produced by the 6-8 year old children in the original experiment were due, at least in part, to the derived properties of the correct responses rather than word length per se.

In summary, therefore, the findings from these studies indicate that the relational repertoires required for perspective-taking appear to follow a distinct developmental trend, and may be comprised of functional relational units of analysis. This latter point has important implications for the design of programs of remediation with populations that display perspective-taking deficits, for example, those on the Autistic Spectrum.

Four RFT training studies have been conducted which have begun to investigate using the perspective-taking protocol to remediate deficits in relational perspective-taking in a number of normally developing young children (Barnes-Holmes, 2001; McHugh, Barnes-Holmes, and Barnes-Holmes, 2004; Heagle and Rehfeldt, 2006; Weil, unpublished doctoral thesis). In the first study, two children were exposed to the perspective-taking protocol with corrective feedback presented after each trial. One seven-year-old female required training on the reversed and double reversed relations in order to complete the entire protocol. A three-and-a-half year old male was exposed only to I-YOU and HERE-THERE trials, and required extensive training across exemplars, also on the reversed and double reversed relations (Barnes-Holmes, 2001). The second study again employed the refined perspective-taking protocol (McHugh et al., 2004), with young participants, that is, a four year old male and a four year old female. The findings of the work with the four year olds indicated that prior to the study they had a sophisticated repertoire with regard to simple I-YOU and simple HERE-THERE tasks and no training was required. However, training simple NOW-THEN tasks required extensive and systematic exemplar training. With regard to training of reversed tasks flexible repertoires in both I-YOU and HERE-THERE were trained efficiently using the training protocol. Even the most complex level of relational responding, that is, double reversed I-YOU and HERE-THERE tasks, were trained with relative ease.

In the third study Rehfeldt and Heagle (2006) employed a multiple probe design in order to train the perspective taking protocol to teach three typically developing children between the ages of 6-11 perspective-taking skills. Generalization tests of perspective taking to new stimuli and real-world conversational topics were also tested. All three children were successfully trained on the perspective taking protocol and performed at high accuracy levels on the generalisation tests.

The final training study that has been conducted to date employed a within-subject multiple probe design to train the perspective taking protocol with three children (Weil unpublished thesis). In this study performance on ToM tasks were tested as the before , during and after the training of the perspective taking protocol in order to determine if training the deictic relations directly improved performance on ToM tasks. The results indicated that all demonstrated evidence of improvement on the ToM tasks. After training in reversed relations improved performance was demonstrated in all second-order levels of ToM (levels 3 through 5). And after training on the Double Reversed relations, all three participants showed improved performance in ToM levels 4 and 5 tasks.

In a subsequent study Rehfeldt et al. (2006) investigated whether children with ASD demonstrated relational learning deficits in a perspective-taking task when compared to their age-matched typically-developing counterparts. Eighteeen children (9 per group) were tested. Additionally, these researchers compared accuracy on the perspective-taking protocol with scores on standardized instruments commonly employed in the assessment of ASD (1), the Vineland Adaptive Behavior Scales – Interview Edition (Sparrow, Balla, and Cicchetti, 1984) and the(2) Social Communication Questionnaire (SCQ) – Current Form (Rutter, Bailey, and Lord, 2004 Findings indicated that that the experimental group made more errors overall on the perspective taking protocol and this distinction was most pronounced on reversed relation test trial types. The researchers correlated scores on the perspective-taking task and the SCQ, overall age equivalence as measured on the Vineland Adaptive Behavior Scales, and age equivalence on the communication, daily living, and socialization domains of the Vineland. A modest correlation between the percentage of errors on the Now-Then reversed relations and the Daily Living Skills domain of the Vineland was found indicating that lower age equivalence in daily living skills was associated with a greater number of errors on the Now-Then reversed relations. Surprisingly, no relationship emerged between the SCQ and the perspective-taking protocol. However, the sample size in the current study was small so future research is needed to further explore the link between social communication, general intelligence and flexible repertoires in responding in accordance with the deictic frames of I-You, Here-There and Now-Then.

Summary and Future Directions

The current chapter provided an overview of the literature on behavioral accounts of the development of understanding other minds and introduced the theory and empirical work thus far on joint attention, social referencing and perspective-taking as a forms of operant behavior. The results of the behavior analytic studies reported suggest that there is some utility in the application of the concepts and predictions from behavioral psychology to our understanding of the development of social interactions and understanding other minds. The importance of the current work is exemplified in the fact that the development of socio-communicative repertoires is an essential milestone in human development. Indeed, this fact is also evident in the many problems that result from socio-communication deficits, such as those that characterise individuals diagnosed with ASD.

Although the majority of behavioral studies outlined in the current chapter were conducted on typically-developing individuals this work is obviously of particular significance to populations who display socio-communicative deficits. More research that employs populations such as those diagnosed on the Autistic Spectrum would ameliorate the utility of learnt operant account of phenomena such as joint attention and understanding other minds. The design of remediation packages that train operant repertoires in joint attention and social referencing and subsequently employing relational training protocols to train a theory of mind would be worthwhile avenues of future research.

Appendix 4.1. Protocol Employed by McHugh et al., 2004

Simple Relations

Simple I -YOU

I have a red brick and you have a green brick.
Which brick do I have?
Which brick do YOU have?

I have a green brick and you have a red brick.
Which brick do YOU have?
Which brick do I have?

Simple HERE-THERE

I am sitting here on the blue chair and you are sitting there on the black chair.

Where am I sitting?
Where are YOU sitting?
I am sitting here on the black chair and you are sitting there on the blue chair.
Where are YOU sitting?
Where am I sitting?

Simple NOW-THEN:

Yesterday I was watching television, today I am reading.
What am I doing now?
What was I doing then?

Yesterday I was reading, today I am watching television.
What was I doing then?
What am I doing now?

Yesterday you were reading, today you are watching television.
What are YOU doing now?
What were YOU doing then?

Yesterday you were watching television, today you are reading.
What were YOU doing then?
What are YOU doing now?

Reversed Relations

Reversed I-YOU:
I have a red brick and you have a green brick. If I was you and you were me.
Which brick would I have?
Which brick would YOU have?

I have a green brick and you have a red brick. If I was you and you were me
Which brick would YOU have?
Which brick would I have?

I have a red brick and you have a green brick. If I was you and you were me.
Which brick would YOU have?
Which brick would I have?

I have a green brick and you have a red brick. If I was you and you were me
Which brick would I have?
Which brick would YOU have?

I am sitting here on the black chair and you are sitting there on the blue chair. If I was you and you were me.
Where would YOU be sitting?
Where would I be sitting?
I am sitting here on the black chair and you are sitting there on the blue chair. If I was you and you were me.
Where would I be sitting?
Where would YOU be sitting?

I am sitting here on the blue chair and you are sitting there on the black chair. If I was you and you were me.
Where would I be sitting?
Where would YOU be sitting?

I am sitting here on the blue chair and you are sitting there on the black chair. If I was you and you were me.
Where would YOU be sitting?
Where would I be sitting?

Reversed HERE-THERE

I am sitting here on the blue chair and you are sitting there on the black chair. If here was there and there was here.
Where would YOU be sitting?
Where would I be sitting?

I am sitting here on the black chair and you are sitting there on the blue chair. If here was there and there was here.
Where would I be sitting?
Where would YOU be sitting?

I am sitting here on the blue chair and you are sitting there on the black chair. If here was there and there was here.
Where would I be sitting?
Where would YOU be sitting?

I am sitting here on the black chair and you are sitting there on the blue chair. If here was there and there was here.
Where would YOU be sitting?
Where would I be sitting?

Yesterday I was sitting there on the blue chair, today I am sitting here on the black chair. If here was there and there was here.
Where would I be sitting now?
Where would I be sitting then?

Yesterday I was sitting there on the black chair, today I am sitting here on the blue chair. If here was there and there was here.
Where would I be sitting then?
Where would I be sitting now?

Yesterday I was sitting there on the blue chair, today I am sitting here on the black chair. If here was there and there was here.
Where would I be sitting then?
Where would I be sitting now?

Yesterday I was sitting there on the black chair, today I am sitting here on the blue chair. If here was there and there was here.
Where would I be sitting now?
Where would I be sitting then?

Yesterday you were sitting there on the blue chair, today you are sitting here on the black chair. If here was there and there was here.
Where would you be sitting now?
Where would you be sitting then?

Yesterday you were sitting there on the blue chair, today you are sitting here on the black chair. If here was there and there was here.
Where were you sitting then?
Where would you sitting now?

Yesterday you were sitting there on the black chair, today you are sitting here on the blue chair. If here was there and there was here.
Where would you be sitting now?
Where would you be sitting then?

Yesterday you were sitting there on the black chair, today you are sitting here on the blue chair. If here was there and there was here.
Where would you be sitting then?
Where would you be sitting now?

Reversed NOW-THEN

Yesterday I was watching television, today I am reading. If now was then and then was now.
What would I be doing then?
What would I be doing now?

Yesterday I was reading, today I am watching television. If now was then and then was now.
What would I be doing now?

What would I be doing then?
Yesterday I was watching television, today I am reading. If now was then and then was now.
What would I be doing now?
What would I be doing then?

Yesterday I was reading, today I am watching television. If now was then and then was now.
What would I be doing then?
What would I be doing now?

Yesterday you were watching television, today you are reading. If now was then and then was now.
What would you be doing then?
What would you be doing now?

Yesterday you were reading, today you are watching television. If now was then and then was now.
What would you be doing then?
What would you be doing now?

Yesterday you were watching television, today you are reading. If now was then and then was now.
What would you be doing now?
What would you be doing then?

Yesterday you were reading, today you are watching television. If now was then and then was now.
What would you be doing now?
What would you be doing then?

Yesterday I was sitting there on the blue chair, today I am sitting here on the black chair. If now was then and then was now.
Where would I be sitting now?
Where would I be sitting then?

Yesterday I was sitting there on the blue chair, today I am sitting here on the black chair. If now was then and then was now.
Where would I be sitting then?
Where would I be sitting now?

Yesterday I was sitting there on the black chair, today I am sitting here on the blue chair. If now was then and then was now.
Where would I be sitting now?
Where would I be sitting then?

Yesterday I was sitting there on the black chair, today I am sitting here on the blue chair. If now was then and then was now.
Where would I be sitting then?
Where would I be sitting now?

Yesterday you were sitting there on the blue chair, today you are sitting here on the black chair. If now was then and then was now.
Where would you be sitting then?
Where would you be sitting now?

Yesterday you were sitting there on the blue chair, today you are sitting here on the black chair. If now was then and then was now.
Where would you be sitting now?
Where would you be sitting then?

Yesterday you were sitting there on the black chair, today you are sitting here on the blue chair. If now was then and then was now.
Where would you be sitting then?
Where would you be sitting now?

Yesterday you were sitting there on the black chair, today you are sitting here on the blue chair. If now was then and then was now.
Where would you be sitting now?
Where would you be sitting then?

Double Reversed Relations

I-YOU/HERE-THERE:
I am sitting here on the blue chair and you are sitting there on the black chair. If I was you and you were me and if here was there and there was here.
Where would I be sitting?
Where would YOU be sitting?

I am sitting here on the blue chair and you are sitting there on the black chair. If I was you and you were me and if here was there and there was here.
Where would I be sitting?
Where would YOU be sitting?

I am sitting here on the black chair and you are sitting there on the blue chair. If I was you and you were me and if here was there and there was here.
Where would I be sitting?
Where would YOU be sitting?

I am sitting here on the blue chair and you are sitting there on the black chair. If I was you and you were me and if here was there and there was here.

Where would YOU be sitting?
Where would I be sitting?

I am sitting here on the black chair and you are sitting there on the blue chair. If I was you and you were me and if here was there and there was here.
Where would YOU be sitting?
Where would I be sitting?
I am sitting here on the black chair and you are sitting there on the blue chair. If I was you and you were me and if here was there and there was here.
Where would YOU be sitting?
Where would I be sitting?

HERE-THERE/NOW-THEN

Yesterday I was sitting there on the blue chair, today I am sitting here on the black chair. If here was there and there was here and if now was then and then was now.
Where would I be sitting then?
Where would I be sitting now?

Yesterday I was sitting there on the blue chair, today I am sitting here on the black chair. If here was there and there was here and if now was then and then was now.
Where would I be sitting then?
Where would I be sitting now?

Yesterday I was sitting there on the blue chair, today I am sitting here on the black chair. If here was there and there was here and if now was then and then was now.
Where would I be sitting now?
Where would I be sitting then?

Yesterday I was sitting there on the black chair, today I am sitting here on the blue chair. If here was there and there was here and if now was then and then was now.
Where would I be sitting then?
Where would I be sitting now?

Yesterday I was sitting there on the black chair, today I am sitting here on the blue chair. If here was there and there was here and if now was then and then was now.
Where would I be sitting then?
Where would I be sitting now?

Yesterday I was sitting there on the black chair, today I am sitting here on the blue chair. If here was there and there was here and if now was then and then was now.
Where would I be sitting now?
Where would I be sitting then?

Yesterday you were sitting there on the blue chair, today you are sitting here on the black chair. If here was there and there was here and if now was then and then was now.
Where would you be sitting then?
Where would you be sitting now?

Yesterday you were sitting there on the blue chair, today you are sitting here on the black chair. If here was there and there was here and if now was then and then was now.
Where would you be sitting then?
Where would you be sitting now?

Yesterday you were sitting there on the blue chair, today you are sitting here on the black chair. If here was there and there was here and if now was then and then was now.
Where would be you sitting now?
Where would you be sitting then?

Yesterday you were sitting there on the black chair, today you are sitting here on the blue chair. If here was there and there was here and if now was then and then was now.
Where would you be sitting then?
Where would you be sitting now?

Yesterday you were sitting there on the black chair, today you are sitting here on the blue chair. If here was there and there was here and if now was then and then was now.
Where would be you sitting now?
Where would you be sitting then?

Yesterday you were sitting there on the black chair, today you are sitting here on the blue chair. If here was there and there was here and if now was then and then was now.
Where would be you sitting now?
Where would you be sitting then?

REFERENCES

Andrews, G., Halford, G.S., Bunch, K.M., Bowden D. and Jones, T. (2003). Theory of mind and relational complexity, *Child Development,* 74, 1476–1499.

Arbib, M.A. (2005). From monkey-like action recognition to human language: an evolutionary framework for neurolinguistics. *Behavior and Brain Sciences,* 28, 105–168.

Bakeman, R. and Adamson, L.B. (1984). Coordinating attention to people and objects in mother-infant and peer-infant interaction. *Child Development*, 55, 1278-89.

Barnes, D., McCullagh, P.D., and Keenan, M. (1990). Equivalence class formation in non-hearing impaired children and hearing impaired children. *Analysis of Verbal Behavior,* 8, 1-11.

Barnes-Holmes, Y. (2001). *Analysing Relational Frames: Studying Language and Cognition in Young Children.* National University of Ireland, Maynooth: Unpublished doctoral thesis.

Baron-Cohen, S. (1989). Are autistic children behaviourists? An examination of their mental-physical and appearance-reality distinctions. *Journal of Autism and Developmental Disorders,* 19, 579–600.

Baron-Cohen, S. (1995). *Mindblindness: an essay on autism and theory of mind.* MIT Press/Bradford Books.

Baron-Cohen, S., Baldwin, D. and Crowson, (1997). Do children with autism use the speaker's direction of gaze strategy to crack the code of language? *Child Development,* 68, 48-57.

Baron-Cohen, S. and Goodhart, F. (1994). The "seeing leads to knowing" deficit in autism: The Pratt and Bryant probe. *British Journal of Developmental Psychology,* 12, 397-402.

Baron-Cohen, S., Leslie, A.M., and Frith, U. (1985). Does the autistic child have a "theory of mind"? *Cognition,* 21, 37-46.

Baron-Cohen, S., Tager-Flusberg, H., and Cohen, D. (2000). *Understanding other minds: Perspectives from developmental cognitive neuroscience (2nd Ed.).* Oxford: Oxford University Press.

Bennet, J. (1978). Some remarks about concepts. *Behavioural and Brain Sciences,* 1, 557-560.

Bretherton, I. (1991). Intentional Communication and the development of an understanding of mind. In In Frye, D.and Moore, C. (Eds.). *Children's Theories of Mind: Mental States and Social Understanding*. Hillsdale, NJ: Lawrence Erlbaum Associates.

Campos, J.J., and Barrett, K.C. (1984). *Toward a new understanding of emotions and their development.* In C.E. Izard, J. Kagan, and R.B. Zajonc, Emotions, cognition, and behavior (pp. 229-263). New York: Cambridge. University Press.

Carpenter, M., Tomasello, M., and Striano, T. (2005). Role reversal imitation and language in typically-developing infants and children with autism. *Infancy,* 8, 253–278.

Chin, H.Y. and Bernard-Opitz, V., (2000) Teaching conversational skills to children with autism: Effect of the development of a Theory of Mind. *Journal of Autism and Developmental Disorders,* 30, 569-583.

Clark, E.V. (1990). On the pragmatics of contrast. *Journal of Child Language,* 17, 417-431.

Corkum, V.L., and Moore, C. (1998). The origins of joint attention. *Developmental Psychology,* 34, 28–38.

Cutting. A., and Dunn, J. (1999). Theory of mind, emotion understanding, language and family background: Individual differences and inter-relations. *Child Development,* 70, 853-865.

Dawson, G. and Fernald M. (1987). Perspective-taking ability and its relationship to the social behavior of autistic children. *Journal of Autism and Developmental Disorders,* 17, 487-498.

de Villiers, J.G. and de Villiers, P.A. (2003). Language for thought: Coming to understand false beliefs. In D. Gentner and S. Goldin-Meadow, (eds) *Language in Mind: Advances in the Study of Language and Cognition.* MIT Press.

de Villiers, P., de Villiers, J., Schick, B., and Hoffmeister, R. (2000). *Theory of mind development in signing and non-signing Deaf children: The impact of sign language on social-cognition.* Paper presented at the Seventh International Conference on Theoretical Issues in Sign Language Research, Amsterdam, The Netherlands.

Diesendruck, G., and Markson, L. (2001). Children's avoidance of lexical overlap: A pragmatic account. *Developmental Psychology,* 37, 630-641.

Diesendruck, G., Markson, L., Akhtar, N., and Reudor, A. (2004). Two-year-olds' sensitivity to speakers' intent: An alternative account of Samuelson and Smith. *Developmental Science,* 7, 33-41.

Dougher, M., J. Auguston, M., R. Markham, M., R. Greenway, D., E. and Wulfert, E. (1994). The transfer of respondent eliciting and extinction functions through stimulus equivalence classes. *Journal of the Experimental Analysis of Behavior,* 62, 331–352.

Dube, W.V., MacDonald, R.P.F., Holcomb, W.L Mansfield, R.C.,. and Ahearn, W.H. (2004). Toward a behavioral analysis of joint attention. *The Behavior Analyst*, 27, 197-207.

Dymond, S., and Barnes, D. (1994). A transfer of self-discrimination response functions through equivalence relations. *Journal of the Experimental Analysis of Behavior,* 62, 251-267.

Dymond, S. and Barnes, D. (1995). A transformation of self-discrimination response functions in accordance with the arbitrarily applicable relations of sameness and opposition. *The Psychological Record,* 46, 271-300.

Dymond, S., and Barnes, D. (1997). Behaviour-analytic approaches to self-awareness. *The Psychological Record,* 47, 181-200.

Fisher, N., and Happe, F. (2005). A training study of theory of mind and executive function in children with Autistic Spectrum Disorders. *Journal of Autism and Developmental Disorders* 35, 757-771.

Flavell, J. H., Green, E. R., and Flavell, E. R. (1986). Development of knowledge about the appearance-reality distinction. *Child Development,* 51, 122–156.

Gerwirtz, J.L., and Pelaez-Nogueras, M. (1992). Infants' separation difficulties and distress due to misplaced maternal contingencies. In T. Field, P. McCabe, and N. Schneiderman (Eds.), Stress and coping in infancy and childhood (pp. 19-46). Hillsdale, NJ: Lawrence Erlbaum.

Gopnik, A., Meltzoff, A. N., and Kuhl, P. K. (1999). *The scientist in the crib: What early learning tells us about the mind.* New York: Perennial.

Green, G, Sigurdardottir, Z.G, and Saunders, R.R. (1991). The role of instructions in the transfer of ordinal functions through equivalence classes. *Journal of the Experimental Analysis of Behavior. 55*, 287–304.

Hale, C.M. and Tager-Flusberg, H. (2003). The influence of language on theory of mind: A training study. *Developmental Science,* 6, 346-359.

Halford, G., Wilson, W., and Phillips, S. (1998). Processing capacity defined by relational complexity: Implications for comparative, developmental and cognitive psychology. *Behavioral and Brain Sciences,* 14, 803 - 831

Harmon, K., Strong, R., and Pasnak, R. (1982). Relational responses in tests of transposition with rhesus monkeys. *Learning and Motivation,* 13, 495-504.

Hart, B. M., and Risley, T. R. (1980). In vivo language intervention: Unanticipated general effects. *Journal of Applied Behavior Analysis,* 13, 243-256.

Hayes, S., Barnes-Holmes, D., and Roche, B. (2001). *Relational Frame Theory: A Post-Skinnerian Account of Human Language and Cognition.* New York: Plenum.

Hayes, S.C., Brownstein, A.J., Devany, J.M., Kohlenberg, B.S., and Shelby, J. (1987). Stimulus equivalence and the symbolic control of behavior. *Mexican Journal of Behavior Analysis,* 13, 361-374.

Hayes, S.C., Kohlenberg, B.K., and Hayes, L.J. (1991). The transfer of specific and general consequential functions through simple and conditional equivalence classes. *Journal of the Experimental Analysis of Behavior,* 56, 119-137.

Heagle, A., and Rehfeldt, R. A. (2006). Teaching perspective-taking skills to typically developing children through derived relational responding *The Journal of Intensive Early Behavioral Intervention,* 3, 8-34.

Hobson, P. (2007). *The Cradle of thought*. New York, Oxford University Press.

Howlin, P., Baron-Cohen, S., and Hadwin, J. (1999). *Teaching Children with Autism to Mind-read: A Practical Guide*. Chichester: Wiley.

Hauser, M., Chomsky, N., and Fitch, W. T. (2002). The language faculty: What is it, who has it, and how did it evolve? *Science,* 298, 1569–1579.

Hughes, C., and Dunn, J. (1997). "Pretend you didn't know": Young children's talk about mental states in the context of pretend play. *Cognitive Development,* 12, 477-499.

Jones, E. A., Feeley, K., M. and Takacs, J. (2007). Teaching children with autism spontaneous responses. *Journal of Applied Behavior Analysis.* 40, 565-570.

Kavale, K.A., Mathur, S.R., and Mostert, M.P. (2004). Social skills training and teaching social behavior to students with emotional and behavioral disorders. In R. B. Rutherford, M. M. Quinn, and S. R. Mathur (Eds.), *Handbook of research in emotional and behavioral disorders* (pp. 446-461). New York: Guilford Press.

Koegel, R.L. and Koegel, L.K. (1995). *Teaching children with autism: Strategies for initiating positive interactions and improving learning outcomes.* Baltimore, MD: Paul H. Brookes Publishing.

Krantz, P.J., Zalenski, S., Hall, L.J., Fenske, E.C., and McClannahan, L. (1981). Teaching complex language to autistic children. *Analysis and Intervention in Developmental Disabilities,* 1, 259-297.

Leaf, R. and McEachin, J. (Eds.) (1999). *A work in progress: Behavioral management strategies and a curriculum for intensive behavioral treatment of autism*. New York, NY: Different Roads to Learning.

LeBlanc, L.A., Coates, A.M., Daneshvar, S., Charlop-Christy, M.H., Morris, C., and Lancaster, B.M. (2003). Using video modeling and reinforcement to teach perspective-taking skills to children with autism. *Journal of Applied Behavior Analysis,* 36, 253-257.

Leekham, S. and Perner, J. (1991). Does the autistic child have a metarepresentational deficit? *Cognition,* 40, 203-18.

Leslie, A. M. and Thaiss, L. (1992). Domain specificity in conceptual development: Neuropsychological evidence from autism. *Cognition,* 43, 225–251.

Liszkowski, U., Carpenter, M., Henning, A., Striano, T., and Tomaselo, M. (2004). 12 month-olds point to share attention and interest. *Developmental Science,* 7, 297-307.

Lovaas, O.I. (1981). *Teaching Developmentally Disabled Children: The Me Book.* Baltimore: University Press Park.

Lovaas, O.I. (2003). *Teaching individuals with developmental delays: Basic intervention techniques*. Austin, TX: Pro-Ed.

Marriage, K.J., Gordon, V., and Brand, L. (1995). A social skills group for boys with Asperger's syndrome. *Australian and New Zealand Journal of Psychiatry,* 29, 58-62.

Maurice, C., Green, G., and Luce, S. C. (Eds.). (1996). *Behavioral intervention for young children with autism*. Austin, TX: PRO-ED.

Maurice, C., Green, G., and Fox, R.(2001). *Making a difference: Behavioral intervention for autism.* Austin, TX: Pro-Ed.

McHugh, L., Barnes-Holmes, Y., and Barnes-Holmes, D. (2004). Developmental trends in perspective-taking. *The Psychological Record*, 54, 115–145.

McHugh, L., Barnes-Holmes, Y., O'Hora, D., and Barnes-Holmes, D. (2004). Perspective-taking: A relational frame analysis. *Experimental Analysis of Human Behaviour Bulletin*, 22, 4-10.

McHugh, L., and Reed, P. (2008). Using Relational Frame Theory to build grammar in children with Autistic Spectrum Conditions. *The Journal of Speech-Language Pathology and Applied Behavior Analysis*, 2.4-3.1, 60-77.

Meltzoff, A.N., and Prinz, W. (2002). *The imitative mind: Development, evolution, and brain bases.* Cambridge, England: Cambridge University Press.

Miltenberger, R.G. (2004) *Behavior modification: Principles and procedures* (3rd Ed). Pacific Grove, CA: Wadsworth.

Nikopoulos, C.K., and Keenan, M. (2004). Effects of video modeling on social initiations by children with autism. *Journal of Applied Behavior Analysis,* 37, 93-96.

Pelaez-Nogueras, M. (1992). Recurrent issues in the study of behaviour development: Meta-models. Behavioral Development, 3, 5 – 6.

Pepperberg, I.M., and Wilcox, S.E. (2000). Evidence for a form of mutual exclusivity during label acquisition by Grey parrots (*Psittacus erithacus*)? *Journal of Comparative Psychology,* 114, 219-231.

Perner, J., Frith, U., Leslie, A.M., and Leekam, S. (1989). Exploration of the autistic child's theory of mind: Knowledge, belief, and communication. *Child Development,* 60, 689-700.

Petursdottir, A., McComas, J. McMaster, K, Horner, K. (2007). The effects of scripted peer tutoring and programming common stimuli on social interactions of a student with Autism Spectrum Disorder. *Journal of Applied Behavior Analysis,* 40, 353-357.

Pratt, C. and Bryant, P. (1990). Young children understand that looking leads to knowing (so long as they are looking into a single barrel). *Child Development,* 61, 973-83.

Ratner, N., and Bruner, J., S. (1977). Games, social exchange and the acquisition of language . *Journal of Child Language,* 5, 391-401.

Rehfeldt, R., Dillen, J. E., Ziomek, M. M., and Kowalchuck, R. (2006).Assessing relational learning deficits in perspective-taking in children with high functioning Autism Spectrum Disorder. *The Psychological Record*, 57, 23-47.

Reed, T. and Peterson, C. (1990). Acomparative study of autistic subjects' performance at two levels of visual and cognitive perspective taking. *Journal of Autism and Developmental Disorders,* 20, 555-68.

Reilly, T., Whelan, R., and Barnes-Holmes, D. (2005). The effect of training structure on the latency responses to a five-term linear chain. *The Psychological Record,* 55, 233-249.

Rizzolatti, G., Arbib, M.A. (1998). Language within our grasp. *Trends in Neuroscience,* 21, 188-194.

Rochat, P. and Striano, T. (1999). Social cognitive development in the first year. In P. Rochat (Ed.), *Early Social Cognition*, Hillsdale, NJ: Erlbaum, 3-34.

Roche, B., and Barnes, D. (1996). Arbitrarily applicable relational responding and human sexual categorization: A critical test of the derived difference relation. *The Psychological Record*, 46, 451-475.

Roche, B., and Barnes, D. (1997). A transformation of respondently conditioned stimulus function in accordance with arbitrarily applicable relations. *Journal of the Experimental Analysis of Behavior*, 67, 275-300.

Roche, B., Barnes-Holmes, D., Smeets, P. M., Barnes-Holmes, Y., and McGeady, S. (2000). Contextual control over the derived transformation of discriminative and sexual arousal functions. *The Psychological Record,* 50, 267-291.

Ross, H. S., and Lollis, S. P. (1987). Communication within infant social games. *Developmental Psychology,* 23, 241–248.

Rutter, M., Bailey, A., and Lord, C. (2004). *SCQ: Social Communication Questionnaire*. Western Psychological Services: Los Angeles, CA.

Savage-Rumbaugh, E.S., Murphy, J., Sevcik, R.A., Brakke, K.E., Williams, S.L., and Rumbaugh, D.M. (1993). Language comprehension in ape and child. *Monographs of the Society for Research in Child Development, 58*(3-4), v-221.

Sheridan, S.M., Hungelmann, A., and Maughan, D.P. (1999). A contextualized framework for social skills assessment, intervention, and generalization. *School Psychology Review,* 28, 84-103.

Sigman, M., and Ruskin, E. (1999). Change and continuity in the social competence of children with Autism, Down syndrome, and developmental delays. *Monograph of the Society for Research in Child Development*. London, England: Blackwell.

Slaughter, V. and Gopnik, A. (1996). Conceptual coherence in the child's theory of mind. *Child Development,* 67, 2967-2989.

Sorce, J.F., Emde, R.N., Campos, J., and Klinnert, M.D. (1985). Maternal emotional signaling: Its effect on the visual cliff behavior of 1-year-olds. *Developmental Psychology,* 21, 195-200.

Sparrow, S.S., Balla, D.A., and Cicchetti, D.V. (1984). *Vineland Adaptive Behavior Scales: Interview Edition, Survey Form Manual*. Circle Pines, MN: American Guidance Service.

Steele, D.L. and Hayes, S.C. (1991). Stimulus equivalence and arbitrarily applicable relational responding. *Journal of the Experimental Analysis of Behavior,* 56,519–555.

Striano, T., and Rochat, P. (1999). Developmental link between dyadic and triadic social competence in infancy. *British Journal of Developmental Psychology,* 17, 551-562.

Suddendorf, T. and Fletcher-Flinn, C. (2002). Theory of mind and the origin of divergent thinking. *Cognition,* 7, 78-113.

Sukhodolsky, D. G., Solomon, R. M., and Perine, J. (2000). Cognitive-behavioral, anger-control intervention for elementary school children: A treatment outcome study. *Journal of Child and Adolescent Group Therapy,* 10, 159-170.

Swettenham, J. (1996). Can children with autism be taught to understand false belief using computers? *Journal of Child Psychology and Psychiatry,* 37, 157-65.

Swettenham, J., Baron-Cohen, S., Gomez, J. C. and Walsh, S. (1996). What's inside a person's head? Conceiving of the mind as a camera helps children with autism develop an alternative theory of mind. *Cognitive Neuropsychiatry,* 1, 73-88.

Taylor, M. (1988). Conceptual perspective taking: Children's ability to distinguish what they know from what they see. *Child Development,* 59, 703-718.

Thiemann, K.S., and Goldstein, H. (2001). Social stories, written text cues, and video feedback: Effects on social communication of children with autism. *Journal of Applied Behavior Analysis*, 34, 425–446.

Tomasello, M. (1995). Joint attention as social cognition. In C. Moore and P. Dunham (Eds.), *Joint attention: Its origins and role in development*. Hillsdale: Lawrence Erlbaum Associates.

Tomasello, M. and Haberl, K. (2003). Understanding attention: 12- and 18-month-olds know what's new for other persons. *Developmental Psychology,* 39, 906-912.

Trevarthen, C. (1978). Secondary Intersubjectivity: confidence, confiding and acts of meaning in the first year. In A. Lock (Ed.), *Action Gesture and Symbol, The Emergence of Language*. London: Academic Press.

Trevarthen, C. (1984). Emotions in infancy. In K. R. Scherer and P. Ekman (Eds), *Approaches to emotions*, (pp. 129–157). Erlbaum, London.

Trevarthen, C. (1994). Infant Semiosis. In W. Nöth (Ed.) *Origins of Semiosis*. Berlin: Mouton de Gruyter.

Wellman, H. (1993). Early Understanding of Mind: The Normal Case. In S. Baron Cohen, H., Tagerflusberg, D. Cohen (Eds.). *Understanding other minds: Perspectives from Autism* (pp. 10-39). Oxford: University Press.

Wellman, H. and Estes, D. (1986). Early understanding of mental entities: a reexamination of childhood realism. *Child Development,* 57, 910-23.

Weil, T. (unpublished doctoral dissertation). *The impact of training deictic frames on perspective taking in young children: A Relational Frame approach to Theory of Mind.* University of Nevada, Reno.

Werker, J.F., Cohen, L.B., Lloyd, V.L., Casasola, M., and Stager, C.L. (1998). Acquisition of word-object associations by 14-month-old infants. *Developmental Psychology*, 34, 1289–1309.

Whelan, R., and Barnes-Holmes, D. (2004). Motivation in applied behaviour analysis. *The Irish Psychologist*, 30, 263-266.

K.G. Wilson and J.T. Blackledge. (2000). Recent developments in the behavioral analysis of language: Making sense of clinical phenomena. In: M.J. Dougher (Ed.) *Clinical behavior analysis* (pp. 27-46). Context Press, Reno, NV, 27–46.

Wimmer, H. and Perner, J. (1983). Beliefs about beliefs: representation and constraining function of wrong beliefs in young children's understanding of deception. *Cognition,* 13, 103-28.

PART 2:
BEHAVIORAL SYSTEMS FOR INTERVENTION IN AUTISTIC SPECTRUM DISORDERS

In: Behavioral Theories and Interventions for Autism ISBN 978-1-60741-165-9
Editor: Phil Reed © 2009 Nova Science Publishers, Inc.

Chapter 5

EARLY INTENSIVE BEHAVIORAL INTERVENTION IN THE TREATMENT OF AUTISTIC SPECTRUM DISORDERS

Geraldine Leader*, Olive Healy and Jennifer O' Connor
National University of Ireland, Galway

A considerable body of research over the past 20 years has suggested that children with Autistic Spectrum Disorders (ASD) can benefit significantly from early intensive behavioral intervention (EIBI) based on the principles of applied behavior analysis (Anderson, Avery, DiPietro, Edwards, and Christain, 1987; Birnbrauer and Leach, 1993; Eikeseth, Smith, Jahr, and Eldevik, 2002; Fiske, Aalenski, Krantz, and McClannahan, 1985; Harris, Handleman, 2000; Howard, Sparkman, Cohen, Green, and Stainslaw, 2005; Lovaas, 1987; Smith, Groen, and Wynn, 2000). Such studies have suggested that the intervention that is offered early and intensively will produce best outcomes (Howard, Sparkman, Cohen, Green, and Stanislaw, 2005). Lovaas' (1987) seminal study demonstrated that children receiving 40 hours of EIBI made substantial gains and maintained these gains at follow-up (McEachin, Smith, and Lovaas, 1993). Despite these findings EIBI research continues to be controversial, as although some children have made substantial gains, results have varied widely across studies. For example Lovaas (1987) reported that up to 47% of children were able to function independently and had cognitive and language scores in the normal range while others have reported more modest gains (Anderson et al., 1987; Smith et al., 2000).

There is widespread consensus that early intervention is a predictor to better long-term outcomes for individuals with ASD. In addition, there are many possible interventions available to consumers and several of these have claimed to produce significant results (e.g., Birnbrauer and Leach, 1993; Dawson and Fischer, 1994; Ramey and Ramey, 1998). Early intervention can be divided into three broad categories: early intensive behavioral interventions; early educational approaches and alternative treatments. This chapter will outline each of these categories and will examine the growing body of evidence to support EIBI as a treatment for ASD.

* Correspondence should be addressed to Geraldine Leader, School of Psychology, National University of Ireland, Galway, University Road, Galway, Ireland.

Early Intensive Behavioral Intervention (EIBI)

There are a substantial number of studies demonstrating that intensive early intervention using the principles and methods of applied behavior analysis (ABA) can produce significant positive outcomes for children with autism (e.g., Anderson et al., 1987; Birnbrauer and Leach, 1993; Fenske, Zalenski, Krantz, and McClannahan, 1985; Lovaas, 1987; Matson, Benavidez, Compton, Paclawskj, and Baglio, 1996; McEachin, Smith, and Lovaas, 1993; Wolf, Risley, and Mees, 1963). The primary objective of ABA intervention is to teach socially significant behaviors to a meaningful degree and to demonstrate that individuals can function independently and successfully in a variety of environments as a result of these interventions. ABA as an educational intervention begins by teaching and focusing on small and measurable units of behavior using discrete trial instruction in a massed trial presentation. Typically, intervention is provided for 20-40 hours per week in one-to-one or small group settings by qualified and experienced behavioral therapists. In addition, prompts taken from the literature are systematically introduced and faded moving the student towards the target objective. Teaching can be delivered in highly structured environments and/or within more natural settings to promote generalization (e.g., incidental teaching, Hart and Risley, 1975). There are however, variations in the application of ABA interventions, and few studies have compared the various applications of ABA. However, there are a number of common features that can be identified across approaches. According to Green et al., (2002), these features include; that treatment is comprehensive in the manner in which all skill domains are addressed at the level of the individual learner's strengths and deficits; the behavioral procedures that are applied are implemented with the target of increasing functional repertoires and reduce ones that interfere with the learner's positive interaction with their environment; as part of the approaches at least one if not more individuals have advanced training in ABA (e.g., Board Certified Associate Behavior Analyst® or Board Certified Behavior Analyst®); selection of objectives are based on normal developmental sequences (e.g., Assessment of Basic Language and Learning Skills- Revised® (Partington, 2006) or the Preschool Inventory of Repertoires for Kindergarten® (Greer and McCorkle, 2003). Parents have an important role to play as co-therapists; initially therapy is delivered in one-to-one settings and students are gradually transitioned to small group settings; teaching sessions vary from 20-30 hours of intensive structured teaching; optimal age for intervention is between 3 and 4 years of age; duration of intervention is for 2 or more years.

The Young Autism Program (University of California at Los Angeles [UCLA]; Lovaas, 1987; Lovaas, Smith, and McEachin, 1989; McEachin, Smith and Lovaas, 1993) is a home-based early intervention program underpinned by the principles of applied behavior analysis. Children on the program receive intensive one-to-one discrete trial training for 40 hours per week. In addition, parents participate on a parent education training program designed to extend the ABA intervention across the entire day. The educational curriculum is broadly divided into three stages with emphasis placed on specific priority areas; Year 1- reduce self-stimulatory and aggression, while increasing compliance, imitation and appropriate toy play; Year 2- expressive language and interactive play with peers; Year 3- development of appropriate emotional expression, pre-academic tasks, and observational learning. Across the entire intervention period, the general approach to the treatment of challenging behavior and self-stimulatory behavior is based on functional assessment and subsequently, the implementation of function-based treatments.

CABAS®- The Comprehensive Application of Behavior Analysis to Schooling is a systems wide approach to all components of the student's education (e.g., Greer, 1997, Greer, Keohane, and Healy, 2002). In contrast to the UCLA Program, CABAS® is a school based service, with an intensive parent-education program to skills within the home setting. The components of the system include pedagogy, curricula, supervision, administration and the roles of students, parents, supervisors and university training programs. The CABAS® system teaches socially and educationally significant skills through a variety of ABA procedures which include the Learn Unit® (Greer and McDonough, 1999) direct instruction, personalized system of instruction and incidental teaching. Children receive no less than 30 hours of intervention weekly. In addition, the system draws on over two hundred different teaching tactics derived from the literature and ongoing research to teach the identified objectives. Emphasis is placed on data collection and strategic analysis of the progression of the individual learner. The curriculum focuses on teaching communication skills, academic literacy, self-management, problem-solving and an expanded community of reinforcers in a positive and intensive teaching environment. A recent body of research has produced a curriculum to induce and expand new verbal capabilities in children with ASD (Greer and Ross, 2008). Protocols are provided to induce pre-requisite verbal developmental cusps (Greer and Ross, 2008; Keohane and Greer, 2005). The emergence of such cusps is built on teaching several component repertoires. The CABAS® system has been developed using an extensive database for ensuring and maintaining quality applications. Those components include: minimal standards of teaching as applied behavior analysis, curricula for teachers and other professionals, research-based tools to train and monitor professionals and, curriculum revisions for students occasioned by research. Initially, the Learn Unit® is delivered in intensive massed trial instruction and as the learner increases their verbal capabilities they learn to participate within group (e.g., Direct Instruction, Becker & Engelmann, 1976, 1978) and independent (e.g., PSI, Keller, 1968) work sessions, in which the learn unit® then becomes enlarged and more flexible.

In addition, the quality of the training program delivered to staff ensures that certain expected standards are met resulting in continued improvement in the quality of the professional service delivered. In this particular case, the CABAS® system for ongoing staff training builds on Keller's Personalized System of Instruction (PSI) approach (Keller, 1968) within a 'rank' training protocol. That is, the components of behavior analytic teaching and supervision are divided into three categories for each rank, and arranged from less difficult to complex. Professionals move through the levels of expertise in an individual fashion.

Lifeskills and Education for Students with Autism and other Pervasive Behavioral Challenges (LEAP; (Hoyson, Jamieson, and Strain, 1984; Strain and Cordisco, 1994) comprises of two educational system levels: integrated preschool program (which includes both typically developing children and children with ASD) and a parent training program in ABA techniques. As the program is based within an integrated preschool setting, peer models are available and form a critical role in teaching the target areas of independent play skills and social interaction. As part of the parent skills training program, parents learn how to manage their child's problem behavior and to teach new skills. The educational curriculum exposes children with ASD to the typical school curriculum and adaptations to this are made only when a student encounters a difficulty and/or demonstrates a specific need for adjustment.

Typically, the curriculum is delivered within a group with students receiving 15hours of instruction per week.

The Verbal Behavior Approach provides evidence-based behavior analytic intervention to individuals with ASD and other developmental disabilities based on the work of Skinner (1957; Sundberg and Michael, 2001). The primary focus of the Verbal Behavior Approach is the development of an effective and functional communication repertoire. This is also a primary focus for other ABA interventions such as CABAS® where the use of verbal behavior instruction plays an important part of the teaching curriculum and overall approach. Within the Verbal Behavior Approach, the objective is to identify the child's naturally occurring motivation, capture it, and use it to teach new verbal operants. The principles of learning and their derived technologies (e.g., prompting, fading, shaping, chaining) provide the foundational guide for the analysis and assessment of the language program for the individual learner. The educational intervention is delivered through an arrangement of teaching environments which aim to establish a framework for daily language that results in the promotion of generalized responding across settings. The approach focuses on the development of each verbal operant (rather than on words and their meanings) and on the independent teaching of speaker and listener repertoires. The intervention supports a variety of teaching strategies such as early mand training; frequent opportunities to mand; contriving and capturing motivational operations; use of multiple control procedures; and use of multiple exemplar training where the primary objective is to teach the learner to acquire new verbal operants from naturally occurring settings. Similarly to the other interventions, there is an initial emphasis placed on one-to-one instruction but this is implemented in a less structured environment and is more focused on the creation of opportunities to teach verbal behavior repertoires within the natural environment.

The May Institute (Anderson, Campbell, and Cannon, 1994; Anderson, Avery, Dipietro, Edwards, and Christian, 1987) offers a developmentally sequenced home and school based program based on the principles of applied behavior analysis. Target curricular areas include fine/gross motor, cognitive, and socio-emotional development. In common with many of the other ABA approaches, parents are offered and encouraged to participate on training programs in an effort to expand teaching and generalisation opportunities to the home setting. In addition, the Institute has developed the 'Positive Schools Program', which offers positive behaviour support to mainstream schools. This is implemented through consultation sessions, staff training and parent involvement.

The Douglass Developmental Disabilities Center Program (Handleman and Harris, 1994; Harris, Handleman, Kristoff, Bass, and Gordon, 1990) provides a preschool based program for children from the age of three. For children under the age of three, intervention is primarily delivered in the home setting for a minimum of ten hours weekly. The preschool is comprised of three different types of classrooms: the "prep" class, the small group class, and the integrated classroom (with typically developing children). The program is primarily based on the Lovaas' model using discrete trial training as the key means of instruction. The "prep" classroom provides intensive one-to-one discrete trial training in a structured environment. The small group classroom maintains a 2:1 child–teacher ratio and focuses particularly on skills that will be needed to function in the integrated classroom. The integrated classroom is based in part on the LEAP model. In addition, parent support includes a bi-monthly visit by a qualified staff member and 'clinic' meetings which involve in-depth discussions of the student's progress and identification of areas of concern.

The Princeton Child Development Institute (PCDI) was founded in 1970 and expanded in 1975 by Krantz and McClannahan to include data based teaching and treatment services for preschoolers and school-aged children, as well as individualized parent support and home programming services. The early intervention begins for children at 24months and can be delivered as a home or center based intervention. This service relies on a parent-professional partnership. There is an important emphasis placed on the role of family in intervention and this is demonstrated through regular home supports/visits and parent training services. Intervention programs focus on teaching learning readiness, language, play, family participation, social interaction, and daily routines such as eating, sleeping, bathing, and toilet training. Intensive, one-to-one teaching sessions alternate with small-group activities which aim to teach children to relate to peers and to participate in social situations. Each child's schedule of learning activities is especially designed to meet his or her unique learning needs with a particular emphasis placed on language development and social interaction. Children receive no less than 30 hours of intervention weekly. In addition, a residential setting is available for those children who may require this service. The residential setting employs a unique family focus where two therapists assume parent roles for the child within this setting. The institute has demonstrated empirical evidence of its efficacy and generated support and advancements in the field of ABA across the years (Fenske, et al., 1985; Fenske, Krantz, and McClannahan, 2001; Krantz, MacDuff, and McClannahan, 1993; Krantz, and McClannahan, 1993).

EARLY EDUCATIONAL APPROACHES

The use of ABA in the treatment of children with ASD has a history of more than 45 years. However, despite the empirical support for ABA approaches, alternatives to ABA interventions for individuals with ASD are widely employed. Traditionally, early educational approaches are based on normal developmental sequences for instruction and often employ integration of children with ASD with typically developing peers as a means to teach social skills. Although many of these approaches have little empirical support, they are often selected as the treatments of choice by governmental agencies and service providers for children with ASD.

TEACCH (Treatment and Education of Autistic and Communication-Handicapped Children; University of North Carolina at Chapel Hill; Lord and Schopler, 1994) was developed by Schopler in 1972 in North Carolina and is the most widely implemented intervention for children with ASD (Jordan et al, 1998). Children can begin intervention as young as 8months of age and the programme is typically delivered in a teacher student ratio of 1:3. TEACCH can be delivered in both school and home settings.

The TEACCH program emphasizes two basic principles: structuring the environment to promote skill acquisition and facilitating independence at all levels of functioning (Lord and Schopler, 1989; Ozonoff and Cathcart, 1998). In contrast to ABA interventions, the ethos of the program is to help individuals with ASD to make the most of the skills they possess rather than to teach them to enter more 'typical' settings (Lord and Schopler, 1994). A strong emphasis is placed on establishing modified environments with the use of visual structures to accommodate student deficits. Children often work alone on tasks as set out by their teacher, at partitioned work stations. Tasks tend to be repetitive, visual-motor activities such as sorting, matching, slotting, sequencing, etc. The workstation is structured to include visual cues to assist the child in the completion of designated tasks. For example, 'start' and 'finished' boxes may be used to designate assigned tasks and their termination. Staff are not trained in any one specific area (e.g. speech and language therapy or music therapy) but rather are typically trained in special education. Parents are expected to extend the program to the home setting through the establishment of similar visual structures, workstations and the use of picture communication strategies within the home. 'TEACCH does not address the autism directly, but provides what might be called a 'prosthetic environment' for people with autism whereby many of their difficulties can be circumvented and they can be enabled to live and learn without undue stress and anxiety' (Jordan et al, p81, 1998). The effectiveness of the TEACCH approach to the treatment of ASD has been demonstrated by a very limited number of studies (Schopler, Mesibov, and Baker, 1982).

Portage Home-Based Model is a home-visiting education service for pre-school children with ASD. Portage is a parent led approach which aims to support the development of young children. Initial and ongoing developmental checklists are taken to identify strengths and future goals. A 'family centered curriculum' is developed to target the areas of play, communication, learning, relationships and integration into the community. Families are supported by a weekly visit from a member of the multi-disciplinary Portage team. Each family is encouraged to select a play activity which the family can practice and enjoy together. Parents may use charts or diaries as a reminder of the activity and a record of what happens between visits. The Portage program principles are that: (a) All children and parents should be valued for their unique qualities; (b) Parents play the key role in supporting their child's development; (c) Services for families are most useful when are delivered in a child's natural environment; (d) focus on the child's strengths. Smith (2000) suggests that Portage can have a positive impact on social development of children with ASD.

In the 1980's Greenspan developed a social-emotional intervention for children with deficits in relating and communicating, known as Developmental Individual Difference Relationship Model (DIR Model). The DIR Model employs three basic principles (a) following the child's lead and engaging in child-mediated interactions which are driven by the child's own interests; (b) semi-structured problem-solving interactions that meet specific language and social goals; (c) motor, sensory and spatial learning activities (Greenspan and Wieder, 1999). DIR aims to teach imitation and to develop awareness of social interactions and reciprocity. Greenspan (1992) further developed the model to include Floortime. This is based on the premise that the child can learn to interact and communicate through 'circles of communication'. To achieve this objective the child must master the six basic developmental milestones for emotional and intellectual growth. These milestones are described as; self regulation and interest in the world; intimacy or a special love for the world of human relations; two-way communication; complex communication; emotional ideas; and emotional thinking. Greenspan argues that children with ASD have difficulty in moving naturally through these milestones due to sensory over- or under-reactions, processing difficulties, and/or poor control of physical responses and that Floortime offers children a means of moving through these milestones at their own comfortable level. Parents play a pivotal role in this approach. The parent's role is to engage the child in a level that is enjoyable, then enter the child's activities, and follow their lead to continue and expand on this interaction. The target is to find mutually shared engagement between parent and child. In essence the parent's role is to move the child toward more increasingly complex interactions, which is known as "opening and closing circles of communication." Floortime does not separate and focus on speech, motor, or cognitive skills but rather addresses these areas through a synthesized emphasis on emotional development.

Relationship Development Intervention® (RDI: Gutstein, 2007) is a parent- based clinical treatment that focuses on the core problems of gaining friendships, feeling empathy, expressing love and being able to share experiences with others. Gutstein (2007) argues that children with ASD have not developed 'Dynamic Intelligence' and this leads to rigidity in behaviour, inability to form relationships and deficits in independent skills. The approach classifies these abilities as follows: (1) Emotional Referencing: The ability to use an emotional feedback to learn from the experiences of others; (2) Social Coordination: The ability to observe and continually regulate one's behavior in order to participate in spontaneous relationships involving collaboration and exchange of emotions; (3) Declarative Language: Using language and non-verbal communication to express curiosity, invite others to interact, share perceptions and feelings and coordinate actions with others; (4) Flexible thinking: The ability to adapt, change strategies and alter plans quickly based upon changing circumstances; (5) Relational Information Processing: The ability to obtain meaning based upon the larger context; (6) Foresight and Hindsight: The ability to reflect on past experiences and anticipate potential future scenarios in a productive manner.

The Boston Higashi School , developed by Kitahara, is a holistic intervention for children and adults with ASD that is based on Daily Life Therapy® that aims to capture the essence of humanity and to reflect the sensibilities and sensitivities, the intellect and the aesthetics of humankind and to attain harmony in all aspects of life. This is achieved through an holistic education of the entire child via three broad foundations; 1) Vigorous physical exercise, 2) Emotional stability, and 3) Intellectual stimulation. This in turn is believed to remediate deficits in a positive manner rather than directing intervention in a piecemeal approach to the remediation of difficulties. Children begin this intervention at 3 years of age. The approach provides a full education through group dynamics, modeling, physical activity, academic activity and vocational training. The curriculum consists of academics, art, music, physical education, computer skills, and social education. The goal of this educational approach is for the child to develop as closely to normal physically, emotionally, intellectually and to achieve social independence and dignity. Exercises are founded upon principles of sensory integration and vestibular stimulation to develop co-ordination and co-operative group interaction. Whereas, academic activities focus on the areas of language, arts, mathematics, social studies and science and are compatible with typical school curricula with the objective of promoting inclusion opportunities. There is also an emphasis placed on art and music which in turn helps the student to gain mastery and an appreciation of aesthetics. In addition, students can learn daily living and social skills within the residential program which runs for 304 days in the year. Parent training is also available as part of the service. There is no empirical evidence in support of the approach.

The Son-Rise Program® or Options Approach (Kaufman, 1976) is an intensive one-to-one intervention which is lead entirely by the child and not directed by a set of target objectives as is typically common within educational approaches. Individuals working with the child interact with him/her through mimicking his/her 'isms' - the activities he/she often repeats. The objective of this exercise is to gain the child's trust. It is believed that as the 'trust' is developed the child will lead the adult into his/her world. Interaction can then become a pleasurable activity and make people more attractive to the child than the objects and obsessions that they hold (MacDonald and MacDonald, 1991). The intervention is typically conducted within a 'distraction-free' play room or similar environment. Furthermore, changes are made to the child's environment to ensure that the child's sensitivities and understanding of their environment remain at a level that is within their ability range. The use of eye contact is seen as a foundation for learning and is an important skill to develop as part of the program. There is a strong emphasis also placed upon dietary intervention (e.g., gluten free, and casein free, diets). The practices of the Option approach has been evaluated but there is no research on the outcomes of the intervention (Jordan, 1990).

The Early Bird Programme was developed by the National Autistic Society (NAS) in the U.K. as a parent-focused early intervention with a premise of building confidence in parenting skills. Six families participate in each three month program. Target areas of skill development include teaching an understanding of ASD, social communication, and to analyze and use structure, to prevent inappropriate behaviors. The Early Bird Program incorporates SPELL (Structure, Positive (approaches and expectations), Empathy, Low arousal, Links) Picture Exchange Communication System (PECS) and TEACCH as primary teaching methodologies. Shields (2001) demonstrated some support for the effectiveness of the program.

The Miller Method ® (Miller, 1963; 1991) is a "Cognitive-developmental systems approach" to education which has been developed over the past 40 years and is linked to the work of developmental theorists such as Piaget (1948) and Vygotsky (1962). The premise is that children with ASD learn more effectively when their entire body is involved in the learning process. More specifically, the approach is based on the belief that children with ASD become trapped at certain developmental stages and progression to further stages becomes incomplete or distorted. Stereotypic patterns of behavior develop in children with ASD from a lack of understanding of the body in relation to the world and these aberrant patterns of behavior continue to interfere with typical development. The Miller Method® uses two major strategies to restore typical developmental progressions: One involves the transformation of children's aberrant systems into functional behaviors; the other is the systematic and repetitive introduction of developmentally relevant activities. In order to remediate the developmental gaps, a series of specific activities are selected. This process is facilitated by narrating the children's actions while they are elevated 2.5 feet above the ground on an Elevated Square and similar challenging structures. It is believed that through elevating the child that sign-word guidance of behavior and body-other awareness as well as motor-planning and social-emotional contact is enhanced. This elevation causes the child to 'organize' their body or be more attentive and in turn this leads to improvements in communication and social skills. Parents also play an integral role in the program by generalizing the child's achievement across home and community settings. There is no empirical support for the effectiveness of the Miller Method (Jordan, Jones, & Murray, 1998)

An 'eclectic intervention' delivers a combination of the methods based on the practices and philosophies of TEACCH, ABA and DIR (Howard, Sparkman, Cohen, Green, and Stanislaw, 2005). Some of the other approaches implemented as part of an eclectic approach can include, sensory-motor therapies, speech and language therapy, PECS, occupational therapy and so on. The 'eclectic' intervention does not follow a specific ethos but a single school may implement a variety of different approaches with students with ASD (Jordan, Jones, and Murray, 1998). This in turn may lead to a wide variation in the delivery of the intervention as any combination of treatments can be implemented. Combining any number of treatments or 'levels' of treatments makes it extremely difficult to ascertain which particular treatment, or combination of treatments, has the potential to be effective. There is little and limited empirical support for the 'eclectic' model due to the nature of the mix and a frequent absence of analysis within the approach. Any gains that have been found when the 'eclectic' model has been compared to an ABA approach fall well below the effects of ABA (e.g., Howard et al., 2005; Magiati et al., 2007; Sallows et al., 1999)

ALTERNATIVE TREATMENTS

Parents of children with ASD often undertake a variety of alternative interventions to educational approaches. Many of these interventions are attempted based on the recommendations by other parents. According to Goin-Kochel, Myers, and MacKintosh (2007) parents will endeavor to introduce between 7-9 different therapies with 4-6 of these based on other parent feedback. The following are a list of alternative treatments: Speech and Language Therapy (including Auditory Integration Training (Beard, 1982); Occupational Therapy (including Sensory Integration Therapy (e.g. Schaaf & Miller, 2005), Auditory Integration Training (Berkell, Malgeri, & Streit, 1996); Facilitated Communication (Biklen, 1990); Psychotherapies (including Psychoanalysis; Bettelheim, 1967); Biological Treatments (following certain and very specific diets; medication, vitamin supplements or high fat diets); Animal Therapies (including horseback riding, swimming with dolphins); Art and music therapies (e.g. Allgood, 2005); Psychosocial interventions such as Holding/Attachment Therapy (Tinbergen & Tinbergen, 1983). These treatments do not represent an exhaustive list and each year there appears a number of new treatment types for individuals with ASD.

Given the complexities of ASD and the lifelong costs (both human and financial) there has been a continuing search for effective treatments to ASD. There has been an abundance of potential 'miracle' treatments for ASD and many of these unfortunately are without an established empirical base (Smith, 1996). It is important therefore to be knowledgeable about the validated effectiveness of the various treatment approaches available.

EARLY INTENSIVE BEHAVIORAL RESEARCH

While research into EIBI was first documented in the early 1960's (e.g., Ferster, 1961; Lovaas, Berberich, Perloff, and Schaeffer, 1966; Wolf, Risley, and Mees, 1964), the most influential study to date was conduced by Lovaas (1987) in the University of California, Los Angeles. This study consisted of three groups of children who were under 4 years of age at intake. The first group (n-19) received 40 hours per week of one-to-one, applied behavior analytic intervention. The control group (n-19) received 10 hours of applied behavior analytic intervention, and was assigned to the minimal control group. A second control group (n-21) was in receipt of a mix of non-behavioral interventions. The results of this study were considered ground-breaking. The average IQ score for children in the experimental group was 83, while children in the control groups scored 52 and 58 respectively. There was also a significant difference in educational functioning with 47% of the experimental group functioning well in typical first-grade classrooms without any special support by the age of 7.

Only 1 child (2%) from the two control groups made similar gains. Furthermore, a follow up study by McEachin, Smith, and Lovaas (1993) revealed that 8 of the 9 children had maintained their treatment gains and had intellectual functioning scores in the normal range. Indeed they were indistinguishable from their peers.

This is one of the most comprehensive and thorough studies to date in the literature. Indeed this study included many methodological strengths. Children were assessed by professionals independent of the study, therapists were trained in ABA to a pre-determined level and were supervised closely, group size was large in comparison to previous studies and outcome measures included measures of IQ, school placement, adaptive behavior measures and behavioral measures (Connor, 1998). However, this study has attracted controversy, and its finding has been disputed. For example, Schopler, Short, and Mesibov (1989) questioned the choice of outcome measures. The authors claim that the inclusion of IQ measures and educational placement was inadequate and that there was no clear measure of social, behavioral or communicative measures. The authors also claimed that the participants in the experimental group had a better prognosis as some children with echolalia were included. Furthermore, they criticized the method for assigning participants to the control group and the non-random assignment of groups. Questions have also been raised to the extent of 'recovery' claimed by Lovaas. Schopler et al. (1989) and Jordan (1991) disputed the use of normal classroom placement as well as large increases in IQ scores as indices of 'recovery'. However one cannot dispute the large difference between the groups on several important and objective measures of outcome.

Anderson et al. (1987), Birnbrauer and Leach (1993), and Sheinkopf and Siegal (1998) conducted partial replications of the study by Lovaas and colleagues. Children in these studies received fewer hours of treatment (18 to 25 hours per week) and these studies were conducted for a shorter duration (2 years). Anderson et al. (1987), used a pre-post design to examine the effects of 1 to 2 years of home-based intensive behavioral intervention with 14 young children (mean age = 43 months) but did not use a control group. Outcome data revealed statistically significant increases in children's functioning in mental ages, language functioning and self-help skills. At post-treatment all of the children continued to need special education services.

Birnbrauer and Leach (1993) demonstrated gains in intellectual, language and adaptive behavior measures for 9 children (mean age = 39 months). In the Sheinkopf and Siegal (1998) study, children who had intensive home-based intervention scored significantly higher IQ scores than the control group. Collectively these studies showed substantial average increases in nonverbal IQ (22 to 29 points), but gains in other areas were smaller than those reported by Lovaas (1987). Also children in these studies did not achieve treatment gains in the normal range or were integrated in regular classrooms. These studies do not allow for straightforward comparisons with the Lovaas studies as children from these studies were slightly older at age of onset and had slightly lower adaptive behavior and intelligence scores (Green, 1996).

Studies by Harris, Handleman, Gordon, Kristoff, and Fuentes (1991) and Harris, Handleman, Kristoff, Bass, and Gordon (1990) used a pre-post design to asses the outcome of one and two years of a centre based program of applied behavior analysis. They reported a 19 point increase in verbal IQ and a 8 point increase in language measures after one year of treatment. The control group did not report any changes in such scores although all treated children demonstrated impairments after treatment.

A study by Weiss (1999) investigated the correlation between initial acquisition rates of learning with later learning rates. This study suggests that children who initially learned quickly (i.e., mean of less that 2 days for acquisition of the first five items) maintained this advantage through 2 years of intervention. These children also showed the greatest changes in ASD severity and in adaptive behavior. In contrast children who struggled with initial skill acquisition, continued to struggle and also exhibited higher rates of autistic behavior and lower adaptive behavior skills.

Fenske, Zalenski, Krantz, and McClannahan (1985) investigated the effects of age of entry into their program. They compared the outcome measures of 9 children who entered the intervention *prior* to 60 months with 9 children who entered the program *after* 60 months of age. All participants received 27.5 hours per week of centre based applied behavior analytic intervention. Six of the 9 participants in the early treated group, as opposed to 1 of 9 in the older group, were placed in mainstream education after two years of intervention.

Collectively these studies demonstrate that early and intensive behavior analytic intervention is an effective treatment for children with a diagnosis of ASD. There were methodological differences across studies and treatment gains also varied. Some demonstrated normal to near-normal functioning while others demonstrated more modest gains. While comparison studies have demonstrated varying degrees of treatment effectiveness it is also important to examine case studies that support the effectiveness of EIBI. While case studies are not formal experiments they contain several noteworthy components that warrant their inclusion.

Case Studies Supporting Early Behavioral Intervention

Although controlled studies demonstrate the most precise tests of the effects of EIBI, important recommendations can be made from individual case studies. Case studies share some important and credible features. Firstly, baseline measures of each repertoire are taken before treatment onset. Secondly, objective measurement of treatment effects repeated over extended periods of time are implemented along with corroboration of diagnosis, baseline measures and follow-up provided by an independent psychologists. Thirdly, intensive ABA is introduced systematically across many repertoires of behaviors producing methodical improvements in skill areas across time. Case studies have been documented in which independent evaluators use objective measurement instruments to track children's progress (Green, Brennan, and Fein, 2002; Perry, Cohen, and De Carlo, 1995). For example, Perry et al. (1995) reported the effectiveness of early intensive behavioral intervention with two siblings with ASD diagnoses. The intervention involved up to 35 hours of intensive 1:1 teaching sessions. Professionals who diagnosed the children evaluated their progress systematically and reported that both no longer met the criteria for diagnosis of ASD.

Green et al. (2002) demonstrated that four years of early intensive applied behavior analysis treatment, provided to a young child who was determined to be at high risk for ASD at the age of 12 months, resulted in significant increases in language, social, cognitive, and daily living skills on standardized tests. No evidence of behavioral problems or developmental deficits was evident at the end of the fourth year of EIBI and the participant was functioning as a typical child in a regular public school kindergarten classroom.

Butter, Mulick, and Metz (2006) provided eight case descriptions of children, aged between 4:2 - 8:8 years, diagnosed with an ASD and intellectual disability who received an average of 2 years and 8 months of EIBI. Following this period all eight children no longer met behavioral criteria for intellectual disability or ASD. The average gain in IQ standard scores was 34.6 points and the average gain in adaptive behavior standard scores was 43 points. Both nonverbal IQ scores and academic achievement standard scores were shown to be within the average range for all cases at the end of the intervention period. Language skills remained impaired for seven children. These case reports support findings of other researchers that learning recovery in ASD and PDD is possible and may be related to EIBI.

Healy, O' Connor, Leader, and Kenny (2007) reported a case study of a 2 years and 10 month old child receiving an early intensive teaching program using the Comprehensive Application of Behavior Analysis to Schooling (CABAS®). Progress was measured using behavioral assessment tools and mastery to preset learning criteria. Standardized assessments were also administered annually over a three year period by an independent psychologist. During the intervention period, the participant made significant gains in all areas of testing including a decrease in autism quotient from 94 to 75. Communication skills increased from an age-equivalent of 1 year at pre-treatment to 5:1 years post-treatment. In addition, the measure of adaptive behavior composite increased from a score of 69 to 75. Following three years of EIBI the participant was integrated with age equivalent peers for two hours daily.

PARENT LED EIBI APPROACHES

In addition a number of studies have been published demonstrating the effectiveness of parent directed EIBI and these will be outlined in the next section.

Smith, Groen, and Wynn (2000) compared the treatment effectiveness of an intensive applied behavior analytic treatment group and a parent-led treatment group. This study included children with a diagnosis of ASD as well as children with pervasive developmental disorder not otherwise specified (NOS). Children were randomly assigned to treatment group. The intensive treatment group (7 with ASD, 8 with pervasive developmental disorder not otherwise specified- NOS) received on average 24.52 hours per week of individual treatment for one year. Treatment was reduced over the next 1 to 2 years. The parent training group (7 with ASD, 6 with pervasive developmental disorder NOS) received two sessions per week (5 hours) of parent training for 3 to 9 months. Both groups received intervention based on Lovaas et al.'s (1981) manual. The intensive treatment group made more gains on measures of intelligence, visual-spatial skills, language, and academics but not on measures of adaptive functioning or behavior problems. An interesting finding in this study was that children in the intensive treatment group with pervasive developmental disorder (NOS) made gains similar to children with ASD.

Luiselli, Cannon, Ellis, and Sisson (2002) conducted a retrospective study that examined the outcome of 16 children who were participating in a home-based behavioral intervention. This study examined specifically whether intensity (hours per week, duration in months, total hours of treatment) and onset of intervention (before or after 3 years of age) had an impact on treatment outcomes. Data revealed that all children made gains on the six domains that were assessed (communication, cognitive, fine motor, gross motor, self-care and social emotional). However, no difference was found between the two groups. Finally duration in intervention (months) was predictive of positive outcomes.

Bibby, Eikeseth, Martin, Mudford, and Reeves (2001) examined data from 66 children who were participating in a parent-led behavioral intervention. The intervention was managed by 25 different early intervention consultants. After a mean of 31.6 months of intervention IQ scores for 22 children had not altered significantly. Examining median age of intervention onset highlighted the importance of this variable as it was revealed that children who started before the age of 43 months made a mean gain 10.8 points, and children who started later lost on average 2.4 points. Further analysis of the data revealed that 27% of children made impressive IQ gains while 33% made gains in adaptive behavior.

Sallows and Graupner (2001) designed a study to investigate whether a community-based program in the absence of high levels of supervision and resources and without the application of aversive strategies could achieve results similar to Lovaas (1987). They also sought to examine whether those children who do reach post-treatment test scores within the average range show any residual symptoms of ASD in follow-up measures. Results were reported for twenty three children with ASD diagnoses between the ages of 24 and 42 months, who were randomly assigned to one of two groups – clinic-directed group or parent-directed group. Children in the clinic-directed group (n=13) received an average of 6-10 hours per week of supervision within the home setting from a senior therapist and weekly consultation from the clinic supervisor of the Wisconsin Early ASD Project designating this the intensive treatment group. The parent-directed group (n=10) received 6 hours monthly from a senior therapist and consultation once every two months from the clinic supervisor and this was designated a less intensive treatment group. All children began treatment between the ages of 35-37 months. Results showed that the average Full Scale IQ increase for all participants was 25 points. Five of the clinic-directed group and three of the parent-directed group achieved an IQ of 85 or higher following 1 year of treatment. Three additional participants from the parent-directed group achieved this IQ following the second year of treatment. Eleven participants showed (5 clinic-directed and 6 parent-directed) showed an increase from a mean of 55 prior to treatment to a mean of 104 post 4 years of treatment and were participating in mainstream classes. Measures of residual symptoms for these participants showed eight demonstrating increases in social skills to the adequate range and three showed problems with inattention. The remaining 12 participants did not demonstrate a significant IQ gain after 4 years. This study demonstrates the effectiveness of EIBI in a clinical setting and shows no differences between clinic- and parent-directed programs after 4 years of intervention.

The studies outlined above demonstrate that EIBI provided by parents can produce measurable gains in language, intellectual functioning and adaptive behavior. These studies were home-based and parent led. Variations in outcomes may be a function in variations between programs. Future research is needed to compare the effectiveness of parent-led and centre based EIBI.

Comparison Studies of Early Intensive Behavioral Intervention and 'Eclectic' or Special Education Provision

There is much empirical evidence to show that early intensive behavior analytic intervention produces significant improvements in the symptoms of ASD. The studies outlined above have documented the effectiveness of behavior analytic intervention for individuals with ASD using both home-based and parent-directed behavioral programs. There is a core body of research that has employed controlled comparisons of different treatment effects within school- and home based settings provided by clinical practitioners. Most notably the treatments involved either EIBI or an 'eclectic' mix of interventions incorporating different elements from multiple treatments such as TEACCH, ABA, PECS, sensory-integration therapy, occupational therapy as well as general methods derived from therapists' own personal training and experience. The following section provides a summary of such studies and their findings. These intensive studies have demonstrated the relevance and importance of EIBI in the treatment of ASD. In addition, these studies have investigated whether age of onset of treatment is an important variable in the outcomes achieved.

Eikeseth, Smith, Jahr, and Eldevik (2002) evaluated intensive treatment for 4-7 year old children with ASD over a period of 1 year. Assignment to one of two groups - intensive behavioral intervention (n = 13) or 'eclectic' treatment (n = 12) - was based on availability of personnel to supervise the treatment type and was not influenced by child characteristics or family preference. Both groups received an average of 28.52 hours per week of intervention within the school setting. Results showed that children in the behavioral treatment group made significantly larger gains on measures of intellectual functioning, visual-spatial skills, language functioning, and adaptive behaviors. For example, 7 of the 13 children in the behavioral intervention group achieved IQ scores above 85, on the Wechsler Preschool and Primary Scale of Intelligence-Revised, compared to 2 in the 'eclectic' treatment group. Following one year of EIBI, on average the EIBI group gained 17 points in IQ, 13 points in language comprehension, 23 points in expressive language and 11 points in adaptive behavior. In contrast, the 'eclectic' group gained an average of 4 points in IQ, but decreased in measures of language comprehension and adaptive behavior. There were no increases or decreases in measures of adaptive behavior. Eikeseth et al. (2002) argue that such between-group differences demonstrated emerged even though the groups appeared similar to each other in the amount of treatment that was delivered and the standard of education held by therapists. The behavioral treatment group also displayed fewer aberrant behaviors and social problems at follow-up. Overall results demonstrate that some children with ASD between the ages of 4-7 can make substantial gains with intensive behavioral intervention. Therefore, this study shows that children who begin EIBI after 4 years of age may benefit as much as younger children.

Howard, Sparkman, Cohen, Green, and Stanislaw (2005) compared 61children across three early intervention groups. All participants in the study met the criterion either for ASD or for Pervasive Developmental Disorder – Not Otherwise Specified (PDD-NOS) and were as young as 48 months at treatment onset. One group received intensive clinic-directed behavior analytic intervention (25-40 hours per week) and two comparison groups, received equally intensive eclectic intervention - ASD educational programming (n=16) and generic educational programming (n=16). Assignment to groups in this study was not randomized but depended on advice from practitioners and parental preference for a particular treatment type. The intensive behavioral intervention group were given instruction that was individualized on a 1:1 teacher-student ratio with frequent instructional learning opportunities through discrete trial instruction. A wide number of behavioral strategies from the published literature were implemented to teach a large number of skills from behavioral curricula. Intensive supervision was provided by staff with a minimum qualification of a master's degrees in psychology. No additional services such as occupational therapy and speech therapy were provided to the children in this group.

Children in the ASD educational group were given instruction on a 1:1 or 1:2 student-teacher ratio depending on individual needs and were attending ASD classes within public schools. The program was supervised by a credentialed special education teacher and included provision of a combination of different interventions (discrete trial training, PECS, sensory integration therapy, group speech therapy, TEACCH interventions and 'circle time' activities). Children in the general educational group were enrolled in local community special education classrooms identified as early intervention or communicatively handicapped preschool programs. Those programs served children with a variety of disabilities, and provided an average of 15 hours of intervention per week, with a 1:6 adult:child ratio. Educational programs emphasized exposure to language, play activities, a variety of sensory experiences, group speech therapy.

This study showed that prior to treatment there were no differences between the intensive behavior analytic group and the two comparison groups combined. In a second analysis of functioning 14 months later, children in the intensive behavior analytic intervention group showed statistically significant higher mean scores in all domains (cognitive, linguistic and adaptive functioning) than the other two groups combined. The intensive behavior analytic group had mean standard scores in the normal range on cognitive, non-verbal, communication, and motor skills, whereas the only mean score in the normal range for the comparative groups was in motor skills alone.

A further study comparing early intensive behavioral treatment with special education classes was conducted over 3 years in a community setting. Cohen, Amerine-Dickens, and Smith (2006) compared 21 children receiving EIBI with the same number of children participating in public school special education classes. Assignment to group was based on parental preference for treatment type. Both groups included children with a diagnosis of ASD and with PDD-NOS diagnoses. Performance after each year was measured and revealed that the EIBI group was significantly higher on outcome measures of IQ and adaptive behavior but not on measures of language or non-verbal skills.

A similar comparison study conducted by Eldevik, Eikeseth, Jahr, and Smith (2006) compared 2 groups of children with a diagnosis of autism and intellectual disability, below the age of 6 years at the beginning of treatment, and receiving either EIBI (n=13) or 'eclectic' treatment (n=15) for an average of 12 hours per week. The groups did not differ significantly at pre-treatment. Following 2 years of intervention, the EIBI group made larger gains than the 'eclectic' group in the areas of intelligence, language, adaptive functioning and maladaptive behaviors. This study demonstrated more reserved gains than previously reported comparative studies (See Table 1). Eldevik et al. argue that the reason for this may be that participants had an average pre-treatment IQ score of 41 whereas other studies have reported average pre-treatment IQ's between 50 and 65 (Eikeseth et al., 2002; Harris and Handleman, 2000; Lovaas, 1987). In addition, the difference in treatment hours compared to Smith et al.

(2000) who provided the EIBI group with an average of 24.52 hours weekly may have accounted for the difference in outcomes.

The studies by Howard et al. (2005), Cohen et al. (2006), and Eldevik et al. (2006) demonstrate that EIBI can produce substantial gains in a number of domains when compared with an 'eclectic' mix of interventions. Results for EIBI groups were superior on measures of cognitive, language, and adaptive behavior deficits associated with autism. However, these studies did not address whether EIBI can impact additional core diagnostic symptoms of ASD such as ratings of autistic symptoms, behavior problems and joint attention behaviors.

Remington et al. (2007) addressed this issue by providing additional outcome measures. The authors identified two groups of pre-school children with a diagnosis of autism. The first group of 23 children received EIBI over a two year period in a home-based setting. The second group of 21 children received their local education authorities' standard provision for children with ASD over the same period. Pre-treatment assessment was conducted for both groups and was repeated following the end of the first and second years. Measures of parental mental health, stress, and positive perceptions of their child were also obtained at these times. Participants were aged between 30 and 42 months at the onset of EIBI. A field effectiveness approach was used which compared children whose parents had opted for EIBI with those whose parents had not. The results of this study demonstrated clear gains for the EIBI group on measures of IQ, mental age, expressive language, language comprehension, and adaptive behavior following 1 year of intervention. Significant changes in motor skills and responses to joint attention were also demonstrated for this group. Additionally, children in the EIBI group showed strong improvements in parental ratings of positive social behaviors but there was no evidence of a similar change in parents' reports of children's behavior problems, or ratings of their autistic behaviors.

Remington et al. (2007) extended previous research by examining parental outcomes. Findings on these measures demonstrated that the results for children in the EIBI group did not impact negatively on parent well-being including stress and mental health measures although paternal measures did report more symptoms of depression over the course of the study.

Eikeseth, Smith, Jahr, and Eldevik (2007) extended the findings of Eikeseth et al. (2002) on the effects of EIBI for children who began intervention between 4-7 years (mean 5.5 years). Outcome measures of IQ, adaptive behavior, social emotional functioning were taken pre- and post-treatment. IQ scores for the EIBI group was the largest gain; an increase of 25 points (from 62 to 87) compared to 7 points (from 65 to 72) in the 'eclectic' treatment group. Gains in adaptive behavior were also greater for the EIBI group than for the 'eclectic' treatment group ranging from 9 points for daily living skills to 20 points for communication. In contrast, mean scores in the eclectic treatment group decreased 6 to 12 points.

Table 5.1. EIBI Approaches

Intervention	Setting	Parent Involvement	Unit of Instruction	Hrs of Intervention	Curriculum Focus	Additional services
UCLA Project (Lovaas, 1987)	Home based	Parent Training	Discrete Trial	40hrs	Individualised Prog	Residential Service
CABAS® (Greer, 1997)	School based	Parent Ed. Program	Learn Unit®	<30hrs	PIRK®	NO
LEAP Strain & (Cordisco, 1994)	School & Home	Parent Training Prog.	Discrete Trial	15hrs	Mainstream Curric. (Changed as required) Life Skills	SLT
PCDI (Krantz & McClannahan)	School or Home	Home prog. Support		<27.5	Individ. Prog with emphasis on play & social skills	
The Verbal Behavior Approach (Sundberg & Partington, 1998)	School	Parent Supports		30	Verbal Behavior	NO

Table 5.2. Outcome Effectiveness Studies for EIBI Approaches

Study	Intervention Methodology	Hours Per Week (Mean)	Age Range At onset of Treatment	IQ at Intake (Mean)	Outcome Measures Used	Diagnostic Criteria	Duration of Treatment
Eikeseth at al. (2002) and	1. Behavioral intervention	28	4-7 years	61.92	Intellectual functioning	Autism	1 year
Eikeseth at al.	2. 'Eclectic' intervention	29.8	4-7 years	65.17	Visual-spatial skills	Service	Second follow-up at 8:2 years (mean)
Follow-up (2007)					Language Adaptive Behaviors		
Howard et al. (2005)	1. Behavioral intervention	25-40	30.86 months	58.54	Cognitive	Autism	M = 14 months
	2. 'Eclectic' intervention	30	37.44 months	53.69	Non-verbal		
	3. Mix methods	15	34.56 months	59.88 (Cognitive Scores)	Receptive and expressive language Adaptive Skills		
Eldevik (2006)	1. Low intensive behavioural intervention	12	53 months	41	Intelligence Language Adaptive skills	Autism	2 years
	2. 'Eclectic' intervention	12	49 months	47.92	Maladaptive behavior		
Remington et al. (2007)	1. Behavioral intervention	25.6	30-42 months	61.43	Intelligence Language	Autism	1 year and 2 years
	2. 'Eclectic' intervention		30-42 months	62.33	Adaptive skills Severity of problem behavior Non-verbal Social communication Parental well-being		
Study	Intervention Methodology	Hours Per Week	Age Range At onset of	IQ at Intake (Mean)	Outcome Measures Used	Diagnostic Criteria	Duration of Treatment

		(Mean)	Treatment				
Reed et al. (2006)	1. High-intensity behavioral intervention	30	42.9 months	57.2	Autism severity Intellectual Educational Adaptive skills	Autism	9.10 months
	2. Low-intensity behavioral intervention	12	40.8 months	49.3 intellectual measure			
Zachor et al. (2007)	1. Behavioral intervention	8	>3 years	79.6	Cognitive Autism severity	Autism	1 year
	2. 'Eclectic'-developmental	8	> 3 years	76.1			

Table 5.3. Description of Four Case Studies Examining the Efficacy of Early Intensive Behavioral Interventions

Study	Intervention Methodology	Age at Onset of Treatment	IQ at intake	Diagnosis	Outcome Measures	Duration	Outcome Data
Butter et al. (1996)	Behavioral Intervention	8 children, aged between 4:2-8.8 years	Mean <49.5 +2.73SD	ASD	IQ & adaptive scores Language scores Autism severity Parent & beh. adjustment academic Achievement	2 years & 8 mths	All eight children no longer met the behavioral criteria for ASD although 7 out of 8 still had impaired language scores
Green et al. (2002)	Behavioral Intervention	12 mths	N/A	ASD	Standardized tests of language, social, cognitive, and daily living skills	4 years	No evidence of behavioral or developmental deficits
Healy et al. (2007)	CABAS® Behavioral Intervention	2yrs 10mths	N/A	ASD Significant learning disability	Adaptive Scores IQ, daily living scores Academic achievement (ABLLS® & PIRK®)	3years	Within the average range No evidence of beh. or dev. deficits Integration within mainstream class
Perry et al. (1995)	ABA intervention Based on Lovaas prog.	2 siblings; 23mths & 25mths	N/A	ASD	Adaptive Scores Beh. & language scores	2yrs	No longer met criteria for autism diagnosis

Table 5.4. Parent Led Early Intensive Behavioral Interventions

Study	Intervention Methodology	Age at Onset of Treatment	Diagnosis	Outcome Measures	Duration	Outcome Data
Smith et al. (2000)	UCLA treatment model	35-45mths	ASD or PDD-NOS	IQ, Adaptive scores language visual-spatial scores academics	(1)1yr (2) 3-9mths	gains made on all outcome measures by group 1
Luiselli et al. (2002)	Home based ABA May Institute (Lovaas)	(1)8 children (mean age 2.63yrs) (2)8 children	ASD PDD PDD-NOS	ELAP LAP	(1) 11.6mths (2)7.12mths	improvements in cog, commun., & socio-emotional scores were predicted by duration of treatment & whether treatment began before or after 3yrs of age
Bibby et al. (2001)	UCLA treatment model	(mean age 3.98yrs) 66 children	ASD	Adaptive Scores IQ Language Behavior scales Parent interview	1-2 years	Children who began before 43mths made a mean gain of 10.8 IQ pts Mean IQ scores were sig. less than outcomes of Lovaas study
Sallows et al. (2001)	(1)Community based ABA prog. limited supervision& resources and (2) Clinic ABA	(1)10 children (2)13 children all began treatment 35-37mths	ASD	IQ Scores	4yrs	Increase for children in both groups was average of 25pts 5 children from group 1 & 6 from group 2 participated in mainstream classes following intervention

The most recent study to demonstrate the effectiveness of EIBI employing a comparative study of two treatment interventions was conducted by Zachor, Ben-Itzchak, and Rabinovich (2007). The authors compared the impact of the 'eclectic-developmental' (ED) approach based on a developmental approach incorporating a combination of methods including the Developmental Individual-Difference Relationship (DIR), The Treatment and Education of Autistic and Related Communication Handicapped Children (TEACCH), and techniques from Applied Behavior Analysis (ABA). Programs differed in the type of professionals involved and strategies used to attain progress. The study addressed whether symptoms within autism impairments can change with treatment and if there are specific manifestations in autism that improve with any type of intervention or only with a specific intervention approach. The ED group contained 19 participants aged 23–33 months. The ABA group contained 20 participants aged 22–34 months. All participants were diagnosed with ASD using the Autism Diagnostic Interview (ADI) and were matched on age, autism severity, cognitive abilities and socio-economic background at pre-intervention. Assignment to group was based on children's place of residence at the time of treatment onset. Pre-intervention (PRI) evaluation (baseline) included the Autism Diagnostic Observation Schedule (ADOS) measuring language, communication and reciprocal social interaction; The Bayley Scales of Infant Development-second edition (BSID-II) for preverbal children and the Stanford-Binet Intelligence Scale-fourth edition was used for verbal children. Pre–post intervention differences in language and communication domain were significant only for the ABA group. Both groups showed significant improvement in reciprocal social interaction domain with the effect size greater for the ABA group. Changes in diagnostic classification were noted in both groups but were more pronounced for the ABA group. Pre-treatment IQ scores were positively related to ADOS scores at pre- and post-intervention times. Change in core autism symptoms was shown to be greater with intervention based on ABA principles in comparison to the ED intervention.

Reed, Osborne, and Corness (2007) demonstrated the effectiveness of home-based EIBI for children who began treatment at 2:6–4:0 years old. Participants were assigned to either a high-intensity (mean 30 hours per week) or low-intensity (mean 12 hours per week) EIBI group based on the availability of resources within their demographic area. All participants were diagnosed with ASD and were studied over 9–10 months. Outcome measures of autistic severity, intellectual, educational, and adaptive behavioral functioning were taken. Findings showed that high-intensity behavioral approaches produced greater gains than low intensity programs. In the high-intensity intervention group, there were greater gains in intellectual functioning, and in educational functioning, relative to those in the low-intensity group consistent with Smith et al. (2002). In contrast, there were no differences in terms of intensity on adaptive behavioral functioning. Findings also showed a failure to demonstrate a change in autism severity rating across treatment. This finding contrasts strongly with that of Lovaas (1987). However, the current study was of a much shorter duration than the latter study, and further study of the programs would be needed before firm conclusions could be drawn on this matter. In addition, the sample used in this study was diagnosed with severe autism at the onset of treatment and this factor may have impacted findings. Although results showed the high-intensity EIBI group made generally greater gains on measures than the lower-intensity group, these differences were not always statistically significant. This is an important finding as it queries the emphasis placed on the temporal input of the program as a key factor in the production of greater outcomes. Reed et al. argue that a closer analysis of the relationship between the temporal input of the program and the overall gains made by children receiving high-intensity EIBI shows no clear pattern between temporal input and the gains made. Although the high-intensity group did show greater gains than the low-intensity group, a within group analysis of the high-intensity EIBI showed an inverse relationship between the temporal input and the gains. This finding implies that the suggested 40 hours per week input may not be optimal, and once over a certain level of temporal contribution, there may be diminishing returns for increasing such input of a program. However, the quality of program delivery (amount and type of supervision, curricula employed, staff training, and combined behavioral technologies) may be a critical variable in the relationship between intervention provided and the temporal intensity of intervention. Further research will be necessary to determine if the quality of program 'type' is a factor in such findings.

Not all comparative studies of EIBI and 'eclectic' interventions have demonstrated such favorable results for EIBI. For example, Magiati, Charman, and Howlin (2007) conducted a study that compared outcomes on cognitive, language, play, adaptive behavior and severity of autism measures for pre-school children with ASD receiving autism-specific nursery provision using 'eclectic' intervention or home-based EIBI in a community setting. Forty-four participants between the age of 23-53 months were assigned to one of the two groups (28 in EIBI and 16 in the autism-specific group). The EIBI group received significantly greater hours of intervention during the study. The degree of change was generally small to moderate for most children in each change category for cognitive, language, play, adaptive behavior, and severity of autism. However, in all areas assessed, the extent of individual variation in progress was evident in both group with intake IQ and language level best predicting overall progress. At follow-up twelve participants from the EIBI group were in attendance at mainstream albeit with limited or full support from an ABA therapist.

Overall these studies substantiate the view that intensive early intervention based on the principles of ABA is a treatment approach that under certain conditions can produce systematic, substantial and durable effects. However, given the disparity in research controls, participant characteristics, baseline and follow-up analyses, treatment duration, treatment integrity measures, etc. across many of the studies, there is a firm need for elaborate investigation into the factors that can produce optimal results using EIBI with children diagnosed with ASD. These factors include the following: duration of treatment; treatment integrity parameters; goal selection and intervention strategy selection processes; diagnostic criteria; pre-entry characteristics of participants; age of onset of treatment; types of baseline and outcome measures; environmental variables that mitigate outcomes including parental involvement. An analysis of each of these factors will be necessary as part of future research to identify key features of EIBI that will result in best outcomes for individuals with ASD. In addition, the challenge remains for behavior analysts in identifying predictor variables, including participant characteristics, that will increase the efficacy of EIBI.

Due to the challenges of EIBI research there is often a disparity between "pure research design" and what is done in practice. In the "real world" studies that implement for example random assignment may in reality be very difficult to implement. Absence of control of such factors is commonplace in typical service settings so the long-term clinical benefit of any intervention depends on its remaining effective in conditions that are less than optimal. Considerations of this kind have given rise to field effectiveness research, in which random assignment to groups and the most rigorous experimental control are traded against a more naturalistic evaluation of service delivery in context. Two recent evaluations of early behavioral intervention for autism (Cohen, Amerine-Dickens, and Smith, 2006; Howard, Sparkman, Cohen, Green, and Stanislaw, 2005) have adopted this approach.

Although the efficacy of Intensive Behavioral Intervention (IBI) for young children with Autism Spectrum Disorders (ASD) has been well documented in small model programs, IBI's effectiveness (i.e., does it work in the ''real world''?) has been less studied and may not be as impressive (e.g. Bibby, Eikeseth, Martin, Mudford, and Reeves, 2002). This study reports on the outcomes of 332 children, aged 2–7 years, enrolled in a large, community-based, publicly funded IBI Program in Ontario, Canada. File review data at intake and exit were compared on a group basis as well as on an individual basis. Results indicated statistically significant and clinically significant improvements: reduction in autism severity, cognitive and adaptive levels, as well as a doubling of children's rate of development. There was a considerable heterogeneity in outcome, as expected, and children were classified into seven categories of progress/outcome, as expected, and children were classified into seven categories of progress/outcome. The majority of children (75%) showed some gains during IBI and 11% achieved average functioning. Although the study has clear methodological limitations (chiefly the lack of a comparison group), it suggests that IBI can be implemented effectively in a large community-based program.

A review of the literature to date reveals that EIBI is the most effective treatment for children with autism. As outlined above future research should incorporate an analysis of each of the variables that will result in best outcomes for individuals with ASD. Finally, we need to strive towards greater scientific rigor to answer these and other questions.

REFERENCES

Allgood, N. (2005). Parents' perceptions of family-based group music therapy for children with autism spectrum disorders. *Music Therapy Perspectives, 23(2), 92-99*

Anderson, S. R., Avery, D. L., DiPietro, E. K., Edwards, G. L., and Christian, W. P. (1987). Intensive home-based intervention with autistic children. *Education and Treatment of Children,* 10, 352–366.

Anderson, S.R., Campbell, S., and Cannon, B. O. (1994). The may center for early childhood education. In S. L. Handleman (Eds.), *Preschool education programs for children with autism* (pp. 15-36). Austin TX: Pro-ed.

Beard, G. (1982). *Audition egale comportment.* Sainte-Ruffine: Maisonneuve.

Becker, W., & Engelmann, S. (1976). Analysis of achievement data on six cohorts of low income children from 20 school districts in the University of Oregon Direct Instruction Follow Through Model (Teachnical Report 76-1). University of Oregon, Office of Education, Follow Through Project.

Becker, W., & Engelmann, S. (1978). Analysis of achievement data on six cohorts of low income children from 20 school districts in the University of Oregon Direct Instruction Follow Through Model (Teachnical Report 78-1). University of Oregon, Office of Education, Follow Through Project

Bettelheim, B. (1967). *The empty fortress: Infantile autism and the birth of the self.* New York Free Press.

Bibby, P., Eikeseth, MS., Martin, N.T., Mudford, O.C., and Reeves, D. (2001). Progress and outcomes for children with autism receiving parent-managed intensive interventions. *Research in Developmental Disabilities,* 23, 81-104.

Birnbrauer, J. S., and Leach, D. J. (1993). The Murdoch Early Intervention Program after 2 years. *Behavior Change,* 10, 63–74.

Butter, E.M., Mulick, J.A., and Metz, B. (2006). Eight case reports of learning recovery in children with pervasive developmental disorders after early intervention. *Behavioral Interventions,* 21, 227-243.

Cohen, H., Amerine-Dickens, M., and Smith, T. (2006). Early intensive behavioral treatment: Replication of the UCLA model in a community setting. *Journal of Developmental and Behavioral Pediatrics,* 27, S145-S155.

Connor, M. (1998). A review of behavioural early intervention programmes for children with autism. *Educational Psychology in Practice,* 14, 109-117.

Dawson, G., and Fischer, K.W. (1994). *Human behavior and the developing brain*, Guilford, New York,Eldevik, S., Eikeseth, S., Jahr, E., and Smith, T. (2006). Effects of low-intensity,behavioral treatment for children with autism and mental retardation. *Journal of Autism and Developmental Disorders,* 36, 211-224.

Eikeseth, S., Smith, T., Jahr, E., and Eldevik, S. (2002). Intensive behavioral treatment at school for 4- to 7-year-old children with autism: A one-year comparison controlled study. *Behavior Modification,* 26, 49–68.

Eikeseth, S., Smith, T., Jahr, E., and Eldevik, S. (2007). Intensive behavioral treatment at school for four to seven year old children with autism: A one-year follow up. *Behavior Modification,* 31, 264-278.

Eldevik, S., Eikeseth, S., Jahr, E., & Smith, T. (2006).Effects of low-intensity behavioral treatment for children with autism and mental retardation. *Journal of Autims and Developmental Disorders, 36* (2), 211-224

Fenske, E.C., Krantz, P.J., and McClannahan, L. E. (2001). Incidental teaching: A not-discrete-trial teaching procedure. In C. Maurice, G. Green, and R. M. Foxx(Eds.), *Making a difference: Behavioral intervention for autism* (pp. 7582). Austin, TX: Pro-ed.

Fenske, E.C., Zalenski, S., Krantz, P.J., and McClannahan, L.E. (1985). Age at intervention and treatment outcome for autistic children in a comprehensive intervention program. *Analysis and Intervention in Developmental Disabilities,* 5, 49-58.

Ferster, C.B., andDeMyer, M.K. (1961). The development of performances in autistic children in an automatically controlled environment. *Journal of Chronic Diseases,* 13, 312-345.

Fenske, Aalenski, Krantz, and McClannahan, (1985). Age at intervention and treatment outcome for autistic children in a comprehensive intervention program. *Analysis and Intervention in Developmental Disabilities,* 5, 49-58.

Green, G. (1996). Early behavioral intervention for autism: What does research tell us? In C. Maurice (Ed.), G. Green, and S. Luce (Co-Eds.), *Behavioral intervention for young children with autism: A manual for parents and professionals* (pp. 29–44). Austin, TX: PRO-ED.

Green, G., Brennan, L.C., and Fein, D. (2002). Intensive behavioral treatment for a toddler at high risk for autism, *Behavior Modification*, 26, 69–102.

Greer, R.D. (1997). The Comprehensive Application of Behavior Analysis to Schooling (CABAS®). *Behavior and Social Issues*, 7, 59-63.

Greer, R. D., Keohane, D. D., and Healy, O. (2002). Quality and applied behavior analysis. *The Behavior Analyst Today,* 3, 120-132. www.behavior-analysttoday.org

Greer, R. D. and McCorkle, N. (2003). *Preschool inventory of repertoires for kindergarten (PIRK).* Yonkers, NY: CABAS® and the Fred S. Keller School.

Greer, R. D., and McDonough, S. H. (1999). Is the learn unit the fundamental measure of pedagogy? *The Behavior Analyst, 20.* 5-16.

Greer, R.D., and Ross, D. (2008). *Verbal behaviour analysis: Developing andexpanding verbal capabilities in children with language delays.* Boston: Allyn and Bacon/Merryl.Kendall, Chu, Greenspan, S.J. (1992). Reconsidering the diagnosis and treatment of very young children with autistic spectrum or pervasive developmental disorder. *Zero to Three,* 13, 1-9.

Greenspan, S.J. (1992). Reconsidering the diagnosis and treatment of very young children with autistic spectrum or pervasive developmental disorder. *Zero to Three, 13*(2), 1-9.

Greenspan, S.J., and Wieder, S. (1999). A functional developmental approach to autistic spectrum disorder. *Journal of the Association for Persons with Severe Handicaps,* 24, 147-161.

Goin-Kochel, R.P., Myers, R. P., & MacKintosh, V.H. (2007). Parental reports on the use of treatments and therapies for children with autism spectrum disorders. *Research in Autism Spectrum Disorders, 1,* 195-209.

Gutstein, S.E. (2007). *The Relationship Development Intervention (RDI®) Program and Education.* Connections Center Publishing.

Handleman, S., and Harris, S. (1994). The Douglass Developmental Disabilities Center. In S. Harris and J. Handleman (Eds.), *Preschool education programs for children with autism (pp. 71-86).* Austin, TX: Pro-ed.

Hart, B., and Risley, T.R. (1975). Incidental teaching of language in the preschool. *Journal of Applied Behavior Analysis,* 8, 411-420.

Harris, S.L. and Handleman, J.S. (2000). Age and IQ at intake as predictors of placement for young children with autism: A four- to six-year follow-up. *Journal of Autism and Developmental Disorders*, 30, 137-142.

Harris, Handleman, Kristoff, Bass, and Gordon, (1990). Changes in language development among autistic and peer children in segregated and integrated preschool settings. *Journal of Autism and Developmental Disorders,* 20, 23-31.

Harris, S. L., Handleman, J. S., Gordon, R., Kristoff, B., and Fuentes, F. (1991). Changes in cognitive and language functioning of preschool children with autism. *Journal of Autism and Developmental Disorders*, 21, 281-290.

Healy, O., O' Connor, J. Leader, G., and Kenny, N. (2008). What is possible- Three years of applied behaviour analysis, a case study. *Journal of Early Intensive Behavioral Intervention.*

Hoyson, F.M., Jamieson, B., and Strain, P.S. (1984). Individualized group instruction of normally developing and autistic children: The LEAP curriculum model. *Journal of the Division for Early Childhood,* 8, 157-172.

Howard, J. S., Sparkman, C. R., Cohen, H. G., Green, G., and Stanislaw, H. (2005). A comparison of intensive behavior analytic and eclectic treatments for young children with autism. *Research in Developmental Disabilities,* 26, 359–383.

Jordan, R, Jones, G. and Murray, D. (1998). *Educational interventions for children with autism: A literature review of recent and current research* (Final report). School of Education, University of Birmingham, England, B15 2TT.

Jordan, R. (1991). "Therapeutic approaches to autism", *National Autistic Society Conference Proceedings*, 3-6 April, University of Durham.

Kaufman, B.N. (1976). *Son-rise.* New York: Harper and Row.

Keller, F. S. (1968). Goodbye teacher.... *Journal of Applied Behavior Analysis,* 1,79-90.

Keohane, D.D. and Greer, R.D. (2005). Teachers' use of a verbally governed algorithm and student learning. *International Journal of Behavioral and Consultation Therapy,* 1, 249-268.

Krantz, P. J., MacDuff, M. T., and McClannahan, L. E. (1993). Programming participation in family activities for children with autism: Parents' use of photographic activity schedules. *Journal of Applied Behavior Analysis*, 26, 137-139.

Krantz, P. J., and McClannahan, L. E. (1993). Teaching children with autism to initiate to peers: Effects of a script-fading procedure. *Journal of Applied Behavior Analysis*, 26, 121-132.

Lord, C., and Schopler, (1994). TEACCH services for preschool children. In S. L. Harris and J. S. Handleman (Eds.), *Preschool education programs for children with autism* (pp. 87-106). Austin TX: Pro-ed.

Lord, C., and Schopler, (1989). Stability and assessment results of autistic and non-autistic language impaired children from preschool years to early school age. Journal of child Psychiatry and Psychiatry, 30.

Lovaas, O. I. (1987). Behavioral treatment and normal educational and intellectual functioning in young autistic children. *Journal of Consulting and Clinical Psychology,* 55, 3–9.

Lovaas, O.I, Smith T, McEeachin, J.J. (1989), Clarifying comments on the young autism study: reply to Schopler, Short, and Mesibov. *Journal Consultant Clinical Psychology*, 57, 165-167.

Lovaas, Berberich, Perloff, and Schaeffer, (1966). Acquisition of imitative speech by schizophrenic children, *Science*, 151, 705-707.

Luiselli, J.K., Cannon, B., Ellis, J.T., and Sisson, R.W. (2002). Families of children with developmental disabilities: Assessment and comparison of self reported needs in relation to situational variables. *Journal of Developmental and Physical Disabilities*, 14, 191-202.

Luiselli, J.K., O'Malley Cannon, B., Ellis, J.T., and Sisson, R.W. (2000). Home-based behavioural intervention for young children with autism/pervasive developmental disorder. A preliminary evaluation of outcome in relation to child and age intensity of service delivery. *Autism,* 4, 426-438.

Magiati, I., Charman, T., and Howlin, P. (2007). A two-year prospectve follow-up study of community-based early intensive behavioural intervention and specialist nursery provision for children with autism spectrum disorders. *Journal of Child Psychology and Psychiatry, 48:8, 803-812.*

Magiati, I., and Howlin, P. A. (2001). Monitoring the progress of preschool children with autism enrolled in early intervention programmes: Problems in cognitive assessment. *Autism,* 5, 399–406.

Matson, J., Benavidez, D., Compton, L., Paclawskyj, J. and Baglio, C. (1996). Behavioral treatment of autistic persons: A review of research from 1980 to the present, *Research in Developmental Disabilities*, 17, 433–465.

McEachin, J. J., Smith, T., and Lovaas, O. I. (1993). Long-term outcome for children with autism who received early intensive behavioral treatment. *American Journal on Mental Retardation,* 97, 359–372.

Miller, A. (1963). Verbal satiation and the role of concurrent activity. *Journal of Abnormal and Social Psychology,* 3, 206-212.

Miller, A. (1991). Cognitive-developmental systems theory in pervasive developmental disorders. In Beitchman and M Konsstantareas (Eds.), *Psychiatric clinics of North America (Vol. 14): Pervasive developmental disorders* (pp. 141-161). Saunders Press.

Ozonoff, S. and Cathcart, K. (1998). Effectiveness of a home program intervention for young children with autism. *Journal of Autism and Developmental Disorders,* 28, 25-32.

Partington, J.W. (2006). *ABLLS-R™ - The Assessment of Basic Language and Learning Skills.* Behavior Analysts Inc.

Perry, R., Cohen, I., and De Carlo, R. (1995). Case study: Deterioration, autism, and recovery in two siblings, *Journal of the American Academy of Child and Adolescent Psychiatry,* 34, 232–237.

Persons, J. B., and Silberschatz, G. (1998). Are results of randomized clinical trials useful to psychotherapists? *Journal of Consulting and Clinical Psychology,* 66, 126-135.

Piaget, J. (1948). *Language and thought of the child.* London: Routledge and Kegan Paul.

Ramey, C.T. and Ramey, S.L. (1998). Early intervention and early experience, *American Psychologist*, February, 109–120.

Reed, P., Osborne, L.A., and Corness, M. (2007). The real-world effectiveness of early teaching interventions for children with autism spectrum disorder. *Exceptional Children,* 73, 1-18.

Remington, B., Hastings, R.P., Kovshoff, H., Espinosa, F.D., Jahr, E., Brown, T., Alsford, P., Lemaic, M. and Ward, N., (2007). A field effectiveness study of early intensive behavioral intervention: Outcomes for children and their parents after two years, *American Journal of Mental Retardation.* 112, 418-438.

Sallows, G. O., and Graupner, T.D. (1999). *Replicating Lovaas' treatment and findings: Preliminary results.* Paper presented at PEACH: Putting Research Into Practice Conference, London.

Sallows, G. and Graupner, G. (2001). *Replicating Lovaas: Results after three years.* Presented at the 27th Annual Convention of the Association for Behavior Analysis, New Orleans, LA.

Sallows, G. and Graupner, G. (2005). Intensive behavioral treatment for children with autism. American Journal on Mental Retardation, 110, 417-438.

Schaaf, R.C., and Miller, L.J. (2005). Occupational therapy using a sensory integrative approach for children with developmental disabilities. *Mental Retardation and Developmental Disabilities Research Reviews, 11*, 143-148

Schopler E, Short A, Mesibov G (1989), Relation of behavioral treatment to "normal functioning": comment on Lovaas. *Journal of Consultant Clinical Psychology* 57,162-164.

Schopler, E., Mesibov, G.B., and Baker, A. (1982). Evaluation of treatment for autistic children and their parents. *Journal of the American Academy of Child Psychiatry*, 21, 262-267.

Seligman, M. E. P., (1995). The Effectiveness of Psychotherapy. *American Psychologist,* 50, 965–974.

Sheinkopf, S. J. and Siegel, B. (1998). Home-based behavioral treatment of young children with autism. *Journal of Autism and Developmental Disorders,* 28, 15–23.

Shields, J. (2001). The NAS EarlyBird Programme. *Autism,* 5, 49-56.

Skinner, B. F. (1957). *Verbal behavior*. New York: Appleton-Century-Crofts.

Smith, C. (2000). *The development and evaluation of additional training for portage workers in addressing the needs of children with complex social and communication difficulties/ autistic Spectrum disorders.* Unpublished doctoral dissertation, University of Southampton, U.K.

Smith, T. (1999). Outcome of early intervention for young children with autism. *Clinical Psychology: Science and practice,* 6, 33-49.

Smith, T. (1996). Are other treatments effective? In C. Maurice, G.Green, and S.C. Luce (Eds), *Behavioral intervention for young children with autism: A manual for parents and professionals* (pp. 45-62). Austin, TX: PRO-ED.

Smith, T., Groen, A. D., and Wynn, J. W. (2000). Randomised trial of intensive early intervention for children with pervasive developmental disorder. *American Journal on Mental Retardation,* 105, 269-285.

Strain, P.S., and Cordisco, L.K. (1994). LEAP Preschool. In S. Harris and J. Handleman (Eds.), *Preschool education programs for children with autism (pp. 225-252).* Austin TX: Pro-ed.

Sundberg, M. L., and Michael, J. (2001). The benefits of Skinner's analysis of verbal behavior for children with autism. *Behavior Modification*, 25, 698-724.

Tinbergen, N., and Tinbergen, E.A. (1983). *Austistic children: a New Hope for a Cure.* London: Allen amd Unwin.

Vygotsky, L. S. (1962). *Thought and language.* Cambridge, MA: The MIT Press.

Weiss, M.J. (1999). Differential rates of skill acquisition and outcomes of early behavioral intervention for autism. *Behavioral Interventions,* 14, 3-22.

Wolf, M., Risley, T., and Mees, H. (1964). Application of operant conditioning procedures to the behaviour problems of an autistic child. *Behaviour Research and Therapy,* 1, 305-312.

Zachor, D.A., Ben-Itzchak, E., Rabinovich, A.L., and Lahat, E., (2007). Change in autism core symptoms with intervention. *Research in Autism Spectrum Disorders*, 1, 304–317.

In: Behavioral Theories and Interventions for Autism
Editor: Phil Reed
ISBN 978-1-60741-165-9
© 2009 Nova Science Publishers, Inc.

Chapter 6

TEACHING VERBAL BEHAVIOR TO CHILDREN AND ADULTS WITH DEVELOPMENTAL DISABILITIES, INCLUDING AUTISM SPECTRUM DISORDER

Patrick McGreevy
Florida Institute of Technology, USA

Since *Teaching Language to Children with Autism and Other Developmental Disabilities* was published (M. L. Sundberg and Partington, 1998), there has been considerable interest among professionals and consumers in what has been called Applied Verbal Behavior, The Verbal Behavior Approach, or ABA-Verbal Behavior. M. L. Sundberg and Partington (1998) described language assessment and teaching procedures based on B. F. Skinner's analysis of verbal behavior (Skinner, 1957), further explication of this analysis by Michael (1982a, 1982b, 1983, 1984, 1985, 1988, 1993), and empirical evidence supporting the use of this analysis to teach communication and language to individuals with developmental disabilities, including Autism Spectrum Disorder (ASD; e.g., Braam and Poling, 1982; Braam and M. L. Sundberg, 1991; Carr, 1979; Carroll and Hesse, 1987; Hall and M. L. Sundberg, 1987; Hart and Risley, 1975; Luciano, 1986; Partington and Bailey, 1993; Sigafoos, Doss, and Reichle, 1989; Stafford, M. L. Sundberg, and Braam, 1988; M. L. Sundberg, 1980; M. L. Sundberg, Michael, Partington, and C. A. Sundberg, 1996; C. T. Sundberg and M. L. Sundberg, 1990; Touchette, 1971; Watkins, Pack-Teixteira, and Howard, 1989; Wraikat, C. T. Sundberg, and Michael, 1991).

ABA-Verbal Behavior is an approach to teaching children and adults with developmental disabilities, including ASD, who exhibit very limited communication and language, and socially-mediated problem behavior. This approach is based on B. F. Skinner's functional analysis of verbal behavior, which more accurately describes and explains significantly delayed or defective language, than traditional, formal accounts of language development. This analysis, when paired with specific behavior analytic procedures, often results in increases in the extent and frequency of expressive language and decreases in the frequency of problem behavior. From the beginning, ABA-Verbal Behavior programs emphasize the learner as a speaker and as a listener, include instruction in the natural environment, and teach the formal units of language as each unit is functional for the learner. Other ABA programs often begin by emphasizing the learner as a listener, providing intensive instruction at a table, and teaching a sequence of formal, structural units of language (e.g., length of utterance, vocabulary, and parts of speech) without regard to the effect of each unit on the learner. While our work is based largely on the applied work of Carbone (2001, 2004), M. L. Sundberg (2008), M. L. Sundberg and Partington (1998), and Partington and M. L. Sundberg (1999), there are similarities between our work and that of Greer and his colleagues (Greer and Ross, 2008).

This chapter will provide a brief description of B. F. Skinner's analysis of verbal behavior and its application, ABA-Verbal Behavior, to the teaching of language to children and adults with developmental disabilities, including ASD. The description of ABA-Verbal Behavior will include: (1) *stimulus control transfer* procedures, fundamental to the effective implementation of an effective ABA-Verbal Behavior program; (2) issues involved in selecting a communication response form for learners with limited-to-no vocal skills; (3) critical elements and components of ABA-Verbal Behavior programs; (4) teaching and data collection procedures, which have enhanced the effects of these programs, and which have been suggested by Carbone (2001, 2004), Greer and Ross (2008), McGreevy (2002), M. L. Sundberg (2007), and M. L. Sundberg and Partington (1998, 2001); and, (5) suggestions for future research. This chapter will not provide a thorough or critical account of Skinner's analysis. Readers are referred to Skinner (1957), the primary source, and Brady, Saunders, and Spradlin (1994), Catania (2007), Donahoe and Palmer (2004), Greer and Ross (2008), MacCorquodale (1969, 1970), Michael (1982a, 1982b, 1983, 1984, 1985, 1988, 1993, 2000), M. L. Sundberg (2007), M. L. Sundberg and Michael (2001), Palmer (2006), and Vargas (1982, 1986), eloquent secondary sources. Further, this chapter will not provide a 'how-to' manual for the implementation of ABA-Verbal Behavior programs. Readers are referred to Greer and Ross (2008) and Sundberg and Partington (1998), or to workshops by Mark Sundberg, Vince Carbone, Patrick McGreevy, Carl Sundberg, and others. Finally, this chapter will provide only brief comparisons between ABA-Verbal Behavior programs and other language programs. Readers will find more detailed comparisons in Kates-McElrath and Axelrod (2006) and LeBlanc, Esch, Sidener, and Firth (2006)

B. F. Skinner's Analysis of Verbal Behavior

Prior to 1998, most language instruction was based on formal or structural accounts of language with presumed biological and cognitive determinants (Brown, 1973; Chomsky, 1957; Piaget, 1926; Pinker, 1994). These accounts emphasize formal units of language (e.g., phonemes, morphemes, words, and sentences) and formal properties of language (e.g., parts of speech, grammar, syntax, and semantics) without regard to the circumstances under which either occurs (Skinner, 1957). When specific units, primarily words, or properties of these words are delayed or defective, these accounts invoke *explanatory fictions* (e.g., processing, apraxia, and memory), which lead to circular reasoning. For example, when Matt, a 17-year-old young man with ASD, responded to questions from his parents by repeating the questions, rather than providing answers, professionals described this phenomenon as echolalia with an auditory processing problem. Then, a few weeks later, auditory processing was offered by these same professionals as an explanation for Matt's responses, even though the only indications of an auditory processing problem were, in fact, Matt's responses. This type of reasoning does not lead to real explanations (Skinner, 1957) and seldom results in effective interventions.

In 1957, B. F. Skinner wrote *Verbal Behavior*, in which he provided a descriptive, functional analysis of language based on the same principles he had used earlier to analyze nonverbal behavior (Skinner, 1938, 1953). This analysis provided explanations in terms of defective or delayed language and directly suggested the shaping of new language to replace that which was defective or delayed. This analysis provided real explanations that could lead to effective interventions (if specific teaching procedures were implemented correctly). For example, with Matt, the problem is a *defective echoic repertoire* and *delayed intraverbal responses*, which suggests, in the short term, the teaching of *mands* using *the echoic-to-mand stimulus control transfer procedure*, and, in the long term, *the gradual transfer of stimulus control from mands to tacts, tacts to intraverbals, and echoics to echoic-intraverbals*. If the author is successful, readers who are unfamiliar with Skinner's analysis will be able to re-read this paragraph with understanding by the end of this chapter.

Rather than the traditional, abstract term, language, Skinner (1957) used a new term, *verbal behavior*, which he defined as the behavior of a speaker, which required the mediation of other persons, an audience, in order to contact reinforcement. The behavior of a listener, which did not require this mediation, and which contacted reinforcement directly, was termed *nonverbal*. For example, '*asking someone to make a peanut butter sandwich for you' is verbal behavior, whereas, 'making a peanut butter sandwich when asked to do so' is nonverbal behavior*. In another example, *saying 'washing dishes' when someone asks what you are doing is verbal behavior, whereas simply 'washing the dishes' is nonverbal behavior.*

Skinner's analysis of verbal behavior represents a functional account of speaker behavior and audience control. In addition to *what people say*, Skinner (1957) was concerned with completing the account of verbal behavior by including *the conditions under which they came to say it*. Rather than formal units (words, sentences, nouns, verbs), he described functional units of verbal behavior, which he called *operants* (Skinner, 1957; Catania, 1973a). These units included what was 'said', *the response form* (a specific spoken word or an equivalent sign, picture, symbol, or printed word), and the conditions under which it was 'said', *the controlling antecedent events and maintaining consequent events*. For example, *saying 'cookie' (or signing cookie, selecting a picture of a cookie, selecting the word cookie, or typing the word cookie) when you want one with a history of receiving a cookie after doing so* is *a mand.* Whereas, *saying 'cookie' (or the aforementioned alternative response forms) when someone else says 'what's your favorite snack'* is an *intraverbal.* Speech-language pathologists will notice the similarity between Skinner's analysis and the study of pragmatics.

Skinner's primary verbal operants were *mand, tact, intraverbal, textual, transcription, and echoic*. Michael (1982) added two other categories, *codic*, which combined *textual* and *transcriptive* responses, and *duplic,* which permitted the inclusion of additional forms of imitation. The revised classification system is described in Table 6.1. The operants are described in ordinary language with their controlling antecedents and maintaining consequences. Behavior analysis terms, terms used by Skinner, and examples of each operant are provided in italics. Vargas (1982) retained the terms *codic* and *duplic* and suggested a more extensive revision of the classification system, which readers may want to examine.

Skinner (1957) also described *a* secondary verbal operant, the *autoclitic*, which only occurs after the primary verbal operants are already occurring frequently.

Table 6.1. The Verbal and Nonverbal Operants

<table>
<tr><td>Primary Verbal Operant</td><td>Antecedent Event</td><td>Speaker's Response</td><td>Consequent Event</td></tr>
<tr><td>Mand
(Request)</td><td>[Motivating operations]
Not having access to a preferred item or activity, warnings, or events that result in 'wanting' or 'wanting to avoid' something or someone...</td><td>pointing, leading, making sounds, saying words, forming idiosyncratic or standard signs, selecting pictures or words, activating switches, writing or typing words, writing Braille, or exhibiting forms of problem behavior...</td><td>[Specific reinforcers]
access to or avoidance of specific items, activities, or people</td></tr>
<tr><td colspan="4">Asking for a cookie when you want one and often receiving one
Hitting someone when you are asked to complete a task and often avoiding or escaping the task</td></tr>
<tr><td>Tact
(Label or Description)</td><td>[Nonverbal stimuli]
Seeing, hearing, touching, tasting, or smelling objects, actions, or events...or experiencing private events...</td><td>saying words, forming signs, writing words, typing words, or writing Braille...</td><td>[Generalized, conditioned reinforcers: GCR]
hearing someone else provide praise</td></tr>
<tr><td colspan="4">Announcing or describing a dog as you see one
Naming or describing a sound as you hear it
Announcing or describing a headache as you are experiencing it
Describing a specific thought or a feeling as you are experiencing it</td></tr>
<tr><td rowspan="4">Intraverbal
(Fill in the Blank, Answer to a question or Response to a Statement)</td><td>[Verbal stimuli without point-to-point correspondence or formal similarity]
Hearing words</td><td>saying different words, forming the same or different signs, or writing or typing different words...</td><td>[GCR]
hearing someone else provide praise</td></tr>
<tr><td>Seeing words</td><td>saying the same or different words, forming the same or different signs, or writing or typing different words...</td><td>[GCR]
hearing someone else provide praise</td></tr>
<tr><td>Seeing or touching signs</td><td>forming different signs, or writing, typing, or Braille writing different words...</td><td>[GCR]
hearing someone else provide praise</td></tr>
<tr><td>Touching Braille</td><td>saying the same or different words, forming the same or different signs, or writing, typing, or Braille writing different words...</td><td>[GCR]
hearing someone else provide praise</td></tr>
<tr><td colspan="4">Responding with '4' when someone counts '1, 2, 3...'
Responding with 'chicken sandwich' when someone asks what you had for lunch yesterday
Responding with 'it's my turn' when someone says 'let's finish the game'
Responding with the sign for 'shoes' when someone says 'what's the sign for shoes'
Responding with '8' (or '7' or '9', etc.) to the problem '4 +4'
Making the sign for 'pencil' in response to the printed word 'pencil' (sign reading)</td></tr>
</table>

Table 6.1. (Continued)

Primary Verbal Operant	Antecedent Event	Speaker's Response	Consequent Event
Codic: Textual (Phonetic Reading)	[*Verbal stimuli with point-to-point correspondence, but without formal similarity:VS PTP*] Seeing words or touching Braille letters	saying words, one phoneme after another...	[*GCR*] hearing someone else provide praise
Saying the word 'farmer' one phoneme at a time in response to the printed word 'farmer' *Saying the word 'farmer' one phoneme at a time in response to the word 'farmer' written in Braille*			
Codic: Transcription (Spelling or Taking Dictation)	[*VS PTP*] Hearing words...	writing, typing, Braille writing, or finger-spelling words...	[*GCR*] hearing someone else provide praise
Writing or spelling the word 'useful' in response to hearing the word 'useful'			
Duplic: Echoic (Vocal Imitation)	[*Verbal stimuli with point-to-point correspondence and formal similarity: VS PTP FS*] Hearing sounds or words...	saying the same sounds or words...	[*GCR*] hearing someone else provide praise
Saying the sound 'b' in response to hearing the sound 'b' *Saying the word 'spoon' in response to hearing the word 'spoon'* *Saying the words 'what's your name' in response to hearing the words 'what's your name'*			
Duplic: Copying Letters or Words	[*VS PTP FS*] Seeing letters or words...	writing the same letters or words...	[*GCR*] hearing someone else provide praise
Writing the letter 'k' in response to seeing the letter 'k' *Writing the word 'table' in response to seeing the word 'table'*			
Duplic: Imitating Signs	[*VS PTP FS*] Seeing finger-spelling or signs...	forming the same fingerspelling or signs...	[*GCR*] hearing someone else provide praise
Making the sign for 'milk' in response to seeing the sign for 'milk'			
Duplic: Imitating Selection Mands	[*VS PTP FS*] Seeing pictures or words selected as mands...	making the same selections...	[*GCR*] hearing someone else provide praise
Selecting a picture of 'juice' in response to seeing someone select a picture of 'juice' as a mand			
Secondary Verbal Operant	Antecedent Event	Speaker's Response	Consequent Event
Autoclitic	[*Primary verbal operants*] Hearing words, seeing signs, seeing words, or touching Braille letters exhibited by herself/himself	adding letters, words, signs, Braille letters, punctuation marks, grammar or syntax, properties of text, tone of voice, or gestures...	[Specific reinforcers] specific audience responses

Table 6.1. (Continued)

Responding with '<I think I'd like> or <I'm sure I want> to go to the movie'			
Responding with 'I see <three> sticker<s>" when someone asks if you found the sticker			
Responding with 'I <am eating now>' or 'I just <ate>' when someone asks if you have eaten lunch			
Responding with <animated signs> while manding for a sandwich			
Responding with '<please> send the <red> sweater' when someone asks which sweater you want			
Responding with 'the ball is <under> the table' when someone says 'where's the ball'			
In the presence of a picture, responding with 'this <is> a cheetah' or 'this <is not> a leopard'			
Nonverbal Operant	Antecedent Event	Listener's Response	Consequent Event
Manded Stimulus Selection or Manded Compliance (Receptive IDs or Receptive Instructions)	[*Verbal stimuli -- Mands*] Hearing words, seeing signs, seeing words, or touching Braille letters which function as mands...	pointing to objects or pictures...or completing activities...	[*GCR*] hearing someone else provide praise
Pointing to a 'cup' in response to hearing someone say 'point to the cup' or 'where's the cup'			
Pointing to a picture of a 'giraffe' in response to hearing someone say 'find the giraffe'			
Giving someone a 'spoon' when someone asks for one			
'Washing your hands' when someone asks you to do so			

Autoclitic responses are often described as 'talking about what you are talking about' (or 'listening to your own verbal behavior and adding grammar, syntax, emphasis, description, quantification, or exclusion'), and, as a result, having a special effect on your audience. Skinner (1957) also described a nonverbal operant, which Michael later termed *manded stimulus selection* or *manded compliance* (Michael, 1985). This operant can be described as responding as a listener to the language of others (i.e., pointing to a named object or completing a named activity when requested to do so). These operants are also described in Table 6.1.

Noam Chomsky's very unfavorable review of *Verbal Behavior* (Chomsky, 1959) resulted in a general lack of acceptance of Skinner's analysis in the fields of education, psychology, and speech and language pathology. The difficulty of the book and the lack of data also resulted in a general lack of response among members of the behavior analytic community. A notable exception, however, was Jack Michael, who began teaching classes in verbal behavior at Western Michigan University in the late 1960s. Others who made significant, early contributions included Catania (1973a, 1973b, 1979), MacCorquodale (1969, 1970), Spradlin (1963), and Vargas (1982). Then, in 1982, Mark Sundberg, founded a new journal, *The Analysis of Verbal Behavior*, following which there was an immediate increase and a rapid acceleration in published articles (Eshleman, 1991). As an examination of the reference list for this chapter will confirm, conceptual papers and research studies based on Skinner's analysis can be found in a substantial number of journals.

Skinner (1957) contended that the operants were independent of one another, at least during acquisition. In other words, if a child began to exhibit a mand for 'cookie', intraverbal responses in the form of 'cookie' would not begin to occur without specific training. This contention has been confirmed by Hall and M. L. Sundberg (1987), LaMarre and Holland

(1985), Twyman (1995), and Williams and Greer (1993). Some evidence of this independence was also provided by Lerman, Parten, Addison, Vorndran, Volkert, and Kodak (2006), and Miguel, Petursdottir, and Carr (2005). Skinner (1957) also suggested that, during or after acquisition, operants often did not occur in a 'pure' form, but instead were multiply controlled. For example, a *mand* for a cookie might occur after someone says 'what do you want'. This *impure mand* would be controlled by motivation [*motivating operations*] and a prior verbal stimulus, making this response *mand-intraverbal.* The occurrence of *multiply controlled operants* suggests that in order for children and adults with significant language deficits to communicate effectively with teachers and parents, they would need to acquire many forms of multiply controlled operants. The independence of the operants and the need for multiply controlled operants strongly suggests that an approach to teaching language based on *operants*, rather than simply 'words', is warranted.

Green (2003, 2004) has suggested that there is insufficient empirical evidence to support teaching language to children with ASD using Skinner's analysis of verbal behavior. In addition to support for the independence of the operants, at least 80 empirical investigations based on Skinner's analysis, between 1975 and 2003, including Braam and Poling (1983), Braam and M. L. Sundberg (1991), Luciano (1986), Rogers-Warren and Warren (1980), Stafford, M. L. Sundberg, et al. (1988), C. T. Sundberg and M.L. Sundberg (1990), M. L. Sundberg, Loeb, Hale, and Eigenheer (2002), Tsiouri and Greer (2003), and Watkins, Pack-Teixteira, and Howard (1989) have provided data indicating the importance of specific variables or the effectiveness of teaching specific operants to children and adults with developmental disabilities, including ASD. Since 2003, there have been at least 40 additional empirical studies, which have supported the teaching of language based on Skinner's analysis to individuals with the aforementioned deficits, including Esch, Carr, and Michael (2005), Sweeney-Kerwin, Carbone, O'Brien, Zecchin, and Janecky (2007), and Yi, Christian, Vittimberga, and Lowenkron (2006). Carr and Firth (2005) have suggested that, while ABA-Verbal Behavior is supported by a moderate amount of research on the acquisition of the operants, long term outcome research is needed. Cautilli (2006) concurred, but suggested that there is already a considerable history of research to support its application.

Williams and Greer (1993) compared a language curriculum based on Skinner's analysis of verbal behavior with a structural, linguistic curriculum (Guess, Sailor, and Baer, 1976). During the acquisition phase, more words were emitted during the verbal behavior training sessions than during the linguistic training sessions. During subsequent training sessions, more words taught during previous verbal behavior training sessions occurred than words taught during linguistic training sessions. During maintenance and multiple maintenance probes, considerably more correct responses were emitted from the verbal behavior curriculum than from the linguistic curriculum. This study provided more direct support for ABA-Verbal Behavior than previous studies based on single verbal operants (e.g., Braam and Poling, 1983). Readers are referred to Oah and Dickinson (1989) and Sautter and LeBlanc (2006) for a review of empirical studies in verbal behavior, to Eshleman (1991) for an examination of the early history of verbal behavior research, to Dymond, O'Hora, Whelan, and O'Donovan (2004) for an analysis of citations to *Verbal Behavior* (Skinner, 1957) in the published literature, and to Greer and Ross (2008) for a list of experimental studies in verbal behavior and seminal studies in the acquisition of verbal behavior and prerequisite skills.

There is also support for Skinner's analysis from neuropsychological data (Donahoe and Palmer, 2004). Some individuals, who suffer from brain damage, experience *alexia*, or the loss of reading skills *[textual responses]*; others suffer from *anomia*, or the loss of naming skills *[tacting]*. Many individuals experience *transcortical aphasia*, which can result in the loss of spontaneous requests *[mands]* and labels *[tacts]*, but in the retention of word repetition *[echoics]* and 'filling in' parts of songs *[intraverbals]*. Other types of *aphasia* result in the preservation of labels *[tacts]*, but in the loss of words that connect the labels *[certain autoclitic tacts]*. The manifestations of these disorders suggest that certain individuals can 'use' or 'respond to' language in some circumstances but not others, and, hence, are compatible with an analysis of *operants*, rather than *words* (Donahoe and Palmer, 2004). Direct observation of the language exhibited by many children and adults with significant language delays or developmental disabilities, especially ASD, also provides support for Skinner's analysis. These commonly observed delays are described with examples in Table 6.2. The conclusion from these observations -- many children and adults with developmental disabilities are 'using' or 'responding to' specific words in some contexts but not 'using' or 'responding to' the same words in other contexts – again suggests that Skinner's analysis may more accurately describe and explain the delayed or defective language, than formal or structural accounts. In other words, what we observe are delays or deficiencies in *operants*, rather than *words*.

Table 6.2. Significant Language Delays Commonly Observed In Children and Adults with Development Disabilities, Including Autism Spectrum Disorder

Language Delay	An Example of the Language Delay
Naming many objects, activities, and events, but answering very few questions when those objects are not present or those activities or events are not occurring [*tact repertoires with almost no intraverbal responses]*	*Saying or signing your teacher's name when you see her, but, later, when your teacher is not present, not responding to the question 'what's your teacher's name?'*
Pointing to named objects, activities, or events, but not providing names when the same objects, activities, or events are present, and not requesting any of those objects, activities, or events when you want one [substantial nonverbal repertoires with almost no verbal responses]	*Pointing to a ball or retrieving a ball when directed to do so, but not saying or signing 'ball' when you see one, and not saying, signing, or selecting a picture of a 'ball' when you want to play with one*
Repeating spoken words, but not making requests, not naming objects, and not answering questions with the same words [*Echoic responses with no mand, tact, or intraverbal responses]*	*Hearing the word 'milk' and saying 'milk', but not saying 'milk' when you're thirsty, when you see it, or when someone says 'what do you like with cookies?'*

Many older children and adults with severe developmental disabilities, especially those with limited-to-no spoken words [*vocal-verbal skills*] or echolalia [*uncontrolled vocal-verbal repetition*], even after intensive instruction in listening skills, have experienced what Skinner described: "...in acquiring the behavior characteristic of a listener, [a person]...does not spontaneously become a speaker" (Skinner, 1957, p. 195). Apparently, with some individuals, the independence of the operants is difficult to overcome and may require very specific teaching procedures.

Carr and Durand (1985) were the first to suggest that socially-mediated problem behaviors in individuals with developmental disabilities and limited language were essentially speaker behaviors (they used the term 'nonverbal means of communication') and functionally equivalent to *mands*. Others have suggested that these problem behaviors function as verbal behavior (M. L. Sundberg and Partington, 1998), and, given control by motivating operations and specific reinforcers, are *mands* (McGreevy, 2002; M. L. Sundberg, 2007).

Carr and Durand (1985) suggested that socially-mediated problem behaviors be replaced with a single, socially-acceptable *mand* (spoken-word, sign, or picture-selection request) for any of several nonspecific items or activities within a category of reinforcers ('attention', ''assistance', 'escape from demands', or 'access to tangible items') estimated, in a functional analysis, to be maintaining the problem behaviors. This line of research and practice, referred to as Functional Communication Training (FCT), continues to demonstrate that teaching socially-acceptable *nonspecific mands* results in a significant decrease in problem behaviors with the same function (Bowman, Fisher, Thompson, and Piazza, 1997; Richman, Wacker, and Winborn, 2001; Winborn, Wacker, Richman, Asmus, and Geier, 2002). Some have suggested, for practical reasons, that *mands for nonspecific reinforcers within categories* be replaced with *mands for specific reinforcers* (e.g., 'cookie', 'push [the swing]', 'hug', or 'tie my shoe') and that *mands for nonspecific reinforcers* (e.g., 'eat', 'come here', 'play', 'take a break') be taught later (Carbone, 2001, 2004; McGreevy, 2002). This suggestion is beginning to receive empirical support (Kahng, Hendrickson, and Vu, 2000) in terms of the effect on problem behavior and the resulting verbal repertoire. The work in Functional Communication Training suggests that Skinner's analysis of verbal behavior, or, at least the *mand,* has an important place in the analysis of problem behavior and delayed language.

ONE OPERANT BECOMES ANOTHER: THE STIMULUS CONTROL TRANSFER PROCEDURES

With *operants* as our unit of analysis, rather than *words*, we begin the task of teaching verbal behavior to a child or an adult with a developmental disability and very little expressive language. In view of the independence of the operants and the need for multiply controlled operants, the task of teaching language would appear many times more difficult and lengthy than it otherwise would have been. Instead of teaching a word and being 'done with it', we must teach each word across operants, that is, as a mand, a tact, an intraverbal, a receptive, a textual, an autoclitic, and as part of many other multiply controlled operants. The task is difficult, and, at times, overwhelming. Consider a child or an adult with ASD who exhibits what is often called 'echolalia'. Each time you say one or more words to this child or even in the general vicinity of the child, she repeats all or the last part of what you said. Then, when she wants a cookie, she exhibits a tantrum near the cookie jar. Or, consider a child or an adult with an unnamed developmental disability who 'walks away from you' whenever you ask a simple question that could be answered with a word or a sign he already exhibits when he sees a specific item or picture. In each of the aforementioned situations, the learner exhibits a word or a sign as one operant and not another. In the first instance, the learner exhibits words as *echoics*, but not as *mands, tacts, or intraverbals*. In the second instance, the learner exhibits words or signs as *tacts, but not as intraverbals.* A teaching procedure that would transfer words or signs (or some other response forms) from one operant to another (i.e., transfer control from one set of antecedent and consequent conditions to another) is needed and is available. This procedure is called a *stimulus control transfer procedure* (Braam and Poling, 1983; Luciano, 1986; Touchette, 1971). In the first instance, the procedure is called the *echoic-to-mand transfer procedure* (M.L. Sundberg and Partington, 1998), while in the latter instance, the procedure is referred to as the *tact-to-intraverbal transfer procedure* (M. L. Sundberg and Partington, 1998). These procedures are described in Tables 6.3 and 6.4.

Table 6.3. The Echoic-to-Mand Transfer Procedure

When a learner exhibits words as echoics reliably, but not as mands,
1. capture or contrive circumstances such that the learner 'wants cookies' and begins to approach a plate of cookies on the table;
2. immediately say 'cookie' (without saying anything else) and wait 1-2 seconds (but no longer);
3. when the learner says 'cookie', provide her with a piece of cookie immediately and wait until she approaches the cookies again; if not, repeat steps 1-3; if she does not begin to say 'cookie', this procedure will not be effective;
4. repeat steps 1-3, each time increasing the time between when she begins to approach the cookies and you say 'cookie', until she says 'cookie' before you do; when she does so, provide her with a larger piece of cookie;
5. gradually fade the presence of the cookies, by covering the plate with a cloth and later removing the covered plate from the table; if the learner approaches the covered plate or the table and says 'cookie', provide her with an even larger piece of cookie; if not, remove the cover from the plate or place the covered plate back on the table and begin the fading process again.
You have transferred 'cookie' from an echoic to a mand; the learner is now saying 'cookie' as a mand (in fact, a 'pure' mand).

Table 6.4. The Tact-to-Intraverbal Transfer Procedure

When a learner exhibits words as tacts reliably, but not as intraverbals,
1. with a learner who likes to play basketball, but does not 'want to' at the moment, place a basketball or a picture of a basketball in the learner's view and say 'what do you like to play when you are outside?';
2. immediately point to the basketball or the picture;
3. when the learner says or signs 'basketball', say 'I do, too'; and something like 'maybe we can play later'; if not, repeat steps 1-3; if he does not begin to say 'basketball', this procedure will not be effective;
4. repeat steps 1-3, each time increasing the time between when you say 'what do you like to play when you are outside?' and you point to the basketball or the picture, until he says or signs 'basketball' before you point to it;
5. gradually vary the form of the question to 'when you are outside, what do you like to do?' to 'what do you like to do when you're outside?' to 'what's your favorite thing to do outside?'; if the learner says or signs 'basketball', say something like 'great, me too'; if not, return to the original form of the question and begin the varying process again.
You have transferred 'basketball' from a tact to an intraverbal; he is now saying or signing 'basketball' as an intraverbal (in fact, a 'pure' intraverbal).

A number of other transfer procedures are also available: mand-to-tact, mand-to-echoic, tact-to-mand, and intraverbal-to-tact, to name a few. The stimulus control transfer procedures, especially the echoic-to-mand, are among the most robust procedures in all of Applied Behavior Analysis, and without which, an ABA-Verbal Behavior program would be completely ineffective. Readers are referred to Greer and Ross (2008) and M. L. Sundberg and Partington (1998) for more detailed descriptions and discussions of these procedures.

SELECTING A COMMUNICATION RESPONSE FORM

Prior to designing an ABA-Verbal Behavior program for a specific learner, it is important to select an appropriate communication response form for that learner. This response form can signficantly effect the eventual response form and the extent of the learner's verbal repertoire. Frequently, 'selecting pictures' and The Picture Exchange Communication System [PECS] (Bondy and Frost, 2001; Frost and Bondy, 1994, 1998) are selected as the primary communication response form and communication program for many children, especially those with ASD who exhibit reliable echoic responses that include many hundreds of words and utterances from 1-5 words in length. In fact, one participant in the first well-controlled empirical investigation of the effectiveness of PECS "...imitated three-word phrases upon request" prior to the beginning of the study (Charlop-Christy, Carpenter, Le, LeBlanc, and Kellet, 2002). If a learner exhibits frequent, clear, single or multiple-word utterances as *echoics*, the learner's communication response form should be 'saying words' [*vocal-verbal*], rather than selecting pictures, and mand training should begin immediately, *not with PECS, but with the echoic-to-mand transfer procedure*. Spontaneous, spoken word mands will begin to occur very rapidly.

If, on the other hand, the learner does not exhibit clear spoken words as *echoics,* some will select 'saying words' as the communication response form and wait for clear spoken words to emerge. Since prompting spoken words is virtually impossible, Carbone (2001, 2004), McGreevy (2002), and M. L. Sundberg and Partington (1998) strongly recommend that an alternative response form -- (1) signs, (2) manual or electronic selection of pictures, symbols, or words, (3) writing, or (4) typing -- be selected and implemented immediately. Without a consistent response form to which an audience can respond effectively, learners must express their needs and wants by leading, gesturing, or exhibiting problem behavior. In addition to providing a method of communication, alternative response forms have been instrumental in the emergence of sounds and spoken words (Carbone, Lewis, et al., 2006; Charlop-Christy, Carpenter, et al., 2002; Tincani, 2004).

While there is empirical support for each alternative response form, there is very little conceptual analysis of response forms and very few empirical comparisons among forms (Shafer, 1993). The selection of alternative response forms for individual learners is often guided by the preferences of therapists and teachers, rather than the learner's current skills and skill deficits (Reichle, Sigafoos, and Remington, 1991). From the perspective of Skinner's analysis of verbal behavior, Michael (1985) has provided a conceptual analysis of response forms and has differentiated two types of forms: topography-based and selection-based. Examples of these forms are described in Table 6.5.

Table 6.5. Communication Response Forms

Topography-based Response Forms	Selection-based Response Forms
saying words forming signs writing words drawing Braille patterns	pointing to or touching items touching textures, shapes, or miniature items pointing to pictures, symbols, or words on a board or an electronic device without voice output selecting pictures, symbols, or words and handing these pictures to another person touching pictures, symbols, or words on an electronic device with voice output activating a switch which selects pictures, symbols, or words on an electronic device with voice output typing letters and words making Braille patterns with a Braille Writer

Among hearing individuals with developmental disabilities or language deficits, the most common alternative, topography-based response form is 'forming signs' (as opposed to sign language). Learners acquire signs from the sign language used in their geographic area with the grammar and syntax of the dominant spoken language. This is the type of signing used by deaf children in the process of learning academic skills. In the U.S., our children and adults learn signs from American Sign Language (ASL) in American English order, sometimes referred to in the U.S. as Signed English. In the U.K., our children and adults learn Makaton or Sign Along, simplified forms of British Sign Language (BSL), and move to signs from BSL in Queen's English order. In Quebec, our children and adults learn signs from La Langue des Signes de Quebec (LSQ) in French or English order, depending on the primary language in their home or residential program. Then, as we prompt our learners to sign, we can model spoken words immediately after the signs, and, this, in turn, will make it more likely that the signs will evoke spoken words from our learners.

The two most common alternative, selection-based response forms are 'pointing to pictures, symbols, or words on a board or an electronic device without voice output' and 'selecting pictures, symbols, or words and handing these pictures to another person', the latter of which is the central feature of the Picture Exchange Communication System (Bondy and Frost, 2001; Frost and Bondy, 1994, 1998). Spoken words are also paired with 'pointing to pictures' or 'picture exchanges'. These response forms, along with 'forming signs', are used primarily, but not exclusively, by ambulatory individuals with at least some fine motor skills.

Other forms are more common with individuals with more severe and more complex disabilities.

Although there is empirical support for both signs (e.g., Bartman and Freeman, 2003; Browder, Morris, and Snell, 1981; Remington and Clarke, 1983) and picture selection (e.g., Charlop-Christy, Carpenter, et al. 2002; Tincani, Crozier, and Alazetta, 2006), few comparison studies have been conducted. Michael (1985) has suggested that selection-based responding may be more difficult, because there is no correspondence between the response form (i.e., what the learner does) and the response product (i.e., what the learner selects), because of the necessity of a scanning repertoire, and because conditional discriminations (discriminations based on two stimuli) are required. In a study with 52 children with severe developmental disabilities, Hodges and Schwethelm (1984) found that sign mand-tacts were consistently acquired more rapidly than graphic symbols. Of 17 children who did not learn to select any symbols, 12 learned one or more signs. C.T. Sundberg and M.L. Sundberg (1990) found that, with four adults with developmental disabilities, in all tact and intraverbal responses trained, the sign response form was acquired more rapidly and formed equivalence classes more readily. Wraikat, C.T. Sundberg, et al. (1991) found that, with 5 of 7 participants, sign tacts and intraverbals were easier to learn and formed equivalence classes more readily.

M.L. Sundberg (1993) provided a conceptual analysis of topography-based and selection-based responding and concluded that signs may have substantial advantages over pointing systems. Shafer (1993) also provided a thorough conceptual analysis, along with a review of the literature. She concluded that signs have substantial advantages over selection systems for many learners.

Adkins and Axelrod (2002) found that, with one participant, PECS resulted in fewer trials to criterion than signs. In a study conducted by Chambers and Rehfeldt (2003), PECS resulted in a faster rate of acquisition of four mands by 3 of 3 participants. Four sign mands were acquired by 2 of 3 participants, but at a slower rate. Setting generality was evident with PECS and signs. Participants were more likely to mand with PECS in the absence of the requested item.

Tincani (2004) found that PECS resulted in more independent mands for 1 of 2 participants, while signs resulted in more independent mands for the other. Setting generality was evident for both signs and PECS. Signs resulted in more vocalizations for both participants.

Although empirical investigations support the acquisition of spoken words with signs (Barrera, Lobato-Barrera, and Sulzer-Azaroff, 1980; Barrett and Sisson, 1987; Kouri, 1988; Sisson and Barrett, 1984; Tincani, 2004) and with pictures (Charlop-Christy, Carpenter, et al. 2002; Kravits, Kamps, Kemmerer, and Potucek, 2002; Tincani, Crozier, and Alazetta, 2006; Yokoyama, Naoi, and Yamamoto, 2006), no significant comparison studies have been conducted.

In sum, the few studies previously cited provide slightly more empirical support for signs as a communication response form than picture selection, but, clearly, more controlled research is necessary. For example, Charlop-Christy, Carpenter, et al. (2002) have suggested that the acquisition of sounds and spoken words by specific participants in their studies with PECS may have been due, in part, to the teaching of mands, the pairing of spoken words with picture exchanges, the use of a delay in the transfer of stimulus control, the use of reinforcers selected by the children, the training in multiple environments, and the presence of vocal and verbal imitation skills in these participants prior to the beginning of the studies. Carbone (2001, 2004), McGreevy (2002, 2005, 2007), McGreevy and C.T. Sundberg (2007), and M.L. Sundberg and Partington (1998) have described advantages of signs and picture selection, from the learner's perspective. These descriptions are summarized in Table 6.6.

Table 6.6. The Advantages of Signs and Picture Selection as Communication Response Forms

Advantages of Signs
(1) simplicity (signs require one response [picture selection requires two responses -- scanning and pointing] and signs require discriminations based on a single stimulus [picture selection requires discriminations based on two stimuli, referred to as *conditional discriminations*]); (2) portability (signs do not require equipment and go wherever the learner goes); (3) availability (signs are immediately available to the learner and can more easily contact reinforcement, so that functional equivalence between aggressive or self injurious behaviors and signs can be established); (4) rapidity (signs can generally be formed much more quickly, especially in succession, than pictures can be selected); (5) continuity (signs can be used easily while participating in other activities); (6) mediation (signs help many learners complete delayed or multiple-step receptive instructions by repeating the sign before following the instruction(s), referred to as *joint control*); (7) linguistic (signs permit a full range of linguistic responses, some of which are not available with picture selection [e.g., picture selection tacts are indistinguishable from picture-to-item matching]); (8) academic (signs provide an observable reading response not available with any form of selection-based response); (9) conversational (it is much easier to carry on a conversation with signs than with picture selection); and (10) motivational (since signs can be formed quickly, there is less tendency for a learner to stop communicating).
Advantages of Picture Selection
(1) fine motor (selecting pictures requires fewer fine motor skills than signing); and, (2) audience (pictures have a much larger audience that does not require new skills to respond; most people do not understand or use signs).

In sum, for many children and adults with developmental disabilities, including ASD, without spoken-word repertoires, signs have many practical advantages and two major disadvantages: signs require more fine motor skills and signs have a much smaller audience. It comes down to this: signs will permit learners to 'learn' more, and to 'say' more, albeit to fewer people (McGreevy, 2005). In consideration of the data from the few comparison studies, the aforementioned practical advantages of signs and picture selection, and the motor skills of a specific learner, we must decide which response form to use with that learner.

We generally do not recommend teaching signs and picture selection at the same time, even when the learner has already acquired specific responses across response forms (e.g., three sign mands and five picture selection mands, three of which 'make the same request' [i.e., result in the same reinforcer] as the signs)[1]. Learning signs and picture selection at the same time requires discriminations and translations (a form of intraverbals) not required when learning one or the other. Our experience also suggests that when multiple response forms are taught simultaneously, no one form is acquired to a level of fluency required to effectively communicate in common, daily interactions.

If we select signs as the response form for a specific learner, it becomes our responsibility, as teachers, therapists, care providers, and parents, to overcome the 'audience problem' by ourselves becoming an effective audience, that is, by acquiring the learner's signs. This requires a sign language dictionary (see Sternberg, 1998, or http://commtechlab.msu.edu/sites/aslweb/browser.htm), but does not require a course in sign language. It does, however, require a commitment, behavior consistent with that commitment, and advocacy. In other words, we must commit to learning signs, to using these signs frequently with the learner, to making certain that the learner's signs are acquired by new teachers, therapists, and care providers, and to making certain that a statement such as the following appears in a prominent place in the learner's individual education or individual program plan (IEP or IPP): [learner's name] communicates with individual signs from American Sign Language in English order (or the sign language common to that geographic area); all individuals who interact with [learner's name] must respect and respond to that form of communication; the learner's primary teachers and therapists must also use that form of communication; no other form will be used without the permission of the IEP [IPP] team.

Specifically, if signs are selected as the response form for a specific learner, we recommend that teachers, therapists, care providers, and parents begin by learning to form the signs they will be teaching to the learner. At the same time, they should function as an audience for these signs by responding appropriately with spoken words and actions. They should continue to speak with the learner and teach the learner to respond to their spoken words with signs and actions. Then, many, but not necessarily all of the teachers, therapists, care providers, and parents, should respond as speakers by intermittently using the learner's signs to communicate with the learner. In other words, as the learner acquires signs, some of those who support the learner will function as listeners and speakers with respect to these signs, and some will function simply as listeners. The learner will respond as 'a speaker' with signs and as 'a listener to spoken words and signs' with signs and actions. While this may sound complicated, we have found this to be a reasonable expectation with most families, schools, and residential programs, and, more importantly, we have experienced this outcome many times.

Many people fear that signs will inhibit the emergence of spoken words. In almost all circumstances, this fear is unfounded. In fact, signs with modeled spoken words sometimes evoke spoken words in the learner (Carbone, Lewis, et al. 2006; Tincani, 2004). As the learner is prompted to sign or forms the sign, we strongly recommend saying the corresponding word. We also recommend saying the word as the specified reinforcer is provided after a mand and immediately after a word of praise is provided following a correct tact or intraverbal (e.g., 'yes, it's a cup' or 'spider, that's right'). If the learner says the word or any part of the word, provide additional reinforcement. In the mand, provide more of the requested item or activity. In the tact, provide additional forms of approval (e.g., picking up or tickling the learner or providing 'high fives'). In the intraverbal, provide an immediate opportunity to mand. As word approximations or words occur more frequently, provide additional reinforcement less often until reinforcement occurs only if the closest

[1] There are a few circumstances in which we would teach sign and picture selection at the same time, but these are beyond the scope of this chapter.

approximation or the word occurs with the sign. *Do not discontinue signs until words are occurring frequently that include most of the major phonemes of the primary spoken language in the initial, middle, and final positions.* You may need a speech language pathologist to help you determine this. Our experience suggests that some signers become 'completely vocal' (vocal-verbal), particularly if you initiate signs at a very early age, if you teach signs as mands, if you provide hundreds of opportunities to mand each day with modeled spoken words, and if they exhibit phonemes when they begin signing or within a few months thereafter.

Many signers, despite early intervention and frequent opportunities to mand, acquire only a few spoken words or none at all (Charlop and Haymes, 1994). If the signer does not exhibit an understandable echoic repertoire or understandable words as mands or tacts by the early teenage years or after 4-5 years of signing, we recommend the introduction of a back-up device, namely, a velcro book (see www.augresources.com) or a small electronic device that can be worn as an attachment to a belt, purse strap, key chain, or lanyard (e.g., an iPhone and some iPod models). This device will serve the same function as a notepad for an individual who is deaf, that is, it will allow the learner to communicate with those who do not understand her signs. The device should contain pictures of items and activities for which the learner currently mands with signs. The learner should be taught to use this device when someone responds to their signs by saying 'I don't understand'. Given the advantages of signs, however, the learner will continue to communicate with signs in the presence of his primary audience. As the learner begins to use the device, we recommend gradually replacing the pictures with printed words (an electronic device with voice output may be preferred, but is not required), and teaching mands, tacts, and intraverbals. If the learner exhibits excellent fine motor skills, we recommend using a keyboard and teaching the learner to type words (this can be done with an iPhone).

While signs are not appropriate for every learner, we recommend that signs be considered the preferred alternative response form for learners without spoken-word repertoires, when the learner exhibits some fine motor skills, and when all those who support the learner are responding to the learner's signs and most are using these same signs to communicate with the learner. Green (2003) indicated that she had never experienced a child with ASD who communicated effectively with signs. Our experience and that of our colleagues has been quite the contrary: we have taught many hundreds of children and adults with Autism Spectrum Disorder and related developmental disabilities repertoires of signs that permit them to communicate quickly and easily with many 'significant others' in their lives (Carbone, 2001, 2004; McGreevy, 2002, 2005, 2007; C.T. Sundberg and McGreevy, 2007; M.L. Sundberg, 2007). Many of these learners have acquired some spoken words while signing and currently exhibit primarily signs, with some spoken words, and picture selection with people who do not understand their signs. Some of these learners have acquired spoken word repertoires while signing and no longer require signs.

When learners do not demonstrate the motor skills necessary to form even simple signs, we often recommend using a selection-based response form. Our first choice is PECS (Bondy and Frost, 2001; Frost and Bondy, 1994, 1998), because it is primarily a manding program and because there appears to be an advantage in exchanging, rather than pointing to the pictures. There are, however, several modifications we would suggest: (1) using a book that is portable from the beginning; (2) checking motivation (which item or activity the learner 'wants') before the selection response occurs, rather than after; and (3) introducing text, not as carrier phrases, but as replacements for pictures (this permits tact and intraverbal responses that will not be confused with matching and receptive responses, respectively).

Some learners with more severe or complex disabilities can also use standard signs or idiosyncratic signs. Others, however, will require other selection-based response forms and supporting devices, a discussion of which is beyond the scope of this chapter.

DESIGNING AND IMPLEMENTING ABA-VERBAL BEHAVIOR PROGRAMS

When language is significantly defective or delayed, *operants and forms within those operants* are the functional units of verbal and nonverbal behavior that you actually observe or that are missing, and these are the units that must be added or replaced. Once we have selected our learner's response form, we begin the task of selecting units to add or replace:

- a defective unit of verbal behavior -- *[the learner] currently mands by leading or pointing to preferred items or screaming and falling to the floor*
- *a replacement unit of verbal behavior -- [the learner] will exhibit single-sign mands for 10 tangible item or activity reinforcers.*

These units specify the operant, *the mand,* and the forms within that operant, *signs corresponding to 10 tangible item and activity reinforcers* (e.g., cookie, juice, pudding, ball, train, video, cup, spoon, swing, and jump).

To determine which units are defective or delayed, we need an assessment instrument based on Skinner's analysis. An initial screening instrument was developed by M.L. Sundberg and Partington (1998) and is included in *Teaching Language to Children with Autism and Other Developmental Disabilities* (pp. 36-38.) This instrument, *The Behavioral Language Assessment,* contains the following domains: Cooperation with Adults, Requests (*Mands*), Motor Imitation, Vocal Play, Vocal Imitation (*Echoics*), Matching-to-sample, Receptive (*Manded Stimulus Selection or Manded Compliance*), Labeling (*Tacts*), Receptive by Function, Feature, and Class, Conversational Skills (*Intraverbals*), Letters and Numbers, and Social Interaction. Five of these domains correspond to the verbal and nonverbal operants. Each domain contains five general units. For example, the labeling (*tact*) domain begins with 'cannot identify any items or actions', followed by 'identifies only 1-5 items or actions', and ends with 'identifies over 100 items or actions and emits short sentences' (M.L. Sundberg and Partington, 1998). *The Behavioral Language Assessment (BLA)* is administered by directly observing and testing the learner or by interviewing an individual who spends a considerable amount of time with the learner. A profile on this instrument that contains scores from 1-3 on most domains will guide the first few steps of an ABA-Verbal Behavior program for a learner with very limited skills. A profile that contains scores from 4-5 or the completion of an Early Learner program will require a more specific assessment instrument.

Partington and M.L. Sundberg (1999) also developed such an instrument based on Skinner's analysis, *The Assessment of Basic Language and Learning Skills (The ABLLS).* This instrument, with respect to language acquisition, includes the following domains: Vocal Imitation (*Echoics*), Requests (*Mands*), Labeling (*Tacts*), *Intraverbals, Receptive Language,*

Spontaneous Vocalizations, Syntax and Grammar, Visual Performance (Match-to-sample and Sorting, Imitation (Motor Imitation), and Cooperation and Reinforcer Effectiveness. Five of these domains again correspond to the verbal and nonverbal operants. Five additional domains support the acquisition and development of verbal and non-verbal behavior. Domains for academic skills, classroom instruction, social and play skills, self-help skills, and gross and fine motor skills are also included. Within each operant or skill domain, specific units are sequenced from the earliest to the latest typically acquired by learners without disabilities or language deficits and from the least to the most complex response or discrimination required. For example, the labeling (*tact*) domain contains 42 units and begins with 'labels reinforcers', followed by 'labels common objects', 'labels common (familiar) people', and 'labels pictures of common items'. This domain proceeds to 'three-component labels with a carrier phrase' (e.g., 'I see a red kite flying'), 'internal events and emotions' (e.g., 'it hurts', 'I'm angry'), and ends with 'labels social interaction behavior' (e.g., 'he's talking with the music teacher'). The *ABLLS* also suggests teaching sequences across operants. The *ABLLS*, which is administered by directly observing and testing the child, also serves as a curriculum and skill-tracking device. This instrument has guided ABA-Verbal Behavior programs all over the planet since its inception.

Recently, the *ABLLS* was revised by one of its original authors (Partington, 2007) to include additional response forms and adjusted sequences within some domains. In our opinion, many more revisions are needed, some of which include: (1) many more functional units within each domain (e.g., mands for several items or activities at the same time and mands to delay a scheduled or preferred activity); (2) guidelines that suggest when specific forms of verbal and nonverbal behavior within operants are functional for a learner (i.e., these forms accomplish something for a learner); (3) additional guidelines that suggest specific sequences across operants; (4) sequences within and across operants that correspond more closely to sequences observed in children without delays or disabilities; (5) units containing conversational exchanges and variables that support those exchanges; and, (6) barriers to successful instruction (e.g., is easily distracted, refuses to respond to any direction, refuses to mand for a known reinforcer when it is made available or presented by someone else, exhibits forms of stereotypic behavior, mands in the form of aggressive or self-injurious behavior). M.L. Sundberg (2008) has recently published an assessment device based on Skinner's analysis, *The Verbal Behavior Milestones Assessment and Placement Program: The VB-MAPP*, which takes into account many of these suggestions.

Once an *ABBLS* or *VB-MAPP* is completed, it's time to plan an initial ABA-Verbal Behavior Program for a specific learner. Many beginning language programs, including many ABA programs, include *Manded Stimulus Selection (Receptive IDs)* as a major component and teach 'pointing to' familiar items presented in an array when each item is named (Lovaas, 1987). The notion, derived from formal accounts of language and influenced by everyday language we use to describe language, is that 'understanding' words is necessary before you can 'use' them, 'you have to learn to be a listener before you can be a speaker', and with learners without spoken word repertoires, 'extensive receptive language training will result in the emergence of expressive language in the form of spoken words'. Some beginning language programs also include *tacts* as a major component, especially if the learner's communication response form is 'saying words' or 'forming signs' (Carr, 1982; Lovaas, 1987). The notion here is that you must 'know the name of things' before you can 'use the names in other contexts'. These notions, which seem to 'make sense', are contrary to our own observations of learners. Many older children and adults with developmental disabilities have extensive receptive repertoires, with little to no spoken words. Very young children begin expressing themselves by requesting (exhibiting *mands*), even before spoken words emerge. The first gestures and noises, and later sounds and words, are *mands* to be picked up, *mands* for a bottle, and *mands* for warmth. Most parents wouldn't expect an infant to point or look toward her bottle, or name the bottle, before she begins requesting it. Hence, ABA-Verbal Behavior programs for learners with very limited repertoires do not include *receptives* or *tacts* as major components.

The remainder of this section will describe six levels of ABA-Verbal Behavior programs and basic recommendations for implementation. These levels range from one for an early learner, with little to no verbal or nonverbal behavior, to one for an advanced learner, who exhibits verbal behavior in conversations and academic skills. These levels serve only as approximate guides for the design and implementation of programs for individual learners. Many learners exhibit units from more than one level and will require targeted units described in more than one level. Descriptions of levels offered by others (Carbone, 2001, 2004; Greer and Ross, 2008; M.L. Sundberg, 2008; M.L. Sundberg and Partington, 1998) should also be consulted.

Our ABA-Verbal Behavior programs are based largely on the applied work of Carbone (2001, 2004), M.L. Sundberg (2008), M. L. Sundberg and Partington (1998), and Partington and M. L. Sundberg (1999). Readers familiar with the work of Greer and his colleagues (Greer and Ross, 2008) will notice similarities, namely, a mand-tact-intraverbal teaching sequence in early learners, specific stimulus control transfer procedures (e.g., the echoic-to-mand transfer procedure), and a stimulus-stimulus pairing procedure (also known as the automatic reinforcement procedure) for conditioning sounds and words as reinforcers. Readers will also notice differences, namely, the content and teaching sequence of verbal behavior milestones, an emphasis on pure and impure operants, and teaching tacts, receptives, and the bi-directional naming repertoire.

An ABA-Verbal Behavior Program for an Early Learner

A learner who exhibits limited to no vocal mands and no alternative method of expressive communication will require an Early Learner program. Some of these learners exhibit echoic skills (sounds or words), others exhibit a few sounds or words, and still others no vocal skills at all. Some of these learners exhibit motor imitation or matching skills, while others do not. Some exhibit a few receptive skills, while others exhibit frequent non-compliance with problem behavior.

Begin by selecting a communication response form (see previous section). Then, determine the learner's most preferred items and activities, that is, items and activities that function as *reinforcers*. You can do this by observing what the learner approaches and by asking someone who spends a considerable amount of time with him. Then, begin to pair yourself with those items and activities by providing free access to the same. This pairing will establish yourself (i.e., your behavior) as a *conditioned reinforcer* and the learner will begin approaching and interacting with you because doing so has resulted in reinforcement.

As soon as the learner is approaching you, looking for reinforcers, begin to implement the major component of an Early Learner program, that is, begin to select and teach mands for those reinforcers throughout the day in as many settings as possible (home, group home, residential program. school, day care, or vocational setting). If spoken words are occurring as echoics, use the echoic-to-mand transfer procedure. If some motor imitations are occurring, use a corresponding stimulus control transfer, imitation-to-mand, to teach sign or picture selection mands. If neither words as echoics nor motor imitations are occurring, teach sign or picture selection mands using hand-over-hand prompts. Remember to begin with mands for specific reinforcers (e.g., crackers, juice, a ball); avoid teaching mands in the form of 'more' or 'please'. These forms should be taught as *autoclitic/mands* at a later time. Provide a minimum of 400-500 opportunities each day for the learner to mand. Use rapid, errorless (most-to-least) prompting (Born-Miller, 2002; Brownjohn, 1988; Moore and Goldiamond, 1964; Terrace, 1963; Touchette, 1971; Walsh and Lamberts, 1979) and rapid prompt-fading, and provide the requested item or activity immediately after the mand response (Heflin and Alberto, 2001). Say the corresponding word when you prompt the sign or the picture selection and again when you provide the requested item or activity. If the learner exhibits any sound from the word or the word itself, provide an additional amount of the item or duration of the activity. If the response form is 'forming signs' or 'selecting pictures', and the learner resists physical prompts, continue the pairing procedure and gradually begin to prompt mands. Readers are referred to Shafer (1994) for a review of procedures to teach mands.

Once the learner is beginning to exhibit 5-10 mands, even if the presence of the requested items is still required, begin intensive instruction in other operant or skill domains. In accordance with the learner's performance on the *BLA*, the *ABLLS*, or the VB-MAPP, select units and response forms within each unit (e.g., imitates initial sounds of words -- 'm' for mom, 'd' for dog, 'u' for up; motor imitation of gross motor movements -- clap, jump, turn around) and conduct brief, intensive teaching sessions, which include several forms within a unit and one or more units from each of the following domains: *Echoics* -- single-sound or single-word echoics - 'm', 'b', and 'd'; or 'mom', 'ball', and 'dog'; *Motor Imitation* -- gross motor movements - 'clap', 'jump', 'turn around'; *Receptive Instructions* -- follow instructions to do a simple motor movement -- 'clap', 'jump', 'turn around', 'sit down; and, *Match-to-sample* -- match identical objects to sample -- 'spoon', 'cup', and 'toothbrush'. Echoics can only be taught if there is already some tendency for the learner to exhibit sounds as echoics, since echoic responses cannot be directly prompted.

In the beginning, intensive teaching sessions should include 1-3 easy tasks which require minimal response effort, followed by an opportunity to mand. We strongly recommend fast-paced presentation with very brief intertrial intervals (Carnine, 1976; Darch and Gersten, 1985; Englert, 1984), interspersed tasks (Billington, Skinner, Hutchins, and Malone, 2004; Dunlap, 1984; Rowan and Pear, 1985), and varied cues (Becker, 1992; Adams and Engelmann, 1996; Horner and Albin, 1988; Tateyama-Sniezek, 1989), *from the beginning,* with errorless prompting and rapid prompt-fading. Easy and effortless tasks, fast-paced presentation, interspersed tasks, and errorless prompting should function as conditioned reflexive motivating operations (CMORs) and reduce or abolish the value of escape as a reinforcer (Carbone, Morgenstern, Zecchin-Tirri, and Kolberg, 2007). These recommendations represent a significant departure from common teaching procedures and may require guidance from someone with considerable experience. If the learner responds without resistance, gradually increase the number of required responses according to a variable schedule (e.g., 4, 4, 5, 3, 4, 3, 2, 5, 4, 6, *a variable ratio schedule, specifically a VR4*). If the learner resists prompts, remain with the learner and continue to prompt until the resistance diminishes or decrease the number of required responses. If the resistance continues or increases in intensity, reinstate the pairing procedure, provide many opportunities to mand, and gradually return to intensive teaching.

Select forms within each unit which are functional for the learner (i.e., immediately useful or necessary for the completion of a task that is useful in the long term). Emphasize mands especially for older children or adults with primarily receptive repertoires.

As the learner begins to exhibit spontaneous mands, begin to teach 'giving up reinforcers', 'waiting for opportunities to mand for reinforcers', and 'accepting no for an answer'. After the learner has acquired 4-5 mands, begin teaching mands with friends and peers. Emphasize the mand repertoire by providing twice as many opportunities to mand as all other targeted units and forms within each unit combined. If the learner is an older child or an adult with a limited skill repertoire, focus almost exclusively on mands and functional receptives (e.g., 'requesting a coke' and 'getting his shoes when asked').

If the learner exhibits problem behaviors, focus almost exclusively on mands for specific items and activities that are very highly preferred and receptives that protect the learner (e.g., 'stand next to me' or 'hold my hand'). Avoid teaching mands for attention or escape, even if these non-specific forms of reinforcement correspond to the estimated functions of the problem behaviors, *UNLESS the behaviors are dangerous or life-threatening (if so, contact an experienced board certified behavior analyst for assistance).* Instead, provide attention, escape (i.e., no demands), and the aforementioned items and activities frequently and *noncontingently* (without required responses) and very gradually begin to prompt mands for specific items and activities. Then, later, just as demands are reintroduced, teach a mand for escape and a two-step mand that includes attention (e.g, 'Ms. Smith, cookie').

If the learner exhibits few or no sounds or words, use the automatic reinforcement procedure [also known as a *stimulus-stimulus pairing procedure*] (Esch, Carr, and Michael, 2005; M.L. Sundberg, Michael, Partington, and C.A. Sundberg, 1996; Yoon and Bennett, 2000). This procedure may increase vocalizations (sounds or words), especially if some sounds are already occurring.

An ABA-Verbal Behavior Program for a Second Step Learner

A learner who has acquired 10-20 mands or mands for all of her favorite items and activities, and who is beginning to acquire motor imitation, match-to-sample skills, and receptive instructions, will require a Second Step Learner program. Begin by teaching tacts for items and activities previous acquired as mands and corresponding receptive IDs during intensive teaching sessions. Also, teach additional motor imitation and match-to-sample skills. In light of the research on joint control (Lowenkron, 1991, 2004, 2006), it is advisable, with learners with single-word echoic responses or excellent motor imitation skills, to teach receptives that correspond to specific tacts after these tacts have been acquired. If spoken words are occurring, gradually increase the length of echoic utterances, and begin to control echoic responding by inserting 'say' in front of each word or phrase you want the learner to repeat (e.g., 'say, cup'). If not, continue teaching sounds. Use the teaching procedures described in the Early Learner program. If the learner resists prompts, use the procedures described in that program. Gradually increase the ratio of required responses to opportunities to mand (*thinning the variable ratio schedule).* Conclude each intensive teaching session with an opportunity to mand.

Continue to provide a minimum of 400-500 opportunities to mand per day, using the procedures described in the Early Learner program. Teach mands for additional items and activities, mands to perform an action, mands for missing items, mands for attention, mands with yes/no, mands for help, and mands to remove an item or stop an activity. Also, teach two word, two-sign, or two-picture mands, which include *autoclitics* (e.g., chocolate milk, video and remote). Prompt the expanding mand repertoire in situations with friends and peers.

Then, select new items and activities that are part of themes which include the learner's reinforcers (e.g., going to McDonalds or snack time), and add tacts and corresponding receptives for these items and activities to the intensive teaching sessions. Gradually insert 'what's this' in front of each word the learner exhibits as a tact (e.g., 'what's this?'...'cup'). Later, insert variations of this question (e.g., 'what do you see?', 'what do you call this?'). Begin teaching corresponding intraverbals using the TFFC (*tact by function, feature, or class*)-to intraverbal transfer procedure. Also, teach immediately functional intraverbals (i.e., intraverbal responses that follow questions that commonly occur in everyday interactions) by using a mand/tact/intraverbal-to-mand/intraverbal-to-intraverbal transfer procedure. Also, teach intraverbals within a contingency that includes opportunities to mand immediately before and after each intraverbal response and that results in withdrawal of the audience when intraverbal responses do not occur and responsiveness to mands when intraverbal responses do occur.

If the learner exhibits problem behaviors, use the procedures described in the Early Learner program. Continue teaching 'giving up reinforcers', 'waiting for opportunities to mand for reinforcers', and 'accepting no for an answer'. If spoken words have not begun to occur, continue with the automatic reinforcement procedure (see the Early Learner program).

An ABA-Verbal Behavior Program for a Missing Steps Learner

A learner who exhibits 50 or more spoken word, sign, 'picture selection', or word selection tacts, many receptive IDs, many motor imitation and match-to-sample skills, and some textual responses, but few mands, few intraverbals, and very little spontaneous expressive language will require a Missing Steps Learner program. Of those who communicate with signs or word selection, some exhibit echoic skills (sounds or words), others exhibit a few sounds or words, and still others no vocal skills at all. Some exhibit frequent non-compliance with problem behavior.

If the learner communicates with sign, picture selection, or word selection, and she exhibits clear, single word echoics, continue to respond to the signs, pictures, or word selection, but gradually change her response form to spoken words and begin teaching mands using the echoic-to-mand transfer procedure.

If the learner exhibits 'picture selection tacts', exchange the pictures for words and change his response form to 'word selection'. This will insure that 'picture selection tacts' are actually tacts, rather than picture to item matches. Depending on the extent of his repertoire and the willingness of parents and professionals, consider changing his response form to signs, so that a full range of linguistic responses, including reading, are available to him.

Then, select and teach mands for the learner's most preferred items and activities as described in the Early Learner program.

In accordance with the learner's performance on the *ABLLS* or the *VB-MAPP*, conduct intensive teaching sessions, which include echoics (if spoken words have not begun to occur and there is already some tendency for the learner to exhibit sounds as echoics), motor imitations, receptive instructions, matches-to-sample, and tacts and corresponding receptive IDs. Begin intensive teaching sessions with 1-3 required responses, followed by an opportunity to mand (see Early Learner program). Use the teaching procedures described in the Early Learner program. If the learner resists prompts, use the procedures described in that program. Gradually increase the ratio of required responses to opportunities to mand (*thinning the variable ratio schedule).* Conclude each intensive teaching session with an opportunity to mand.

Gradually add tacts and corresponding receptive IDs for new items and activities that are part of themes which include the learner's reinforcers (see Second Step Learner program). Begin teaching corresponding intraverbals using the procedures described in the Second Step Learner program.

If the learner exhibits problem behaviors, use the procedures described in the Early Learner program. Teach 'giving up reinforcers', 'waiting for opportunities to mand for reinforcers', and 'accepting no for an answer'. If spoken words have not begun to occur, continue with the automatic reinforcement procedure (see the Early Learner program).

An ABA-Verbal Behavior Program for a Third Step Learner

A learner who exhibits spontaneous mands for almost all preferred items and activities, 200 or more tacts and corresponding receptive IDs, many motor imitation and match-to-sample skills, many textual responses, only a few intraverbals, and very little conversation will require a Third Step Learner program. If the learner is a child, consider introducing her to mainstream education for about one hour per day, beginning with non-academic activities.

Then, begin combining mands, tacts, and intraverbals that have been taught within themes into conversational modules, such as the one described in Table 6.7.

Do not teach a module from a script; simply use the module as a guide. Vary the cues, prompt variation in the targeted responses, and insert new exchanges as it seems possible to do so. Teach 2-3 modules at a time, with specific words and phrases occurring within several operants and across modules.

Begin to teach mands for information. Also teach additional autoclitic mands. Continue to teach mands with friends and peers, and gradually add other learners to the conversational modules, including learners without disabilities. Also, begin to teach grammar and syntax within the modules.

In accordance with the learner's performance on the *ABLLS* or the *VB-MAPP*, continue to conduct intensive teaching sessions, which include motor imitations, matches-to-sample, many tacts and corresponding receptive IDs which include functions, features, and classes of items, activities, and events, and some corresponding intraverbals of gradually increasing difficulty. Continue to gradually increase the ratio of required responses to opportunities to mand (*thinning the variable ratio schedule) and c*onclude each intensive teaching session with an opportunity to mand or an opportunity for another session.

Table 6.7. A Conversational Module

Theme: Eating Cheetos and Watching Vidoes
Mand, tact, receptive, and intraverbal targets: Cheetos bag of Cheetos eat Cheetos Could I have some Cheetos video watch a video may I watch a video napkin may I have a napkin Bowl
Teacher -- [brings a bag of Cheetos] "look what I have"… Learner -- [reaches toward bag] "(could I have some) Cheetos" *MAND* Teacher -- "yes; could you get something to put the Cheetos in" Learner -- gets a bowl *RFFC* Teacher – "what do you want" Learner -- "Cheetos" *MAND/INTRAVERBAL* Teacher -- [provides Cheetos and puts a video on the table] "when you're eating Cheetos, what else do you like to do?" Learner -- "(watch a) video" *TACT/INTRAVERBAL* "(may I watch a) video" *MAND/TACT* Teacher -- [puts the video in the player and turns on the player] Teacher -- [no napkin in view] "look, your hands are messy; what do you need" Learner -- "(a) napkin" *MAND/INTRAVERBAL* "(may I have a) napkin" *MAND* Teacher – [hands the learner a napkin] [After the video is over and the video and the Cheetos have been put away] Teacher -- "Tell me again -- when you're eating Cheetos, what else do you like to do?" Learner -- "(watch a) video" *INTRAVERBAL*

With effective instruction, the learner's tacts and receptives will gradually increase in length and complexity. In other words, in the presence of items, activities, and events within the environment, and features of the environment, the the learner will 'respond to' and "describe' what he sees or experiences with single words, a few words, and many words forming sentences. Then, through stimulus control transfer, corresponding intraverbals will begin to occur. In other words, the learner will 'respond to' these words with actions and 'exhibit' these same words in response to questions and statements, when the items, activities, events, and features are not present.

Teach additional social skills, including 'appropriate intraverbal responses' and 'task completion' after transitions, after unexpected changes in the schedule, and after unexpected responses from other learners or other adults.

An ABA-Verbal Behavior Program for a Fourth Step Learner

A learner who exhibits spontaneous mands for information, many hundreds of tacts and corresponding receptive IDs that include functions, features, and classes of items, activities, and events, along with an increasing number of corresponding intraverbals, many complex motor imitation and match-to-sample skills, textual responses in sentences, 1-3 intraverbal and receptive responses between opportunities to mand, and brief, but sustained conversations will require a Fourth Step Learner program. If the learner is a child, consider increasing time in mainstream education to 1-2 hours per day, including some time in academic activities.

Continue to teach and combine increasingly complex mands, tacts, and intraverbals into conversational modules. Recycle older modules with the more complex operants. Gradually add more learners to the conversational modules, especially friends and learners without disabilities.

Continue to prompt and correct grammar and syntax within the modules. In accordance with the learner's performance on the *ABLLS* or the *VB-MAPP*, continue to conduct intensive teaching sessions which include advanced tacts and intraverbals. Continue to gradually increase the ratio of required responses to opportunities to mand (*thinning the variable ratio schedule)* and conclude fewer intensive teaching sessions with an opportunity to mand and more with brief breaks and additional sessions. Continue emphasizing appropriate intraverbal responses and the completion of assigned tasks after transitions, after unexpected changes in the schedule, and after unexpected responses from other learners or other adults.

Begin to teach academic skills. For example, for learners whose communication response form are spoken words, transfer stimulus control from multiple, partial-word echoics to 'phonetic reading' or from fluent tacts to 'sight-word reading'.

For learners whose response form is signs, transfer stimulus control from tacts to 'sight-word sign reading'. With regard to mathematics, transfer stimulus control from intraverbal counting sequences (rote counting) to tacting numerals in sequence along a number line. Then, place identical objects next to the numerals along the line while counting in sequence, and fade the numerals along the line. Then, proceed to addition and subtraction, by counting forward and backward. Begin to teach 'copying letters' and transfer stimulus control to transcription (i.e., writing dictated letters), and later to spelling.

Teach tacts for private events. Begin by teaching tacts for physical sensations within the learner (e.g., itching) when, because of accompanying public events (e.g., scratching), it is probable that these sensations are occurring.

Then, proceed to painful sensations in the same manner, followed by a mand for assistance or relief. Later, proceed to teaching tacts for emotions in the learner and transferring control to the public behavior and physical appearance of the learner. Then, begin to teach empathy for others by comparing the public behavior and physical appearance of the learner to the behavior and appearance of others. Readers will notice that this sequence, which begins with our learner's private events, is very different from that which is commonly used, which often begins with pictures of faces or the public behavior or appearance of other learners.

An ABA-Verbal Behavior Program for an Advanced Learner

A learner who exhibits many hundreds of complex mands, tacts and corresponding receptives, and intraverbals, many complex motor imitation and match-to-sample skills, 20+ intraverbal and receptive responses in everyday interactions, academic tasks between opportunities to mand, sustained conversations, many textual responses, including entire stories, and math skills to include counting and addition of objects, will require an Advanced Learner program. If the learner is a child, consider increasing time in mainstream education to 3-4 hours per day, including considerable time in academic activities.

Continue to teach and combine increasingly complex mands, tacts, and intraverbals into conversational modules and recycle older modules with the more complex operants. Continue to include friends and learners without disabilities in these modules and continue to prompt and correct grammar and syntax.

Continue to teach language, academic, and social skills. We recommend the following programs, which are supported by empirical research and often result in very productive outcomes: (1) for teaching additional language -- *Language for Learning* (www.sraonline.com) and *Language for Thinking* (www.sraonline.com); (2) for sight word reading -- *Edmark Reading* (www.riverdeep.net); (3) for phonetic reading -- *Reading Mastery* (www.sraonline.com and *HeadSprout* (www.headsprout.com); (4) for math -- *Touch Math* (www.touchmath.com) *or Distar Arithmetic* (www.sraonline); (5) for social skills – *Skillstreaming* (www.skillstreaming.com).

For learners in an Advanced Learner program, as well as all other learners, continue to emphasize mands, 'giving up reinforcers', 'waiting for opportunities to mand for reinforcers', 'accepting no for an answer', and 'exhibiting appropriate intraverbal responses and completing assigned tasks, especially after transitions, after unexpected changes in the schedule, and after unexpected responses from other learners or other adults'.

DATA COLLECTION, FLUENCY, MAINTENANCE, AND SKILL TRACKING

Many ABA programs include massed trials with the same verbal cue and the same response form, along with the collection of trial-by-trial data. These data include information about the physical properties of each response and the ratio of correct to incorrect responses.

These data, however, do not include the amount of time from the end of the verbal cue to the beginning of each of the learner's responses (*latencies*) or from the beginning to the end of the responses (*durations*), which are fundamental dimensional quantities of single responses (Johnston and Pennypacker, 1993). These data also do not include the amount of time from the beginning of the first cue to the end of the last response, which, when combined with the number of correct responses, would result in a measure of *frequency* (also called *rate),* the fundamental dimensional quantity of a collection or class of responses (Johnston and Pennypacker, 1993; Skinner, 1938). These dimensional quantities include measures of time and are necessary in order to measure fluency, that is, accuracy and speed of performance (Binder, 1996). Fluency is a strong predictor of skill retention (Ritseman, Malanga, Seevers, and Cooper, 1996; Shirley and Pennypacker, 1994), endurance [i.e., attention span] (Binder, Haughton, and Van Eyk, 1990), and ease of transfer to more complex skills (Haughton, 1972).

With intensive teaching sessions that include interspersed tasks, fast-paced instruction, and rapid, errorless prompting, it is virtually impossible to record latency, occurrence, prompts, and duration for each response. Frequency data, which would provide a measure of speed and accuracy for the specific set of units, would require sessions or recording intervals within sessions of constant duration and would be difficult to record even with videotape. Also, the sets of units would be difficult to categorically distinguish from similar sets.

With learners with limited repertoires, the probability of very specific, functional response forms becomes as important as the frequency of large classes of units or operants of which these response forms are members. In other words, the fact that a learner 'exhibits a sign tact for cup within one second from the time the teacher points to a cup' is as important as the same learner 'exhibiting 30 sign tacts in 1 minute'. As Skinner (1957) suggested "we must move on from the study of frequencies to a consideration of the probability of a single event (p. 28)". In consideration of the importance of these single events, along with the importance of retention, endurance, and transfer with respect to these events, we strongly recommend teaching to fluency by establishing single-response fluency criteria, and using probe data collection with units and response forms taught in intensive teaching sessions.

Specifically, we recommend selecting a fluency criterion for most response forms. We have found 'within one second from the end of the cue' (in the mand, 'within one second from the time the learner's behavior suggests he wants something) to be quite useful. We recommend that, prior to conducting intensive teaching sessions each day, a single probe trial be presented on each unit and response form. This trial serves as a test trial, during which prompting is delayed and provided in a least-to-most manner. The response is recorded with the level of prompt required as described earlier in this section. If no prompt is required, that is noted on the data sheet. If an unprompted response occurs within one second from the end of the cue, it is recorded as fluent. After probe trials are conducted, intensive teaching sessions begin and no more data are collected on these response forms that day. If a fluent response occurs on a probe trial three consecutive days, that response form is removed from intensive teaching sessions. Probe maintenance checks are then conducted once per week for three weeks and once per month for three months.

In order to insure the provision of 400-500 opportunities to mand per day and to monitor the progress of manding, we strongly recommend counting prompted and unprompted mands. We also recommend two cumulative graphs, one for 'mands typically exhibited without prompts' and 'units [not including mands] demonstrated as fluent three consecutive days".

Suggestions for Further Research and Instructional Development

In the last ten years, much has been learned about verbal behavior and how to teach verbal repertoires to children and adults with developmental disabilities, including ASD. We concur, however, with Carr and Firth (2005), who suggest that additional empirical investigations of the following types are necessary: (1) published case studies, (2) published outcome data for multiple cases, and (3) experimental and quasi-experimental treatment comparisions. Our experience suggests the following topics for these studies: (1) replacing mands in the form of severe problem behaviors with mand repertoires (i.e., many mands for specific items, activities, and events), rather than generalized mands for attention and escape; (2) teaching sign mands to older children and adults with severe developmental disabilities, including Autism Spectrum Disorder, who exhibit no formal mand responses, and who are considered, by many, to be incapable of expressive language; (3) teaching conversational intraverbal responses that follow commonly-occurring questions or statements; (4) transferring mands and mand/tacts to intraverbals; (5) teaching learners to exhibit intraverbal responses in order to retain an audience for mands; (6) teaching autoclitic mands and tacts; (7) examining elements of successful conversations; (8) teaching specific forms of verbal behavior (e.g., 'I want', 'please', 'and', 'when', 'in', 'I can', 'red') within and across operants when these forms accomplish something for the learner (i.e., are functional for the learner), rather than simply add to the length of the response[2]; (9) using signs to teach delayed and multiple-step receptive responses, and (10) transferring tacts to generalized intraverbals by systematically varying cues.

ACKNOWLEDGMENTS

I would like to acknowledge the influence of Jack Michael, Ogden Lindsley, John Eshleman, Carl Binder, Vince Carbone, Mark Sundberg, and Carl Sundberg in the writing of this chapter, much of which was first uttered as echoic responses in their presence or as textual responses in the presence of their work. I would also like to thank Mark Sundberg and Carl Sundberg for reviewing parts of this chapter and for providing valuable suggestions.

Correspondence can be sent to drmcg@attglobal.net.

REFERENCES

Adams, G.L. and Engelmann, S. (1996). *Research on Direct Instruction: 25 Years beyond Distar.* Seattle: Educational Achievement Systems.

Adkins, T. and Axelrod, S. (2002). Topography-based versus selection-based responding: A comparison of mand acquisition in each modality. *The Behavior Analyst Today*, 2, 259-266.

Barrera, R.D., Lobato-Barrera, D., and Sulzer-Azaroff, B. (1980). A simultaneous treatment comparison of three expressive language training programs with a mute autistic child. *Journal of Autism and Developmental Disorders*, 10, 21-37.

Barrett, R.P. and Sisson, L.A. (1987). Use of the alternating treatments design as a strategy for empirically determining language training approaches with mentally retarded children. *Research in Developmental Disabilities*, 8, 401 – 412.

Bartman, S., and Freeman, N. (2003). Teaching language to a two-year-old with autism. *Journal on Developmental Disabilities*, 10, 47-53.

[2] The carrier phrase 'I want' is often added to an existing mand for 'cookie' to increase the length of utterance. A learner experiences more effort with a similar outcome. Consider a situation, however, in which a learner has acquired the word or sign for 'cookie' as a mand and a tact. Now, the learner may say or sign 'cookie' in a situation in which it is not clear to the audience whether this response was a mand or a tact (as might happen when the learner and a teacher walk past a plate of cookies on a table). When this happens, the learner will need a response form, such as 'I want', that helps to clarify the operant as a mand (if it was one) and produce the desired outcome (cookie) for the learner. When this response form within the mand is taught after mands and tacts have been acquired, it is functional for the learner.

Becker, W.C. (1992). Direct Instruction: A twenty year review. In R. P. West and L. A. Hamerlynck (Eds.). *Designs for excellence in education: The legacy of B. F. Skinner* (pp. 71-112). Longmont, Colorado: Sopris West.

Billington, E.J., Skinner, C.H., Hutchins, H.M., and Malone, J.C. (2004). Varying problem effort and choice: Using the interspersal technique to influence choice towards more effortful assignments. *Journal of Behavioral Education*, 13, 193-207.

Binder, C. (1996). Behavioral fluency: Evolution of a new paradigm. *The Behavior Analyst*, 19, 163-197.

Binder, C., Haughton, E. and Van Eyk, D. (1990). Increasing endurance by building fluency: Precision Teaching attention span. *Teaching Exceptional Children*, 22, 24-27.

Bondy, A., and Frost, L. (2001). The picture exchange communication system. *Behavior Modification*, 25, 725-744.

Born-Miller, K.L. (2002). The use of an errorless teaching procedure to teach children with autism for whom trial-and-error teaching has failed. *ProQuest Information and Learning. Dissertation Abstracts International: Section B: The Sciences and Engineering*, 63(4-B), 2088.

Bowman, L.G., Fisher, W.W., Thompson, R.H., and Piazza, C.C. (1997). On the relation of mands and the function of destructive behavior. *Journal of Applied Behavior Analysis*, 30, 251-265.

Braam, S.J., and Poling, A. (1983). Development of intraverbal behavior in mentally retarded individuals through transfer of stimulus control procedures: Classification of verbal responses. *Applied Research in Mental Retardation*, 4, 279-302.

Braam, S.J., and Sundberg, M.L. (1991). The effects of specific versus non-specific reinforcement on verbal behavior. *The Analysis of Verbal Behavior*, 9, 19-28.

Brady, N.C., Saunders, K.J., and Spradlin, J.E. (1994). A conceptual analysis of request teaching procedures for individuals with severely limited verbal repertoires. *The Analysis of Verbal Behavior,* 12, 43-52.

Browder, D.M., Morris, W.W., and Snell, M.E. (1981). Using time delay to teach manual signs to a severely retarded student. *Education and Training of the Mentally Retarded*, 16, 252-258.

Brown, R. (1973). *A first language*: *The early stages*. Cambridge, MA: Harvard University Press.

Brownjohn, M.D. (1988). Acquisition of makaton symbols by a young man with severe learning difficulties. *Behavioural Psychotherapy*, 16, 85-94.

Carbone, V.J. (2001). Teaching language to children with developmental disabilities, including autism. *Guided notes from ABA-Verbal Behavior workshops*, from introductory to advanced levels, presented to audiences in the U.S. and many other countries.

Carbone, V.J. (2004). Teaching language to children with developmental disabilities, including autism. *Guided notes from ABA-Verbal Behavior workshops*, from introductory to advanced levels, presented to audiences in the U.S. and many other countries. Valley Cottage, NY: The Carbone Clinic.

Carbone, V.J., Lewis, L., Sweeney-Kerwin, E.J., Dixon, J., Louden, R., and Quinn, S. (2006). A comparison of two approaches for teaching VB functions: Total communication vs. vocal-alone. *Journal of Speech-Language Pathology and Applied Behavior Analysis*, 1, 181-191.

Carbone, V. J., Morgenstern, B., Zecchin-Tirri, G., and Kolberg, L. (2007). The role of the reflexive conditioned motivating operation (CMO-R) during discrete trial instruction of children with autism. *Journal of Early and Intensive Behavioral Intervention*, 4, 658-680.

Carnine, D.W. (1976). Effects of two teacher-presentation rates on off-task behavior, answering correctly, and participation. *Journal of Applied Behavior Analysis*, 9, 199-206.

Carr, E.G. (1979). Teaching autistic children to use sign language. *Journal of Autism and Developmental Disorders*, 9, 345-359.

Carr, E.G. (1982). Sign language. In R. Koegel, A. Rincover, and A. Egel (Eds.), *Educating and understanding autistic children* (pp. 142–157). San Diego, CA: College-Hill Press.

Carr, E.G., and Durand, V.M. (1985). Reducing behavior problems through functional communication training. *Journal of Applied Behavior Analysis*, 18, 111-126.

Carr, J.E., and Firth, A.M. (2005). The verbal behavior approach to early and intensive behavioural intervention for autism: A call for additional empirical support. *Journal of Early and Intensive Behavioral Intervention*, 2, 18-27.

Carroll, R. J., and Hesse, B. E. (1987). The effects of alternating mand and tact training on the acquisition of tacts. *The Analysis of Verbal Behavior*, 5, 55-65.

Catania, A.C. (1973a). The concept of the operant in the analysis of behavior. *Behaviorism*, 1, 103-116.

Catania, A.C. (1973b). The psychologies of structure, function, and development. *American Psychologist,* 28, 434-443.

Catania, A.C. (1979). *Learning.* Englewood Cliffs, NJ: Prentice-Hall.

Catania, A.C. (2007). *Learning* (interim 4th ed.). Cornwall-on-Hudson, NY: Sloan Publishing.

Cautilli, J. (2006). Validation of the verbal behavior package: Old wine new bottle –A reply to Carr and Firth (2005). *The Journal of Speech-Language Pathology and Applied Behavior Analysis*, 1, 81-92.

Chambers, M., and Rehfeldt, R.A. (2003). Assessing the acquisition and generalization of two mand forms with adults with severe developmental disabilities. *Research in Developmental Disabilities*, 24, 265-280.

Charlop, M.H., and Haymes, L.K. (1994). Speech and language acquisition and intervention: Behavioral approaches. In J.L. Matson (Ed.), *Autism in children and adults: Etiology, assessment, and intervention* (pp. 213–240). Pacific Grove, CA: Brooks/Cole.

Charlop-Christy, M.H., Carpenter, M., Le, L., LeBlanc, L.A., and Kellet, K. (2002). Using the picture exchange communication system (PECS) with children with autism: Assessment of PECS acquisition, speech, social-communicative behavior, and problem behavior. *Journal of Applied Behavior Analysis*, 35, 213-231.

Chomsky, N. (1957). Syntactic structures. The Hague: Mouton and Company.

Chomsky, N. (1959). A review of B. F. Skinner's Verbal Behavior. *Language*, 35, 26-58.

Darch, C., and Gersten, R. (1985). The effects of teacher presentation rate and praise on LD students' oral reading performance. *British Journal of Educational Psychology*, 55, 295-303.

Donahoe, J.W., and Palmer, D.C. (2004). *Learning and complex behavior*. Richmond, MA: Ledgetop Publishing.

Dunlap, G. (1984). The influence of task variation and maintenance tasks on the learning and affect of autistic children. *Journal of Experimental Child Psychology*, 37, 41-64.

Dymond, S., O'Hora, D., Whelan, R., and O'Donovan, A. (2006). Citation analysis of Skinner's Verbal Behavior: 1984-2004. *The Behavior Analyst*, 29, 253-267.

Englert, C.S. (1984). Effective direct instruction practices in special education settings. *Remedial and Special Education*, 5, 38-47.

Esch, B.E., Carr, J.E., and Michael, J. (2005). Evaluating stimulus-stimulus pairing and direct reinforcement in the establishment of an echoic repertoire of children diagnosed with autism. *The Analysis of Verbal Behavior*, 21, 43-58.

Eshleman, J. (1991). Quantified trends in the history of verbal behavior research. *The Analysis of Verbal Behavior*, 9, 61-80.

Frost, L.A., and Bondy, A.S. (1994). *The picture exchange communication system training manual.* Cherry Hill, NJ: Pyramid Educational Consultants.

Frost, L.A., and Bondy, A.S. (1998). The picture exchange communication system. *Seminars in Speech and Language*, 19, 373–389.

Ganz, J.B., Simpson, R.L. (2004). Effects on communicative requesting and speech development of the picture exchange communication system in children with characteristics of autism. *Journal of Autism and Developmental Disorders*, 34, 395-409.

Granzin, A.C., and Carnine, D.W. (1977). Child performance on discrimination tasks: Effects of amount of stimulus variation. *Journal of Experimental Child Psychology*, 24, 332-342.

Green, G. (2003). *The "Verbal Behavior" approach to autism: Where are the data?* An invited address to the annual meeting of the Florida Association for Behavior Analysis, St. Petersburg, FL.

Green, G. (2004). *The "Verbal Behavior" approach to autism: Where are the data?* An invited address to the annual meeting of the Experimental Analysis of Behavior Group, London, England.

Greer, R.D., and Ross, D. (2007). *Verbal behavior analysis: Inducing and expanding new verbal capabilities in children with language delays*. New York, NY: Pearson Education, Inc.

Hall, G., and Sundberg, M.L. (1987). Teaching mands by manipulating conditioned establishing operations. *The Analysis of Verbal Behavior*, 5, 41-53.

Hart, B., and Risley, T.R. (1975). Incidental teaching of language in the preschool. *Journal of Applied Behavior Analysis*, 8, 411-420.

Haughton, E.C. (1972). Aims: Growing and sharing. In J. B. Jordan and L. S. Robbins (Eds.), *Let's try doing something else kind of thing*. Arlington, VA: Council on Exceptional Children.

Heflin, L.J., and Alberto, P.A. (2001). Establishing a behavioral context for learning for students with autism. *Focus on Autism and Other Developmental Disabilities*, 16, 93-101.

Hodges, P., and Schwethelm, B. (1984). A comparison of the effectiveness of graphic symbol and manual sign training with profoundly retarded children. *Applied Psycholinguistics*, 5, 223-253.

Horner, R.H., and Albin, R.W. (1988). Research on general-case procedures for learners with severe disabilities. *Education and Treatment of Children*, 11, 375-388.

Johnston, J.M., and Pennypacker, H.S. (1993). *Strategies and tactics of behavioural research* (second edition). Hillsdale, NJ: Lawrence Erlbaum Associates.

Kahng, S. W., Hendrickson, D. J., and Vu, C. P. (2000). Comparison of single and multiple functional communication training responses for the treatment of problem behavior. *Journal of Applied Behavior Analysis,* 33, 321-324.

Kates-McElrath, K., and Axelrod, S. (2006). Behavioral intervention for autism: A distinction between two behavior analytic approaches. *The Behavior Analyst Today*, 7, 242-252.

Kouri, T.A. (1988). Effects of simultaneous communication in a child-directed treatment approach with preschoolers with severe disabilities. *Augmentative and Alternative Communication,* 4, 222 – 230.

Kravits, T. R., Kamps, D. M., Kemmerer, K., Potucek, J. (2002). Brief report: Increasing communication skills for an elementary-aged student with autism using the picture exchange communication system. *Journal of Autism and Developmental Disorders*, 32, 225-230.

LaMarre, J., and Holland, J.G. (1985). The functional independence of mands and tacts. *Journal of the Experimental Analysis of Behavior*, 43, 5-19.

LeBlanc, L. A., Esch, J., Sidener, T. M., and Firth. A. M. (2006). Behavioral language interventions for children with autism: Comparing Applied Verbal Behavior and Naturalistic teaching approaches. *The Analysis of Verbal Behavior*, 22, 49-60.

Lerman, D.C., Parten, M., Addison, L.R., Vorndran, C.M., Volkert, V.M., and Kodak, T. (2005). A methodology for assessing the functions of emerging speech in children with developmental disabilities. *Journal of Applied Behavior Analysis*, 38, 303-316.

Lovaas, O.I. (1987). Behavioral treatment and normal educational and intellectual functioning in young autistic children. *Journal of Consulting and Clinical Psychology*, 55, 3–9.

Lowenkron, B. (1991). Joint control and the generalization of selection-based verbal behavior. *The Analysis of Verbal Behavior*, 9, 123-128.

Lowenkron, B. (2004). Meaning: A verbal behavior account. *The Analysis of Verbal Behavior,* 20, 121-126.

Lowenkron, B. (2006). An introduction to joint control. *The Analysis of Verbal Behavior*, 22, 123-127.

Luciano, M. C. (1986). Acquisition, maintenance, and generalization of productive intraverbal behavior through transfer of stimulus control procedures. *Applied Research in Mental Retardation*, 7, 1-20.

MacCorquodale, K. (1969). B. F. Skinner's Verbal Behavior: A retrospective appreciation. *Journal of the Experimental Analysis of Behavior*, 12, 831-841.

MacCorquodale, K. (1970). On Chomsky's review of Skinner's Verbal Behavior. *Journal of the Experimental Analysis of Behavior*, 13, 83-99.

McGreevy, P. (2002). Teaching language to children and adults with developmental disabilities, including autism. *Guided notes from ABA-Verbal Behavior workshops*, from introductory to advanced levels, presented to audiences in the U.S., the U.K., Canada, The United Arab Emirates, and India. Winter Park, FL: Patrick McGreevy, Ph.D., P.A. and Associates.

McGreevy, P. (2005). Teaching signs and sign language to children and adults with developmental disabilities, including autism. *Guided notes from a workshop* presented to audiences in the U.S. and Canada. Winter Park, FL: Patrick McGreevy, Ph.D., P.A. and Associates.

McGreevy, P. (2007). Teaching signs and sign language to children and adults with developmental disabilities, including autism. A pre-conference workshop presented to the annual meeting of the Association for Behavior Analysis, San Diego, CA.

McGreevy, P., and Sundberg, C.T. (2007). Teaching signs and sign language to children and adults with developmental disabilities, including autism. A pre conference workshop presented to the annual meeting of the California Association for Behavior Analysis, San Francisco, CA.

Michael, J. (1982a). Distinguishing between discriminative and motivational functions of stimuli. *Journal of the Experimental Analysis of Behavior*, 37, 149-155.

Michael, J. (1982b). Skinner's elementary verbal relations: Some new categories. *The Analysis of Verbal Behavior*, 1, 1-3.

Michael, J. (1983). Evocative and repertoire-altering effects of an environmental event. *The Analysis of Verbal Behavior,* 2, 19-21.

Michael, J. (1984). Verbal behavior. *Journal of the Experimental Analysis of Behavior*, 42, 363-376.

Michael, J. (1985). Two kinds of verbal behavior plus a possible third. *The Analysis of* Verbal *Behavior,* 3, 1-4.

Michael, J. (1988). Establishing operations and the mand. *The Analysis of Verbal Behavior*, 6, 3-9.

Michael, J. (1993). Establishing operations. *The Behavior Analyst*, 16, 191-206.

Michael, J. (2000). Implications and refinements of the establishing operation concept. *Journal of Applied Behavior Analysis*, 33, 401-410.

Miguel. C. F., Petursdottir, A.I., and Carr, J.E. (2005). The effects of multiple-tact and receptive discrimination training on the acquisition of intraverbal behavior. *The Analysis of Verbal Behavior,* 21, 27-41.

Moore, R., and Goldiamond, I. (1964). Errorless establishment of visual discrimination using fading procedures. *Journal of the Experimental Analysis of Behavior*, 7, 269-272.

Oah, S., and Dickinson, A.M. (1989). A review of empiricial studies of verbal behavior. *The Analysis of Verbal Behavior*, 7, 53-68.

Palmer, D.C. (2006). On Chomsky's appraisal of Skinner's Verbal Behavior: A half century of misunderstanding. *The Behavior Analyst*, 29, 253-267.

Partington, J.W. (2007). *The assessment of basic language and learning skills: The ABLLS-R Protocol.* Pleasant Hill, CA: Behavior Analysts, Inc.

Partington, J.W., and Bailey, J.S. (1993). Teaching intraverbal behavior to preschool children. *The Analysis of Verbal Behavior*, 11, 9-18.

Partington, J. W., and Sundberg, M. L. (1999). *The assessment of basic language and learning skills: The ABLLS*. Pleasant Hill, CA: Behavior Analysts, Inc.

Piaget, J. (1926). *The language and thought of the child.* London: Routledge and Kegan Paul, Ltd.

Pinker, S. (1994). *The language instinct*. New York: William Morrow and Company.

Reichle, J., Sigafoos, J., and Remington, B. (1991). Beginning an augmentative communication system with individuals who have severe disabilities. In B. Remington (Ed.), *The challenge of severe mental handicaps*. Chichester, NH: Wiley and Sons.

Remington, B., and Clarke, S. (1983). Acquisition of expressive signing by autistic children: An evaluation of the relative effects of simultaneous communication and sign-alone training. *Journal of Applied Behavior Analysis*, 16, 315-327.

Richman, D. M., Wacker, D. P., and Winborn, L. (2001). Response efficiency during functional communication training: Effects of effort on response allocation. *Journal of Applied Behavior Analysis*, 34, 73-76.

Ritseman, S.K., Malanga, P.R., Seevers, R.L., and Cooper, J.O. (1996). Immediate retelling of current events from Channel One by students with developmental disabilities and its effect on their delayed retelling. *Journal of Precision Teaching*, 14, 18-34.

Rogers-Warren, A., and Warren, S. (1980). Mands for verbalization: Facilitating the display of newly trained language in children. *Behavior Modification*, 4, 361-382.

Rowan, V. C., and Pear, J. J. (1985). A comparison of the effects of interspersal and concurrent training sequences on acquisition, retention, and generalization of picture names. *Applied Research in Mental Retardation*, 6, 127-145.

Sautter, R.A., and LeBlanc, L.A. (2006). Empirical applications of Skinner's analysis of verbal behavior with humans. *The Analysis of Verbal Behavior*, 22, 35-48.

Shafer, E. (1993). Teaching topography-based and selection-based verbal behavior to developmentally disabled individuals: Some considerations. *The Analysis of Verbal Behavior,* 11, 117-133.

Shafer, E. (1994). A review of interventions to teach a mand repertoire. *The Analysis of Verbal Behavior*, 12, 53-66.

Shirley, M.J., and Pennypacker, H.S. (1994). The effects of performance criteria on learning and retention of spelling words. *Journal of Precision Teaching*, 12, 73-86.

Sigafoos, J., Doss, S., and Reichle, J. (1989). Developing mand and tact repertoires with persons with severe developmental disabilities with graphic symbols. *Research in Developmental Disabilities*, 11, 165-176.

Sisson, L.A., and Barrett, R.P. (1984). An alternating treatment comparison of oral and total communication training with minimally verbal retarded children. *Journal of Applied Behavior Analysis,* 17, 559 – 566.

Skinner, B.F. (1938). *The behavior of organisms*. New York, NY: Appleton-Century Crofts.

Skinner, B.F. (1953). *Science and human behavior*. New York, NY: MacMillan.

Skinner, B.F. (1957, 1992). *Verbal Behavior*. Acton, MA: Copley Publishing Group and the B.F Skinner Foundation.

Skinner, B.F. (1974). *About behaviorism*. New York, NY: Random House.

Spradlin, J.E. (1963). Assessment of speech and language of retarded children: The Parsons language sample. *Journal of Speech and Hearing Disorders Monograph*, 10, 8-31.

Spradlin, J.E. (1985). Studying the effects of the audience on verbal behavior. *The Analysis of Verbal Behavior*, 3, 5-9.

Stafford, M.W., Sundberg, M.L., and Braam, Steven J. (1988). A preliminary investigation of the consequences that define the mand and the tact. *The Analysis of Verbal Behavior*, 6, 61-71.

Sternberg, M.L.A. (1998). *American sign language dictionary*. New York, NY: HarperCollins Publishers.

Sundberg, C.T., and McGreevy, P. (2007). Teaching signs and sign language to hearing children and adults with developmental disabilities including autism. A pre-conference workshop presented at the annual conference of the California Association for Behavior Analysis.

Sundberg, C.T., and Sundberg, M.L. (1990). Comparing topography-based verbal behavior with selection-based verbal behavior. *The Analysis of Verbal Behavior*, 8, 31-41.

Sundberg, M.L. (1980). Developing a verbal repertoire using sign language and Skinner's analysis of verbal behavior. Unpublished doctoral dissertation, Western Michigan University.

Sundberg, M.L. (1993). Selecting a response form for nonverbal persons: Facilitated communication, pointing systems, or sign language. *The Analysis of Verbal Behavior*, 11, 99-116.

Sundberg, M.L. (2007). Verbal behavior. In J. O. Cooper, T. Heron, and W.L. Heward (Eds.), *Applied Behavior Analysis* [2nd ed.] (p. 526-547). Upper Saddle River, NJ: Pearson Education, Inc.

Sundberg, M.L. (2008). *The Verbal Behavior Milestones Assessment and Placement Program: The VB-MAPP*. Concord, CA: AVB Press.

Sundberg, M.L., Loeb, M., Hale, L., and Eigenheer, P. (2001-2002). Contriving establishing operations to teach mands for information. *The Analysis of Verbal Behavior*, 18, 15-29.

Sundberg, M.L., and Michael, J. (2001). The benefits of Skinner's analysis of verbal behavior for children with autism. *Behavior Modification*, 25, 698-724.

Sundberg, M.L., Michael, J., Partington, J.W., and Sundberg, C.A. (1996). The role of automatic reinforcement in early language acquisition. *The Analysis of Verbal Behavior*, 13, 21-37.

Sundberg, M.L., and Partington, J.W. (1998). *Teaching language to children with autism or other developmental disabilities*. Pleasant Hill, CA: Behavior Analysts, Inc.

Sundberg, M.L., and Partington, J.W. (2001). *QuickTips: Behavioral teaching strategies*. Pleasant Hill, CA: Behavior Analysts, Inc.

Sweeney-Kerwin, E.J., Carbone, V.J., O'Brien, L., Zecchin, G., and Janecky, M. N. (2007). Transferring control of the mand to the motivating operation in children with autism. *The Analysis of Verbal Behavior*, 23, 89-102.

Tateyama-Sniezek, K. M. (1989). The effects of stimulus variation on the generalization performance of students with moderate retardation. *Education and Training in Mental Retardation,* 24, 89-94.

Terrace, H.S. (1963). Errorless transfer of a discrimination across two continua. *Journal of the Experimental Analysis of Behavior*, 6, 223-232.

Tincani, M. (2004). Comparing the picture exchange communication system and sign language training for children with autism. *Focus on Autism and Other Developmental Disabilities*, 19, 152-163.

Tincani, M., Crozier, S., Alazetta, L. (2006). The picture exchange communication system: Effects on manding and speech development for school-Aged children with autism. *Education and Training in Developmental Disabilities*, 41, 177-184.

Touchette, P.E. (1971). Transfer of stimulus control: measuring the moment of transfer. *Journal of the Experimental Analysis of Behavior*, 15, 347-354.

Tsiouri, L., and Greer, R.D. (2003). Inducing vocal verbal behavior in children with severe language delays through rapid motor imitation responding. *Journal of Behavioral Education* 12, 185-206.

Twyman, J.S. (1996). The functional independence of impure mands and tacts of abstract stimulus properties. *Analysis of Verbal Behavior*, 13, 1-19.

Vargas, E.A. (1982). Intraverbal behavior: The codic, duplic, and sequelic subtypes. *The Analysis of Verbal Behavior*, 1, 5-7.

Vargas, E.A. (1986). Intraverbal behavior. In L. J. Parrot and P. Chase (Eds.), *Psychological aspects of language* (p. 128-151). Springfield, IL: Thomas Publishing.

Walsh, B.F., and Lamberts, F. (1979). Errorless discrimination and picture fading as techniques for teaching sight words to TMR students. *American Journal of Mental Deficiency*, 83, 473-479.

Watkins, C. L. Pack-Teixteira, L., and Howard, J. S. (1989). Teaching intraverbal behavior to severely retarded children. *The Analysis of Verbal Behavior*, 7, 69-81.

Williams, G., and Greer, R. D. (1993). A comparison of verbal behavior and linguistic curricula. *Behaviorology,* 1, 31-46.

Winborn, L., Wacker, D.P., Richman, D.M., Asmus, J., and Geier, D. (2002). Assessment of mand selection for functional communication training packages. *Journal of Applied Behavior Analysis*, 35, 295-298.

Wraikat, R., Sundberg, C.T., and Michael, J. (1991). Topography-based and selection-based verbal behavior: A further comparison. *The Analysis of Verbal Behavior*, 9, 1-17.

Yi, J.I., Christian, L., Vittimberga, G., and Lowenkron, B. (2006). Generalized negatively reinforced manding in children with autism. *The Analysis of Verbal Behavior*, 22, 21-33.

Yoon, S. and Bennett, G. M. (2000). Effects of a stimulus-stimulus pairing procedure on conditioning vocal sounds as reinforcers. *The Analysis of Verbal Behavior*, 17, 75-88.

Yokoyama, K., Naoi, N., Yamamoto, J. (2006). Teaching verbal behavior using the picture exchange communication system (PECS) with children with autistic spectrum disorders. *Japanese Journal of Special Education*, 4, 485-503.

In: Behavioral Theories and Interventions for Autism
Editor: Phil Reed
ISBN 978-1-60741-165-9
© 2009 Nova Science Publishers, Inc.

Chapter 7

CABAS® CONTRIBUTIONS TO IDENTIFYING, INDUCING AND SEQUENCING VERBAL DEVELOPMENT

R. Douglas Greer and Dolleen-Day Keohane
Columbia University Teachers College and Graduate School of Arts and Sciences, USA

THE FUNCTIONS OF CABAS® SCHOOLS: LEARNER DRIVEN RESEARCH AND DEMONSTRATION CENTERS

CABAS® (Comprehensive Application of Behavior Analysis to Schooling) was originated to develop a science of teaching. Our first credo was to develop schools based entirely on the use of scientific procedures for classroom management, pedagogy, curriculum design, staff training, and parent education. Moreover, the second credo of our educational model was to make education learner driven. Our experience with schools convinced us that they were driven by professional guilds, and if learning did not occur in school the blame was placed on children and their parents. Only Skinner and behavior analysts seemed to think that the practices might be improved by scientific applications (Skinner, 1984; 1968). Thus, we wanted to develop measurement-based, individualized education for entire classrooms and entire schools driven by what worked for each individual child.

We did not target a particular type of child or subject area. Indeed, our first models of education were for bands, choruses, orchestras, and college music courses that were based on a decade of research in the operant psychology of music (Greer, 1980). That work is still used in Japan (a 1990 Japanese translation of Greer, 1980). Our next goal was to establish regular education for economically disenfranchised children. However, this proved to be politically difficult since there was a great deal of anti-behavioral sentiment in the seventies and eighties and even afterward (Brophy, 1983; Greer, 1983a. 1983b; Skinner, 1984). Critics stated that while "behavior modification" might work for individuals and for some classroom problems, applying it to all aspects of education simply was not possible. Brophy (1983), a leading educational researcher, stated, "... despite its success in the laboratory and in certain other settings, the effect of applied behavior analysis on teaching and learning is limited, *and always will be*." (Brophy, p. 12). We set out to find out if it was possible for behavior analysis to be the basis of a science of teaching in schools for all children. The current evidence appears to substantiate our efforts.

While regular education administrators were not interested in what we had to offer, special education was. Special education in the USA was just beginning in a serious way, and behavior analysis proved very useful. Thus, our learners in our learner-driven model became special education students. We began in 1982 with a residential school for students with developmental disabilities, ASD, and serious assaultive or self-injurious behaviors—students that regular education simply could not teach (Greer, McCorkle, and Williams, 1989). In this setting we had free rein to build what became a behavioral systems approach to all aspects of education.

In 1986, at the request of local county agencies we opened the first publicly funded and privately run preschool in New York State based entirely on applied behavior analysis (i.e., The Fred S. Keller School). There were other treatment centers for ASD in New York State like the one at the University of New York at Binghamton but *we were a school, not a treatment center*, and our initial target population were preschoolers from low income families with diagnoses of emotional disturbance, behavioral disorders, learning or language delays. A few children with ASD did also began to show up. We taught all aspects of the curriculum including academic literacy (reading, mathematics, language arts), self-management, problem solving, and an enlarged community of reinforcers and developed ways to measure all responses to all instruction. Our teachers needed to be experts in curriculum as well as pedagogy and behavior management. We wanted our children to be fluent in reading, writing, speaking, listening and armed with classroom behaviors that would ingratiate typically trained teachers when they left us. Most of our students in the preschool then were economically disenfranchised children with diagnoses of emotional disturbance or learning disabilities. Over 75% of those children went to kindergarten reading and doing math at the first or second grade level. Thus our application of behavior analysis to education is best described as *Teaching as Applied Behavior Analysis*, where all instruction is driven by educational standards, regardless of the students' psychological or demographic characteristics. Our focus was on building a science of teaching and learning that was made possible by a science of the behavior of the individual—one that worked for all children in individualized ways. As behavior analysis became more sought after by parents of children with Autism Spectrum Disorders (ASD), our schools were in much demand and it was no longer allowable for poor children to receive services for learning disabilities—more serious disabilities took priority as a result of legislation.

Unlike pioneers in the treatment of ASD, we were concerned more with the teaching procedures and not with a psychological or therapeutic treatment for ASD. For example, Lovaas (1977, 1987) was interested in treating children with ASD primarily. He incorporated behavior analysis after he had spent some time using other less successful approaches. For Lovas and other clinical psychologists ASD was the focus. For us, the goal was accelerated learning based on scientific procedures that provided a comprehensive education for all the categories of children who were our students.

Serendipitously, it turns out, at least in our opinion, the reason behavior analysis is successful with children and youths with ASD is that it is a powerful teaching methodology. Children with ASD vary a great deal, require extraordinary teaching efforts, and require professionals who can manage behavior that other professionals cannot. Reinforcement, shaping, the systematic development of stimulus control, and other behavioral principles and tactics worked for ASD children when other "therapeutic" approaches did not.

What we learned proved to be beneficial for children and youth with ASD and simultaneously what we learned from developing a science of teaching children with ASD was a better understanding of how to teach children with a range of abilities and deficits. In fact our major efforts are now in elementary education classes that include children with ASD; however, our focus is equally on children for whom English is a second language, children from minority populations, children from low SES homes, and upper middle class children—preferably in the same class (see Greer, 2007 for some of the outcomes of that effort). Most of our children receive 30 hours of instruction in our schools weekly—simply because those are the number of hours that schools are mandated to provide for all children. For a description of one of our classes from a journalists view see: http://www.tc.columbia.edu/news/article.htm?id=6100. The costs are the same as those of any regular education class that includes children with special needs.

The educational model that became the Comprehensive Application Behavior Analysis to Schooling (CABAS®) began over 25 years ago (Greer, 1991) and its foundations over 38 years ago (Greer, 1980). Our mission was to find out if a learner driven and science-based approach to teaching was possible, practical, financially feasible, and effective (Greer, 1991). We endeavored to develop schools for educating the "whole child" (i.e., all of the curricula) and *all children* based entirely on a science of behavior within the constraints of public school funding. CABAS® schools were to be centers of excellence for children, parents, professionals, and university graduate training programs. They incorporated the university as a key player in the system, where the university program was to be responsive to the educational needs of the children. CABAS® schools were to provide the kind of rigorous control found in laboratory settings—settings that would result in superior educations, the advancement of a science of complex human behavior, and revisions in university training based on what worked in the schools. We will briefly describe the status in achieving those goals, and the findings of one of our research programs that led to the identification and induction of verbal developmental cusps.

CABAS® System Training

CABAS® schools are closely aligned with the Programs in Behavior Analysis at Teachers College and the Graduate School of Arts and Sciences of Columbia University. As a part of that affiliation, the schools serve as sites to train all of our MA students (currently there are 51 of them) and our PhD students (currently there are 16 of them). The schools are scientifically rigorous settings for applying what we know, as well as settings for finding out what we don't know, need to know, and ways to go about finding out. We train all of our graduate students, postdoctoral students, and many from other universities, including those from other countries in the CABAS® schools. Our graduate students are in paid positions and have instructional responsibilities commensurate with their expertise and pay. Graduate students progress from serving as teaching assistants (in their MA training) to teachers, to master teachers during their doctoral work. After finishing the PhD, some assume university positions, others supervisory positions in schools, and a few become fulltime researchers. Our

MA graduates are certified (i.e., "licensed") in the State of New York (with reciprocal certification in most other states) as teachers of children *with and without disabilities* from birth to Grade 7 and receive a Masters of Arts is in "Teaching as Applied Behavior Analysis." Students who complete the MA and who excel in their Masters work may apply for admission to the PhD program. All students who complete our PhD must first complete the MA and the relevant teacher certifications and CABAS® Board Certification in Teaching as Applied Behavior Analysis (www.CABAS.com). In some of our schools, like the Jigsaw School in England, the training is the same but occurs at a distance. In these cases training in pedagogy, curriculum, behavior management, and the organizational behavior management components are taught via several yearly visits and distance learning employing PSI. Thus, these teachers are trained on the job as are our masters students and CABAS® supervisors and professors provide the instructional leadership.

One of the key criteria that we look for in professionals who wish to work in our schools or to be admitted to our graduate programs is that the candidate enjoys working with children and can assume the important responsibilities of both teaching and looking after children. They must also have strong academic undergraduate training and a keen interest in the science. University students spend their day in CABAS® schools, rotating placements to encompass teaching both regular and special education students (all types of children from 18 months to grade six) and attend graduate courses in the evening. The behavior analytic content in our university courses (nine courses in the MA program) is tied to what they do in the schools and simultaneously tied to both the basic and applied branches of behavior analysis. Research based method and curriculum courses are all related to the science of behavior. This has allowed us to train graduate students in exemplary settings-- settings that are devoted to teaching as a science where the relation between university instruction and application is immediate. Some of our graduates have stayed on to work in the CABAS® programs in which they did their internships, providing models of advanced expertise for novices. All of our recent PhD students have worked their way through their masters' degrees and have at least a CABAS® Board Certification of Master Teacher (the third level of certification in a nine tier system). Our teachers are also scientists and have constant contact with research and publish widely in refereed scientific journals. By the time they are ready to do their dissertations they have conducted over a dozen experiments. Many of the professionals in our schools were not students in our graduate program. That is they were trained in our schools exclusively, and have worked with us for years, some for over two-decades. They have acquired the same levels of expertise as our MA graduate students (i.e., they must pass the same requirements); however, the time they require for obtaining that expertise is much more prolonged. The system is designed to provide continuous advanced training in teaching as applied behavior analysis and we provide a multi-tiered and criterion referenced board certification in teaching as applied behavior analysis to ensure continued study (www.CABAS.com).

There is considerable evidence that the level of *behavior analytic teacher expertise* predicts success with children. We first found high and statistically significant correlations between progression in teacher ranks and success with children in Greer, McCorkle, and Williams (1989); that is, the higher the teacher rank, the better were the learning outcomes in terms of educational objectives achieved. Each of the nine ranks requires progressively higher levels of criterion-referenced mastery of direct measures of teaching, mastery of verbal behavior about the science, and scientific rule-governed responding.

Subsequent studies provided experimental tests of levels of expertise in learn unit presentations, by teachers or computers (Emurian 2004; Emurian, Hu, Wang, and Durham, 2000; Greer and McDonough, 1999; Hogin, 1996; Ingham and Greer, 1994) and student's achievement. Other studies experimentally demonstrated that levels of expertise in teachers' use of our data based decision protocol predicted teacher effectiveness (Keohane and Greer, 2005). Components of each of the CABAS® board certified ranks include learn unit performance and scientific rule-governed or the following of scientific algorithms. In daily practice teachers must follow the research based scientific algorithm (Keohane and Greer) involving identifying the learning problem scientifically, selecting the relevant tested tactic, and using the data based tactics reliably, and they must show the achievement of objectives relative to those interventions. If objectives are not attained other relevant tactics are used or, if the analysis warrants, a developmental intervention is done. Coincidentally, this appears to be the first experimental analysis of Skinner's (1957) treatment of the behavior of the scientist. These decisions are measured directly and monitored for accuracy by supervisors with advanced board certification for all children for all instructional objectives in all schools (See Keohane and Greer for the evidence and the procedure). This is done for each child across all curricular areas. See Greer (2002) Chapter 4, and Greer and Ross (2008) Chapter 2 for detailed instruction in how to do this. Hence, there is a continuous usage of measurable expertise in day-to-day practice.

Finally, we reported on an application of the entire system, including levels of expertise, that was more effective than control conditions in a multiple baseline across classes for an entire school for children who were blind and developmentally disabled (Selinske, Greer, and Lodhi, 1991). In the latter study children learned four to seven times more educational objectives after they received the system than before. These differences were replicated in an independent and standardized test assessment by the New York City Board of education (Greer, 1998) for a separate school using CABAS®. We have consistently shown that it is teachers' use of tested procedures along with continuous application of the scientific method to teaching each child that predicts student achievement. New trainees are supervised in making decisions and teaching until they acquire the level of expertise to function independently, but always with data based supervision. Professionals with the rank of Master Teacher® supervise Teacher I® and Teacher II® rank teachers and teacher assistants, and behavior analyst supervisors with the ranks of Assistant®, Associate®, and Senior Behavior Analyst® supervise Master Teachers. CABAS® senior consultants monitor the accuracy of senior behavior analysts and provide peer review.

Components of the CABAS® System for Teaching as Applied behavior Analysis

In our schools, all teaching is *applied behavior analysis*, and this provides a setting that often results in research contributions to both the basic and applied sciences. We measure and graph all responses of students to instruction, all teaching interactions, all scientific pedagogical decisions, critical supervisory interactions, mastery of rank performance, and the outcomes and processes of parent education (Greer Keohane, and Healy, 2002). These measures, in turn, are combined with the research derived decision algorithm (described above), that is itself part of the measurement system, to ensure that the data works for the benefit of the student. In our view, education that is based entirely on the use of scientifically reliable procedures is *the most effective and the most ethically defensible way to educate all children*. We cannot insist that everyone follow this credo, after all, one cannot mandate that people believe in natural selection or behavioral selection. However, we do believe that *publicly funded and science-based schools should be part of the options available to parents in democratic societies*. We provide an example of how this can be done and why it is measurably cost-effective.

The more than 200-data based procedures that we use in CABAS® schools, including those that we developed, are available in the literature and in several books for all to use (Greer, 1980; Greer, 2002; Greer and Keohane, 2004; Greer, Keohane, and Healy, 2002; Greer, McCorkle, and Williams, 1989; Selinske, Greer and Lodhi, 1991; Sulzer-Azaroff, Drabman, Greer, Hall, Iwata, and O'Leary, 1988). Tactics from Precision Teaching, verbal behavior analysis, and curricula from Direct Instruction and the Morningside Model, noon-coercive approaches to "bad behavior" or performance management, are part of the armada of procedures: they are not competing approaches. One of the byproducts of our work has been the development of procedures that can be used by teachers who are trained in teaching as applied behavior analysis. Teaching as applied behavior analysis is a specialized expertise in behavior analysis and requires specialized training, just as behavior therapy is a specialized application of behavior analysis. Mastering the basic principles and learning how to manage behavior is simply the beginning (Greer, 2005). Advancing this specialization through research and demonstration is our mission. We seek to further a science of learning and teaching and its dissemination.

However, in our particular approach we did not accept the constraint that teaching operations must follow the typical school arrangement. Rather our approach places the learner on center stage and we design the teaching process and the organization of the school around what is most effective for the student, even if traditionally trained teachers find the procedures scientifically sophisticated. Thus, our model is designed around what works best for the student, even if that requires a radical rearrangement of typical schooling environments, and even if teachers have to work harder and have to master sophisticated repertoires in teaching as a strategic scientist. That's not to say that there isn't a great deal of excellent and important behavior analytic work designed to be user friendly to the teacher in traditional schools; however, our particular mission is to design schooling around optimum student learning using replicable scientific procedures regardless of the sophistication of the pedagogy. We reserve the CABAS® name for schools that meet our accreditation standards (www.cabas.com) for serving as research, demonstration, and training sites that are learner-driven demonstration centers.

We are limited in the number of communities and schools that we can serve because of the levels of expertise that are needed. Hence, CABAS® is not interested in increasing the numbers of CABAS® schools because they are designed to be state of the science centers for innovations—demonstration sites. It is our hope that other schools, and ASD treatment centers will adopt and adapt our work. CABAS® is not an entrepreneurial enterprise as in the case of for-profit companies that are designed to be charter school franchises. We find no fault with those efforts for they can be helpful, too; rather our model was developed as a way provide measurably effective education using a systems science—teaching our children in an exemplary fashion using *replicable procedures*. A close relationship with a university is key to the long-term survival of what we do. However, it is critically important to note that the CABAS® Schools were not designed as places *to do research*; rather, they were designed as *schools to drive applied and basic research that is needed to make education optimally effective*. All of our educational programs are learner driven, and all research is designed to meet that objective. To paraphrase Skinner and Keller, the student knows best and we strive to arrange the contingencies in our system to follow that advice. Good applied and basic science often accrues.

EFFECTIVENESS AND THE COSTS OF CABAS®

The schools are no more costly than other educational models serving comparable schools. Indeed, many of our classrooms are in typical public schools and our teachers are employees of those schools working under the CABAS® model right next door to teachers running classrooms based on eclectic approaches. We have shown that the CABAS® approach is more cost-effective than standard educational models that serve the range of children (Greer, 1994; Greer, et al., 2002) when the educational outcomes are factored in the formula. Greer (1994) compared the numbers of learn units in a non-CABAS® school with a comparable school for children with disabilities. The tuition costs were the same, but the numbers of learn units and educational objectives were significantly higher in the CABAS® School. When costs per learn unit was calculated, CABAS® was significantly more cost-effective.

In our regular education classes with mainstreamed students with ASD (23% of the class) the teacher assistants are assigned to the children with ASD (the typical arrangement in some states in the USA); however, they work on individualizing instruction for all children. The children in our first cohort of regular education classes performed in reading, language and math significantly above grade level at the end of the second grade after two years of CABAS® (84th percentile nationally on the Terra Nova Achievement Test). Children with ASD performed at the third grade level, children for whom English was not the language spoken in the home performed at the fifth grade level, children who were from low SES homes performed at the sixth grade level, minority students performed at the sixth grade level, and upper middle class children at the eighth grade level (Greer, 2007). The costs were the same as that for other classes in the school that had mainstreamed children with special education diagnoses but the outcomes for the CABAS® class were significantly better—statistically significant and educationally significant.

Designed Contingencies for Our System

We have used existing evidence and our own research programs to develop a set of organizational contingencies to achieve our objectives. Some of these contingencies include the following.

Extensive measurement. In order to ensure that the schools are learner driven, we measure and graph all of our students' responses to all instruction including the achievement of state and international educational standards. We also measure the performance of teachers and supervisors as a means to improve our effectiveness, and our research has repeatedly tied the level of data based expertise of our professionals to student outcomes (Greer, et al., 1989; Keohane and Greer, 2004; Selinske et al., 1991). These data are available at all times for parents and professionals in posted graphs in our schools. *The fact that these data are public provides the students with the power to continuously vote for or against what we are doing.* In this way we arrange the contingencies such that the students, not the professions or bureaucracies control the schools (Bushell and Baer, 1994).

All instruction is scientifically derived. All instruction of children, teachers, mentors, related disciplines, and parents is based entirely on scientific procedures drawn from the *basic and applied sciences of the behavior of the individual.* While the science of behavior has provided the brunt of effective procedures, to date, any scientific evidence that assist the students may be used (Greer, 2002; Greer and Keohane, 2004; Sulzer-Azaroff, Drabman, Greer, Hall, Iwata, and O'Leary, 1988).

A behavior analytic systems approach to administration. When CABAS® is responsible for the administration of the school, we use organizational behavior analysis for administrative functions.

Happy places to learn and work. The schools and classrooms use contingencies such that positive procedures are used for management and instruction and the use of coercive procedures is avoided providing students, professionals, and parents a happy and productive environment in which to function. See http://www.tc.columbia.edu/news/article.htm?id=6100 for a description. One of our objectives is for the school to provide a sense of community. This is particularly important in a multicultural country where parents are often separated from their extended family. We strive to provide that community by involving parents and professionals who provide a small village to support the educational progress and well being of *our* children.

Public school funding and service. Funding for the schools and programs is based entirely on local school funding. We do this by design. This provides for our model to become part of existing educational budgets. Often, when grants are part of educational models, when the grant expires the model expires too. None of our programs, or research to date has been funded by grants. What this means for our research is that our work can be driven by the needs of children and the leads that our research identifies, rather than the research agendas of governments or foundations.[1] Research that is driven by the agenda of foundations and governments is important, too. However, the fact that research programs may be done by universities and schools and that the research provides a direct service function simply leads to different types of inquiries. Variability in types of research and funding for that research is the stuff of identifying best practice and a stronger science.

Centers of inquiry. Our schools are designed to be centers of inquiry for the applied and basic sciences of behavior as the sciences are used to serve the needs of the students.

[1] We do have two exceptions to our rule of avoiding external funding. That is, in our preschool, parents of children who do not have disabilities pay tuition or receive scholarships to attend our regular education integrated classrooms in the Fred S. Keller school because there is no public funding for children this young who are not identified as having a delay or who are no eligible for Headstart. Moreover, our current plans to develop a preschool for economically disenfranchised 2-year olds to bridge the educational gap between impoverished and well-to-do may entail seeking extramural funding. We will have to resort to seeking grant funds simply because there are no existing public funding mechanisms for two-year olds without native disabilities or special education diagnoses for the level of service we propose.

Research efforts follow the lead of the students. Good science determines what works best for both the short and long term.

Continuous evolution. Our programs are constantly being changed as a function of new evidence and the needs of students. As others and we develop new research findings, we implement those as quickly as possible. This has made it possible to very quickly apply what is new to any child who might benefit. This means that essentially we have replicated most if not all of the existing tactics from the field. While this kind of continuous change is exciting for many of our professionals, it also means that they must be continuously involved in learning new procedures. Not all professionals find such rapid change gratifying. More traditional schools move at a more gradual pace.

Components of CABAS® and Verbal Behavior Analysis

In developing our schools we have built on and incorporated the foundations of the basic science and applied models such as: relational frame theory, stimulus equivalence, molar and molecular analyses, verbal behavior, observational learning, higher order operants, the Morningside Model, Programmed Instruction, Direct Instruction, Personalized System of Instruction, the corpus of applied behavior analysis for performance (classroom management, organizational management) and teaching (e.g., class-wide peer tutoring, token economies, yoked contingencies, learn units opportunity to respond, response cards, and Precision Teaching tactics) (Greer and McDonough, 1999). See Greer (1991) for the different and compatible uses of each of these in the development of CABAS®. In effect, the entire corpus of behavior analysis served as the foundation for CABAS® schools.

The findings of all of the literatures consist of procedures that are designed for a range of specific uses, but *no scientific system existed* to provide a way to *scientifically* apply those to providing a total education. The CABAS® systems science described above grew out of the need to provide an organizational model to fit individual scientific tactics to both performance and learning goals derived from teaching the entire curriculum. Also we needed a systems science to see that professionals provided measurably and consistently effective instruction, supervision, and parent education day in and say out throughout the school year. In essence we developed a behavior analysis of practicing behavior analysis (Greer and Keohane, 2004). However, *the systems application of what existed was still not enough.* One of the components that were missing was a curriculum for, and an adequate treatment of, complex human behavior that is the very core of what education needs to provide—language functions. Skinner's theory of verbal behavior (Skinner, 1957) filled this void as the research on applications of that theory developed. This work not only made for a data driven approach to complex behavior but also furthered a basic science of verbal behavior including the development of operants and higher order operants or classes (Catania, 2007; Greer, 2002; Greer and Ross, 2008; Hayes, Barnes-Holmes, and Roche, 2000; Horne and Lowe, 1996; Sidman, 1983).

When one operates under *the constraints of using only scientific procedures for instruction*, all of the existing literature must be used, when the findings of any part of that literature are relevant. In the process of using all of the existing tactics and strategies, and developing an applied science of the analysis of professionals doing behavior analysis, certain distinctions between aspects of the existing science became apparent (Greer, 2005). We came to distinguish between research and applications of behavior analysis for: (a) management of performance (e.g., motivating quality of instruction and supervision for the fidelity of treatment, finding and fixing sources for bad behavior), (b) learning or the acquisition of and teaching of new operants (e.g., pedagogical operations that are the source for new operants such as verbally governed mathematical operations), (c) the acquisition of new capabilities to develop higher order operants (e.g., the induction of speaker functions, Naming, transformation of stimulus function across saying and writing, speaking and listening), and (d) curriculum design (the identification of units to be taught such as tacts rather than vocabulary).

Skinner's (1938) book on the behavior of organisms and the ensuing decades of research in the basic and applied sciences provided the basis for performance management. That is much of the subject matter of Skinner's 1938 book and years of subsequent basic science was devoted to the contingencies surrounding performance such as schedules of reinforcement or molar and molecular analyses. This work led to many important applications such as how to have children behave well, engage in well being practices, buckle seat belts, and the development of performance components of organizational behavior analysis.

His book on *A Science and Technology of Teaching* (1968) provided the basis for research on teaching and learning new operants. What was needed differed from the practices that grew from his 1938 book. He needed to develop procedures to teach new operants such as reading, doing math, and learning a new language; he could not simply rely solely on the material from *The Behavior of Organisms* because the objective was now learning not performance. The procedures that were used to shape the pigeons' responses were often laboratory lore and not part of the published work. What resulted for the 1968 book was the teaching machine and programmed instruction, where prompts and models with reinforcement *and corrections* were needed (i.e., learn units or programmed instruction frames).

Finally, *Verbal Behavior* (1957) provided the basis for the real educational units to be taught—functional curriculum (Williams and Greer, 1993). That is rather than teaching requests (a linguistic term), adjectives and adverbs (structural components of language) or receptive and expressive speech (psychological constructs), we now knew that verbal operants like the mand, the tact, and other independent repertoires needed to be the objectives. Also verbal behavior suggested that listener or speaker responses and the joining of these were the units to be taught. That is, verbal behavior introduced verbal function in a way that made the goals of progressive education espoused by Dewey, Pierce, and James possible (i.e., operants needed to be taught under the relevant motivating conditions). Structure is taught too, but structure follows function. Finally, for us, the research on verbal behavior serendipitously led us to the means to induce behavioral developmental cusps or new capabilities (Greer and Keohane, 2005, 2006; Greer and Ross, 2008). The work in verbal behavior simply changed everything!

Skinner's verbal behavior theory and the subsequent research base for that theory led to the redesign of most if not all of our curricula, including curricula for: (a) our 18-month to 5-year olds with and without diagnoses of ASD or related disabilities, (b) our typically developing first, second, and third grade classrooms (senior infants and class 1 and 2), (c) our second through 4th grade classes for children with diagnoses in regular public schools, and (d) our middle school for economically disenfranchised pre-adolescents and adolescents.

One of our first efforts involved early interventions and the founding of the Fred S. Keller School. Since we could not locate a scientifically adequate way to determine our preschoolers existing repertoires and to identify the sequence of educational goals, we developed our own assessment or *inventory of repertoires* that also served as a curriculum, or set of educational standards for pre-school students. This curriculum and criterion-referenced curriculum based assessment now consists of a comprehensive treatment of the entire range of repertoires that we believe to be foundational for success. If children enter junior infant (kindergarten) with all of these repertoires they will be at least a year more advanced than most upper middle class children are at the time they enter kindergarten. We now call this particular inventory/curriculum the *CABAS® International Curriculum and Inventory for Children from Pre-School to Kindergarten* (Greer and McCorkle, 2003). We initially referred to it as the PIRK. It is designed to provide students with the means to be competent independent learners as early as possible. In fact our regular education program is called the Accelerated Independent Learner CABAS® Model or AIL. As CABAS® began to take on more advanced grade levels we developed and are developing similar tools for the more advanced grades. In the latter cases we drew on standard published educational standards in the USA, England, and Ireland.

We converted New York and New Jersey State educational standards and other state and national educational standards (England's *Excellence in Education*) into *functional educational objectives* anchored to Skinner's 1957 theory of verbal behavior. For example, we teach writing by using tested procedures that require the writer to affect the behavior of the reader and the mastery of this objective, in turn, leads to both *functional and structural mastery* of the standards as our curricular targets (Madho, 1997; Reilly-Lawson and Greer, 2006). Most educational standards only specify the structural goals of education. Other examples of incorporating function into educational goals include goals like "appreciation of literature" are expanded to include and to measure children choosing to read certain books in exchange for their tokens, or observing responses to books in free play (Tsai and Greer 2006). Mathematics is taught as functional production and selection responses consistent with verbal functions (Gautreaux, Keohane, and Greer, 2003). We do this by *providing intensive instruction that incorporates the natural controls of learning by design* rather than waiting for teaching moments to occur in the natural environment (natural moments). Because our model is an educational behavioral model rather than a clinical psychology model, we are with the children throughout the day and we provide the entire learning model as a daily diet. In clinical psychological applications, waiting for the natural moments is important; however, in educational settings, educators can create those moments as the very core of pedagogy (i.e., the design of motivation operations as in establishing conditions where writing to affect the behavior of the reader is part of what is learned). In all cases establishing operations, or what Dewey (1916) viewed as "the need to know," are contexts in which operants are taught. More recently we have developed ways for children to learn from indirect contact with instructional contingencies (Greer, Singer-Dudek, and Gautreaux, 2006) and the means to induce behavioral developmental cusps (Greer and Keohane, 2005). The entire range of curricula is viewed through a verbal behavior lens.

After 25 years, the range of applications clearly shows that schools like these are possible, pragmatic, cost-effective and that the benefits are substantial for children's education as well as the advancement of a systems science of teaching and a more sophisticated science of behavior and learning (Greer and Keohane, 2004). While our schools serve the range of children, a large number of the children we have served have come to us with diagnoses of autism spectrum disorders. Having experience with the range of children proved particularly advantageous to our students with ASD because children with autism spectrum diagnoses have the range of repertoires found across all children. Indeed, the schools that we developed in Ireland and England were restricted to children with ASD diagnoses by the governments. While what we have to say applies to all children, we trust that those who work with children with autism, the audience for this book, will find our work on inducing and expanding complex language functions useful. Thus, we chose to focus on this aspect of what we have learned to share with the audience of this book. We hope that our findings in verbal behavior will have extensive benefits for professionals and the children that they serve.

VERBAL DEVELOPMENTAL CUSPS

Behavior analytic approaches to development concentrate on experimental identifications of the environmental sources of development or how experiences contribute to development. For them age is an empty variable; that is age alone doesn't identify the experiences that make development possible. One of the most important contributions in this field has been the identification of a developmental phenomenon called behavioral developmental cusps.

"*A cusp is a change that (1) is often difficult, tedious, subtle, or otherwise problematic to accomplish, yet (2) if not made, means little or no further development is possible in its realm (and perhaps in several realms); but (3) once it is made, a significant set of subsequent developments suddenly becomes easy or otherwise highly probable which (4) brings the developing organism into contact with other cusps crucial to further, more complex, or more refined development on a thereby steadily expanding, steadily more interactive realm.*" (Rosales-Ruiz and Baer, 1996, p. 166).

Rosales-Ruiz and Baer (1996) introduced the construct of the behavioral developmental cusp. Their cusps are critical behavioral stages, such as walking or crawling. When the children acquire them they come in contact with contingencies that they could not come in contact with prior to their attainment. While the stimuli were present somewhere in the environment, they were not part of the stimulus control for the child because they did not have the capability to contact those contingencies. Once the cusp or capability is present new contingencies are contacted and children can make progress in realms they could not prior to their attainment.

In recent years we have identified *verbal* developmental cusps, some that are *verbal capabilities* (Greer and Ross, 2004, 2008). Many of these are higher order operants/frames, or alternately *prerequisite observing stimulus control* that lead to the emergence of higher order classes, accelerated rates of learning, or new ways of learning (e.g., learning by indirect contact with instruction and Naming). See Chapter one of Donahoe and Palmer, 2004 for a comprehensive theoretical treatment of the observing responses and see Greer and Ross (2008) for the relation of observing responses to verbal development. These capabilities are always cusps, but not all cusps are capabilities. Verbal developmental capabilities allow children to learn in different ways such as indirect contact with learn units or simply observing when the capability of Naming is acquired. Capabilities also accelerate rates of learning and prepare children for achieving still more advanced capabilities.

Our work (Greer, and Keohane, 2005; Greer and Ross, 2008) identified several critical verbal developmental capabilities and cusps. The attainment of capabilities, or several of these cusps, allows the child to acquire educational goals that they could not attain prior to acquiring these capabilities or they result in accelerated rates of learning. Moreover, the attainment of certain capabilities allows the subsequent development of more complex verbal development, without which further progress is not possible. Before we identified these as developmental cusps we incorporated them as curricular goals; however, we quickly came to the realization that they were not curricular goals but rather developmental milestones. Hence the interventions are developmental interventions.

We now treat these cusps, and the protocols to develop them, as a separate set of developmental objectives that we distinguish from educational objectives. The verbal capabilities are essentially developmental verbal cusps that are induced by *protocols* derived from our research and that of others. We distinguish between *protocols* that induce new capabilities and *tactics* that result in new operants (i.e., the teaching of educational standards using standard behavioral tactics) or tactics for managing performance. Each of the developmental cusps determines what, if, how, and when we can teach certain educational goals, and when and if we can develop more sophisticated verbal capabilities. The objective of this paper is to outline those verbal capabilities and sources for the procedures that can induce the missing capabilities; space does not allow for a detailed description of the procedures. A book that provides detailed explanations of the capabilities and how to use the tested protocols that induce them was released in May of 2007 (Greer and Ross, 2008).

An Empirically Driven Theory of Verbal Development

The verbal developmental cusps involve both listener and speaker capabilities and the joining of those capabilities *under the skin of the individual* as well as in the social relationships between different individuals. *The verbal capabilities involve all of the senses and the manner in which language function relates these disparate senses.* We shall first outline our developmental scenario of how we believe these capabilities evolve naturally in many children and then we shall explain how our endeavors to induce these missing capabilities led us to protocols to do so, and subsequently, our developmental scenario for the typically developing child. While this is a developmental theory, we did not set out to propose such a theory. Rather, we researched how to develop verbal capabilities in children who were missing them. As our work progressed the findings suggested an empirically derived developmental theory that, in turn, came to guide our subsequent efforts to identify when and if certain protocols were needed.

Applied Ramifications

What are the applied implications? The result of this work allows well trained professionals to advance children in ways that were not possible, or not possible to the degree, before the capabilities or cusps and protocols to induce them were known. Just a few of these include: induction of real verbal listening skills including the capability to be reinforced as listener, induction of vocal verbal speech with more children, development of culturally conditioned controls for social behavior, acquisition of the reinforcement effects that are necessary for true tacts, multiplication of the emission of spontaneous speech, acquisition of the ability to learn from observing others being instructed, acquisition of the wherewithal to acquire vocabulary incidentally (Naming), acquisition of Naming as a facilitator of categorization and abstractions, induction of functional self-talk and speaker as own-listener responding, acquisition of correspondence between saying and writing, acquisition of comprehension as joining of print to Naming, acquisition of effective functional writing and self-editing, acquisition of the production of untaught verbal tenses and suffixes, acquisition of metaphorical responding, and acquisition of complex algorithm control to solve problems. As children acquire these cusps they can learn things they could not learn before, and learn from types of instruction that they could not learn from before. Note that these are not simply expansions of what the children knew how to do as in the expansion of repertoires; for this we use behavior analytic teaching tactics (Greer and Keohane, 2004). Rather, the inductions of these allow children to learn by types of instruction that they could not learn from before. Some of the capabilities allow children to learn incidentally when they could not learn incidentally before. Moreover, the foundational observing capabilities result in accelerated learning and the prerequisite observational responding that makes the learning of discriminated operants possible.

We believe also that these findings validate the basic research and behavioral theories concerning the identification of emergent behavior and the environmental controls for emergent behavior that is verbal (i.e., research in stimulus equivalence, Relational Frame Theory, and Skinner's theory on language as behavior per se). The combined findings and data based theories of this corpus of evidence suggests that learning and complex human behavior is now in the microscope of behavior analysis and that complex language and behavior need no intervening psychological constructs. Moreover, they set the stage for meaningful research beneath the skin using f/MRI.

When the capabilities that we describe below do not occur naturally and incidentally as it does in most typically developing children whose sense are intact, the developmental interventions that have been identified make it possible to instate them. An understanding of the empirically driven verbal development theory is key. The following section is a brief and broad strokes description of some key components of that theory. An in depth treatment of each of the capabilities and how and when they can be induced is found in Greer and Ross (2008) and a more detailed explanation of the theory is found in Greer and Keohane (2005).

Verbal Development

Verbal development begins when the child is in the uterus. As the child receives nourishment in the womb the mother's voice, along with a host of other stimuli, is paired with the feeding. (i.e., conditioned reinforcement for attending to the mother's voice) When the child is born she orients towards her mother's voice—the listener observing response is reinforced by the mother's voice (Decasper and Spence, 1987). After birth, when the infant is fed, the mother's voice is paired with nourishment also, as the child acquires vision and the face of the mother becomes a reinforcer for visually observing the mother's face. The conditioned reinforcement of the voice is paired with the mother's face and movement). Subsequently the mother's touch and the corresponding touch (a production response) involve reciprocal automatic reinforcement relations between observing and producing responses (Luciano, Barnes-Holmes, and Barnes-Holmes, 2002). *See and do* is established at the fundamental level (Meltzoff and Moore, 1983). Simultaneously and independently, the infant emits phylogenetically derived vocal sounds just as they emit various movements that are non-vocal in nature—the movement of legs, arms, and swimming motions for examples (See Donahoe and Palmer, 2004). These producing and observing responses are *independent of each other initially* and their automatic reinforcement is not entirely different than that maintaining stereotypy—the reinforcement that accrues from correspondence between observing and producing. These movements probably provide practice for future functional uses of the movements and muscular strength. The vocal sounds and the non-vocal movements acquire automatic reinforcement effects. Some of those phylogenetically derived sounds, like crying, also begin to have mediation functions; that is the crying leads to caretakers mediating between the behavior of the child and her environment. Crying results in changing diapers, being fed and, most importantly for later verbal functions the caregiver's attention acquires conditioned reinforcement effects—a critical developmental cusp in itself.

From observing the mother's voice, the infant acquires correspondence between the mother's vowel-consonant blends and this leads to auditory matching in which the infant learns correspondence between the infant's vocal sounds and those of the mother—these vowel consonant aspects of the auditory stimulus acquire abstract stimulus control within the range of acoustical stimuli and automatic reinforcement (i.e., infants do not match the frequency or timbre of their mothers voices, perhaps because they cannot) (See Meltzoff, 1996). When these initial parroting responses lead to functional outcomes (i.e., "MAMA" results in a great deal of attention) the echoic function is induced (Sundberg, Michael, Partington, and Sundberg, 1996). When and if the parroting leads to echoic verbal functions, the listener to speaker verbal operant is born *and is itself a higher order operant*. This is why we believe that Skinner's echoic is a speaker operant. See Barnes-Holmes, Barnes-Holmes, and Cullinan, 2001 for an argument for why it is not an indication of being verbal a point on which we agree. However, the speaker operants specified by Skinner are part of the road to becoming verbal.

At either an earlier, or a simultaneous stage, the *see and do* relation of generalized imitation results in still another higher order operant—the duplic class (Vargas, 1982). When see and do joins a common class with hear and say the foundation for much of what we learn is in place. See Greer and Ross (2008) for how to induce these joint observing and producing functions when they are missing.

The capacity for sameness accrues as relations between the sameness of tastes, smells, sounds, and tactile stimuli are joined in an arbitrary class of sameness. This is still another critical component of verbal development, and makes behaving verbally a means for categorization—an arbitrarily applicable relation that is language (Keohane, Greer et al. 2006a). While the speaker and listener are initially independent, the functional effect of the echoic-to-mand and the echoic-to-tact produces a relation between the speaker and listener—but at this point it is basically a speaker function—listening converted to speaking that results in a different listener mediating the environment for the speaker. The tact, mand, and supplementary speaker operants grow with language experiences between the mother or caregiver and the child (Hart and Risley, 1995). See Greer and Ross (2008) for detailed instructions in how to induce these missing capabilities.

The joining of the speaker and listener occurs when the children have say and do correspondence and self-talk involving speaker as own listener conversational units (Lodhi and Greer, 1989). At age two only a few upper middle-class children have acquired the NAMING capability but by age three children from this advantaged educational and economic class have naming for three-dimensional objects (Gilic, 2005). However, Naming for three-dimensional stimuli can be induced in two-year olds as a result of brief but intensive multiple exemplar experiences (Feliciano, 2006; Fiorile and Greer, 2006; Gilic; Greer, Stolfi, Chavez-Brown, and Rivera-Valdes, 2005; Greer, Stolfi and Pistoljevic, in press). Naming with two-dimensional stimuli does not appear to be fully in place for many typically developing first-graders at the beginning of the year, but many do have it at the end of the year apparently as a function of experiences with books and print (Greer and O'Sullivan, 2006). Currently we believe this is a function of conditioned reinforcement for observing responses for two-dimensional print and picture stimuli (Dinsmoor, 1983; Tsai and Greer, 2006). We know that say and do correspondence and conversational units in self-talk are present in typically developing five-year olds (Lodhi and Greer, 1989), although they probably occur initially at a much earlier age.

The joining of the independent speaker and listener responses within the skin occurs as the child acquires Naming (Greer, Stolfi, et al., 2005), say and do correspondence (Paniagua, and Baer, 1982), and self-talk involving conversational units in which the child functions as both speaker and listener during solitary play (Lodhi and Greer, 1989). Once Naming is present and the child acquires print control in which the sounds of printed words are textually emitted, and the child has the tact repertoire and listener repertoire, reading comprehension can accrue (Lee Park, 2005). If, in turn, the child has transformation of dictation stimulus control across saying and writing, the writing response accrues from the auditory experience alone. In the latter case derived relations between the sounds of letters and writing the letters makes the transformation of stimulus control possible after relevant multiple exemplar experiences (Greer, Yuan, and Gautreaux, 2005). We suspect, from the data that we have accrued to date, that naming for two-dimensional stimuli is a critical predictor of school success and may be one of, if not the, biggest obstacle facing children from low socioeconomic backgrounds (Greer and O'Sullivan, 2006). See Greer and Ross (2008) for detailed instructions for when and how to induce Naming and correspondence between saying and writing.

Still other verbal capabilities are part of what has been treated in some literatures as evidence of a language acquisition device that is proposed as the sole source of the spontaneous emission of untaught verb endings and suffixes (Pinker, 1999). Those who hold to that theory believe that children do not learn these through natural environmental teaching experiences. However, we found that the productive formation of verb endings and suffixes or affixes could be brought about as a function of multiple exemplar experiences—a particular instructional history that we provided. That is when children who did not form regular past tenses from context control or creative uses of the irregular past tense (e.g., he "singed" last night), they came to do so after a brief but intensive experience with one or more exemplar contextual control sets (Greer and Yuan, 2006). Moreover the same effect from multiple exemplar experiences led to the production of untaught suffixes (Speckman-Collins and Greer, 2006). Indeed this is how these children learned "the darnedest things." In the case of these children the "creative" verbal behavior did not just develop from a hypothetical language acquisition device; rather it was a higher order operant that accrued from contact with the basic principles of behavior across exemplar contexts and this resulted in the formation of a higher order stimulus control. In such cases novel production need not require direct reinforcement since the responses are part of a higher order operant and in the cases of these endings the source was a particular *history* of reinforcement. In these cases the instructional control was experimentally isolated and induced.

The more advanced capabilities of *affecting the behavior of a reader by writing* and also *being affected by the writing of others as a reader* builds on the prerequisites described above, placing emphasis on the listener capability. A reader is a listener and an effective writer listens as a target audience would listen. Eventually, one can follow complex verbally governing algorithms or write them such that others may follow them. These capabilities make advanced scientific and aesthetic repertoires possible. This is a brief synopsis of the progression with many of the components necessarily omitted (See Greer and Ross, 2008 for the complete range of components). After providing the synopsis, we show how this progression is important to developing language functions and the particular procedures that have led to the induction of those capabilities when they are not present.

How Children with Language Delays Helped Us to Identify the Cusps and Induce New Capabilities.

How did we arrive at this scenario, and how does the identification of them relate to inducing and expanding verbal capabilities in those who are missing them? Over the last two decades research in verbal behavior analysis (Greer and Keohane, 2005; Greer and Ross, 2004; Greer and Ross, 2008) and related work in Relational Frame Theory (Hayes, Barnes-Holmes, and Roche, 2000), stimulus equivalence (Sidman, 1986) and Naming (Horne and Lowe, 1996; Lowe, Horne, Harris, and Randle 2002) has led to the identification of and the development of procedures to identify and induce verbal developmental cusps and related cognitive capabilities in children who were missing them. Once children acquired these cusps, "a significant set of subsequent developments suddenly [*became*] easy or otherwise highly probable." (Rosales-Ruiz and Baer, p. 166). These included the emergence of productive or generative verbal behavior or acceleration in learning across a range of realms. To wit, as described above, the production of untaught suffixes (Speckman-Collins and Greer, 2006) or verb endings (Greer and Yuan, 2006) were shown to be a function of certain multiple exemplar experiences. While much remains to be done, we believe the accumulated findings and the possibilities they suggest are robust enough that they should be reported to the behavior analysis community at large for applications and independent replications.

Early Listener Capabilities

Some children who enter our schools are pre-listeners, who for various reasons (i.e., ontogenetic, phylogenetic sources or a combination) missed those early pairings described above. That is, the vowel consonant blends and all of their permutations (consonant-vowel-consonant, etc.) in words do not direct the actions of these children, although some are very good at discriminating visual cues simply because that is the only means they have to operate in their world. In fact they often get better and better at visual cues and *more adept at avoiding auditory stimulus control,* perhaps because of repeated drills in which the child simply gets better at visual controls or simply receives a variable schedule of reinforcement for guessing. But before we can treat the lack of auditory control and as a first step the child must come under the reinforcement control of the adult who is teaching him or her. Even if the speech of the teacher is simply background noise, children quickly learn to discriminate contingencies provided in programs requiring them to sit, sit still, make eye contact, and do as others do (generalized imitation or components of generalized imitation) (Greer and Ross, 2008). When speech does not control responding but the child picks up sequence or visual cues because of the reinforcement control of the teacher, we attempt to teach them basic listener literacy. We now have their attention and can now focus on developing auditory control or listener responding. The most fundamental evidence of basic listener literacy occurs when two or more words with different vowel-consonant blends acquire differential discriminative control of the child's non-verbal responses. Our first protocol to induce this is a procedure we call "listener emersion." This procedure involves stopping most instruction until basic listener literacy is in place. The protocol is a sequence of interventions that involve teaching the child responses to several sets of vocal commands that include a nonsense command, to which the child cannot and should not respond, until the child can follow these instructions at 100% accuracy solely as a function of the *teacher's vowel consonant blends.* The interventions are arranged such that the *only way* that a child can accrue reinforcement is from following the speech of the teacher, including not responding when the teacher introduces nonsense commands. All sets are taught simultaneously, but as each set is mastered, the child is taught to respond to the commands to a rate criterion (e.g., 30 responses per minute). Once they can do this reliably, *we record a mixture of the commands* with different voices and the child must master responding to the recorded commands. When the child is able to do this, we return to all other instruction. Children who achieve the capability from this protocol learn from four to ten times faster (Greer, Chavez-Brown, et al., 2005). When the child masters this capability we refer to them as having acquired *basic listener literacy.* They can learn responses to new vowel consonant sounds because new ones for which they have no response for are discriminated from those they can. This sets the stage for them to learn stimulus control for the new vowel-consonant blends that can accrue from either direct or *indirect contact* with the contingencies of the learn unit (See Greer, Singer, Gautreaux, 2006 for distinctions between direct and indirect control of learning and the importance of acquiring the capability to learn from indirect contact with instructional contingencies).

When Listener Literacy is Not Forthcoming

However, some children cannot meet the objectives of the listener emersion protocol *because they are missing prerequisite developmental cusps.* When they cannot, we believe that vowel consonant blends are simply not functioning as discriminative stimuli because the observing control (listening is an observing response) of voices is not present. In these cases, we condition voices as reinforcers for observing responses via stimulus-stimulus pairings.

The conditioned reinforcement control of voices that typically developing children have at birth is missing and we attempt to condition voices as reinforcers for the listener observing response. We use auditory reproduction devices that contain recordings of the mother's and teachers' voices reading nursery rhymes or stories. The child depresses a switch on a tape recorder or places her finger on a disc on the table, and as long as the button is pressed or disc is touched the child can hear the recorded voices. When the button is released, or the child removes her finger from the disc, the tape stops and the recorded voices can no longer be heard. When a child does not respond by listening to this arrangement of conjugate reinforcement, we use a protocol to condition voices that involves stimulus-stimulus pairings using the same device until the child selects the voices for 5-minutes in a "free operant" setting (See Greer and Ross, 2008 and Tsai and Greer, 2006 for how to do this). Once a child does so, she is returned to the listener emersion protocol and is typically able to meet the listener emersion objective of basic listener literacy. Once the observing response is in place the components of vowel consonant blends in words can acquire discriminative control (Dinsmoor, 1983; Keohane, Greer, and Ackerman 2006c).

Another protocol that we frequently use at the same time, if not first, is one devoted to conditioning tabletop visual stimuli as reinforcers for observing. This is particularly relevant if the child has difficulty matching visual stimuli or does not attend to tabletop stimuli. In this protocol we provide stimulus-stimulus pairings until the child reliably attends to pages with various abstract stimuli or follows rotated objects on the table. This too is a stimulus-stimulus pairing procedure that acts to condition tabletop stimuli as reinforcement for visual observation. For children like these, the accrual of reinforcement for observing that occurs in typically developing children is simply not in place and must be induced.

Still another capability that is foundational to discrimination learning is what we refer to as *the capacity for sameness*. We remind the reader that verbal behavior involves all of the senses. The capacity for sameness is fundamental to discrimination and language function--the development of *the arbitrarily applicable relations* of verbal behavior. In the protocol to induce a foundational capacity for sameness, we attempt to build capacity for sameness across the five senses (Keohane, Greer, and Ackerman, 2006c). In this case we are attempting to build what may be a fundamental pre-requisite for language as an arbitrarily applicable relation. The child rotates learn units across matching olfactory stimuli, auditory stimuli, textural stimuli (rough and smooth), and gustatory stimuli. When the child masters these rotated stimuli they have a fundamental capacity for sameness across senses. Since sameness across senses is an arbitrarily applicable relation, it too is a higher order operant. We currently believe that the capacity for sameness is one of the first steps toward verbal categorization that is made possible by language.

Once one, or more of these capabilities are in place, children's learning is accelerated in one or more realms and they are now capable of achieving basic listener literacy. As soon as a child has basic listener literacy other and more advanced capabilities become possible.

Early Speaker Capabilities

As we proceed with the listener component, *we work simultaneously on the speaker component*. If a child acquires the echoic-to-mand and the echoic-to-tact repertoires we progress with expanding those repertoires (see Greer and Ross, 2008; Ross and Greer, 2003;

Tsiouri and Greer, 2003; Williams and Greer, 1993 for how to do this). We do not typically shape separate speech sounds; rather entire words are taught. Most children respond readily to this procedure including the tandem feature that requires a tact response in order to have the *opportunity to mand*, thereby arranging the generalized reinforcement effects for the tact operant. If the basic procedure for expanding these repertoires, described in Greer and Ross (2004; 2008) or Williams and Greer (1993), is not successful there are several protocols that are used based on the child's instructional history or existing capabilities. One of the protocols we use joins see and do to hear and say. As a prerequisite for this protocol, the child must be fluent in generalized imitation.

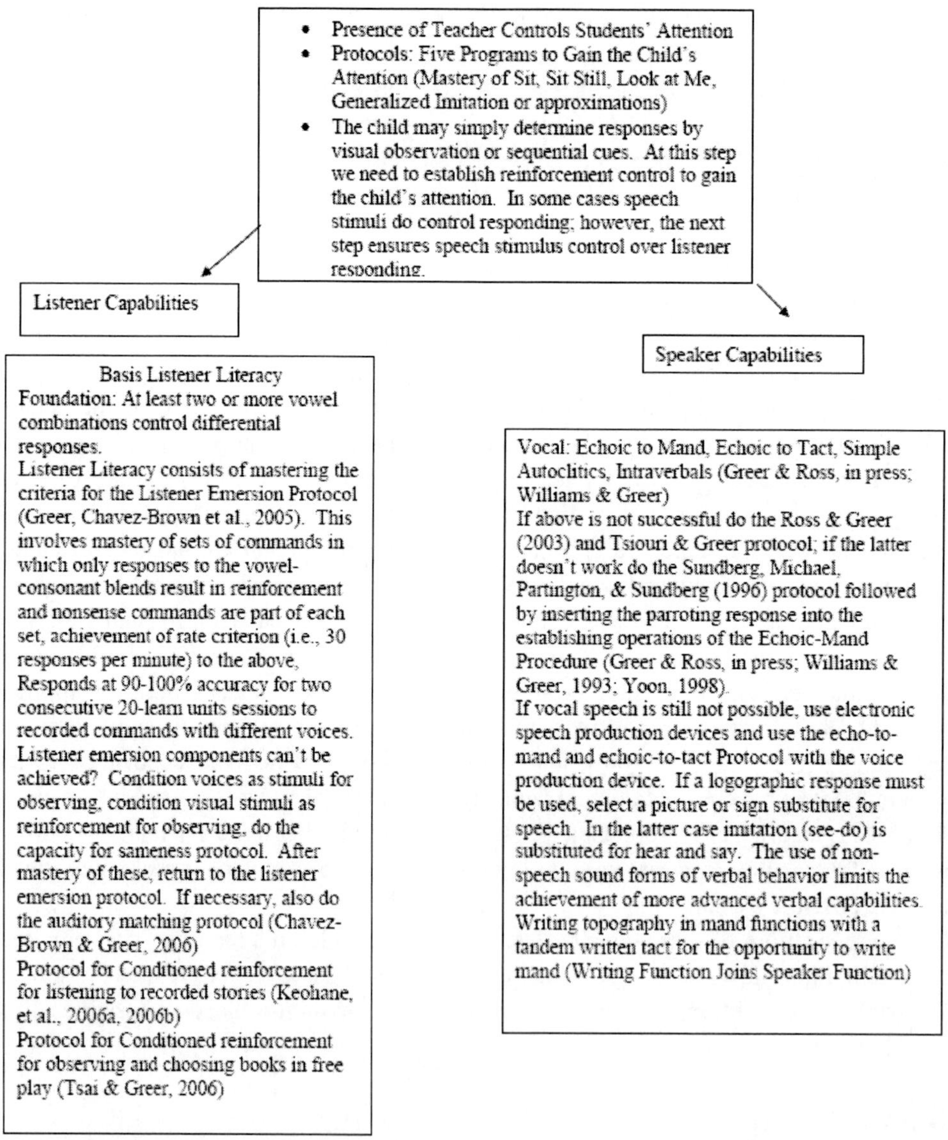

Figure 7.1. First Sequence: Inducing the Speaker and Listener Capability.

First we briefly deprive the child of preferred items and require that the child rapidly imitate a series of responses going from large motor imitations (clap hands, touch knees, stand up, turn around) to fine grained responses, progressively focusing on the face mouth and the lips (touches face, chin, lips, tongue). When the child is clearly working for the item under deprivation, we position the item in front of the child and suddenly insert saying the word for the item (i.e., coke). This protocol has resulted in first instances of speech for some children (one as old as nine) and once this occurs we have expanded mands (Ross and Greer, 2003) and tacts (Tsiouri and Greer)—verbal operants that have been maintained in one instance over years (Greer and Ross, 2003). Finally if this is unsuccessful we use a stimulus-stimulus pairing procedure to develop parroting (Sundberg, Michael, Partington, and Sundberg, 1996). When the parroting is in place, we use the parroting response in the echoic-to-mand protocol (Greer and Ross, 2008; Williams and Greer, 1993) to convert the parroting response into a true verbal operant--the echoic to mand or echoic to tact verbal operant (Yoon, 1998). That is, the establishing operations for the mand are introduced and result in delivery of the item. In many cases this leads to the relevant establishing operation control that converts the parroting into a true verbal operant.

If speech is not forthcoming at this point, we use electronic speaking devices, using the device to replace speech because these devices allow the continual development of the listener component. If this is successful, we can retain the benefits of spoken language that plays a key role in subsequent verbal capabilities and sometimes leads to vocal verbal behavior. Finally, if vocal simulators are not available we use logographic stimuli such as pictures or signs (See Robinson, 1995 and McGuiness, 2004 for the reasons why logographic stimuli are inferior to phonogram stimuli in terms of more advanced cognitive capabilities).

Still another protocol, that has either induced incipient echoics or clarified inaccurate echoic responding, is an auditory matching protocol (Chavez-Brown, 2005; Chavez-Brown and Greer, 2006). This protocol requires the child to emit selection responses (i.e., speech reproduction buttons) for matching sounds and successively matching target words against non-target words until the child can master matching novel word sets on first presentation. When this auditory matching capability is in place we have induced first instances of echoics and drastically improved children's pronunciation of echoics. This procedure is also helpful for assisting children who cannot achieve basic listener literacy to do so. Use of this to replace faulty intraverbal behavior, echolalia, has been successful in a few cases. That is the child selects matching buttons that do not have point-to-point correspondence.

Transformation of Establishing Control for the Emission of Untaught Functions for the Same Topography

Each of the protocols above and their resulting capabilities serve to enhance listener and speaker repertoires and the foundation for joining those different capabilities. Once basic listener literacy is in place and the basic speaker operants (mands, tacts, intraverbals and autoclitics) are present we also want to ensure that the child acquires transformation of establishing operations across mand and tact functions. The independence of the mand and tact functions in early development has been documented in several studies (Lamarre and Holland, 1985; Twyman, 1996a, 1996b; Williams and Greer, 1993; but, also see Petursdottir, Carr, and Michael, 2005 for related evidence).

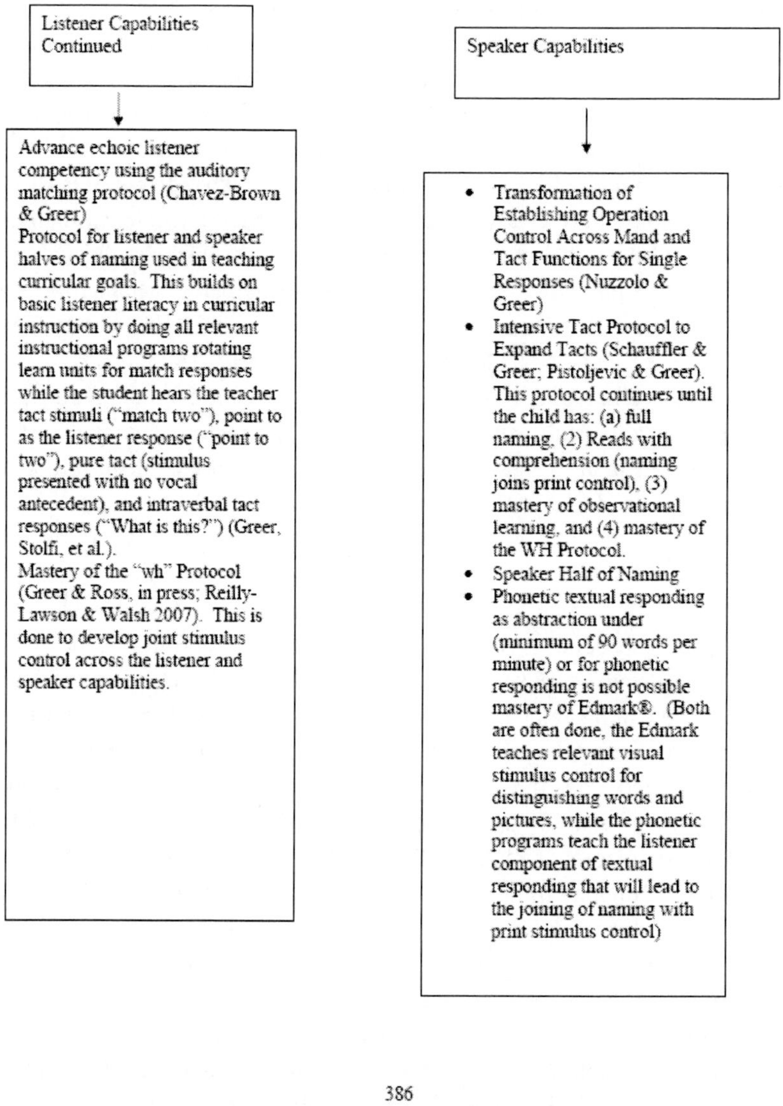

Figure 7.2. After the Listener and Speaker Capabilities are Present, Advance Listening and Speaking Repertoires.

When learning a tact or mand function with a word or words does not automatically result in the untaught function for the same word, this capability can be induced by a protocol tested by Nuzzolo and Greer (2004).

In this protocol the provision of rotated multiple exemplar experiences across mand and tact establishing operations for the same forms resulted in untaught emission of functions with novel responses. This means that teaching a child either a mand or tact function automatically results in an untaught response when the relevant establishing operations are present.

Emergence of Untaught Verb Endings and Suffixes

When children cannot emit regular past tenses in autoclitic functions, rapid alternation of tense contexts (i.e., multiple exemplars) for a subset of verbs resulted in the emission of untaught past tenses for autoclitic functions (Greer and Yuan, 2006). These same children also emitted "creative" irregular verbs ("singed" for sing) as a result of the multiple exemplar experience with regular verbs. These data suggest the apparent developmental trajectory of most children. Subsequent experiences that correct the incorrect irregular responses are probably not different in substance from the distinctions that phonemic readers come to acquire for words that are not phonemic. That is multiple exemplar experiences with special case distinctions probably results in the reliable emission of those distinctions. The same outcomes were found for children's untaught usages of suffixes (Speckman and Greer, 2006).

Verbal Episodes between Individuals

Verbal episodes between individuals involve the rotation of speaker listener exchanges, sometimes referred to as turn taking. Children function as listeners for each other and as speakers in rotated fashion (Donley and Greer, 1993). When a single exchange results in an individual functioning as both a speaker and a listener in a rotated fashion and the individual is reinforced as both speaker and listener the individual has participated in an interlocking verbal episode called a conversational unit. This marks the acquisition of a significant verbal cusp and is a valid measure of socialization. The reinforcement for the speaker is mediated by the behavior of the listener. Equally important, and perhaps even more difficult to obtain, is the acquisition of the reinforcement effects for the listener. The reinforcement for listening is having one's senses extended ranging from (a) avoiding getting wet by bringing an umbrella after hearing it is raining to (b) the phenomenon often described as empathy (Reilly-Lawson, and Walsh, 2006). We use a protocol involving yoked contingencies to induce listener reinforcement in children missing that capacity. In this protocol, pairs of children participate in a series of games and instructional programs in which joint reinforcement accrues as a function of listening to what each member of the pair says. This protocol has resulted in children emitting conversational units in non-instructional settings and emitting more "wh" questions. The yoked contingency games make the reinforcement effects of listening salient.

Joining of Speaker and Listener in the Speaker as Own Listener Capabilities

The listener and speaker verbal functions are different. When one acquires a second language, the way in which one learns that language can result in very different speaker and listener repertoires. Learning the language through conversation has different outcomes than learning the language by the process of learning to "translate from text. One may read phonetically in a new language but not "understand." That is, one may speak the text but not listen to the text they speak. Similarly, children with language delays may become relatively capable as a speaker or listener and not have the other components. The two differ along the dimensions of responses, stimulus discriminative control, establishing operation control and consequent control and most likely evolutionary sources. Terms like receptive and expressive speech contribute to the belief that language is somehow a single entity that has two components—receptive speech and expressive speech. We believe that this commonly accepted psychological construct has disguised the independence of the two capabilities. The result is that deficits in either are seen as a "language deficit." A more parsimonious approach is to treat the two as separate capabilities. Nevertheless, effective verbal behavior requires the joining of the two. The points at which these merge into multiple responses to the same stimuli are key, however, to the more complex functions of verbal behavior such as editing, verbally governed responding, and verbally governing responding. Perhaps, each of us has inconsistencies in our speaker and listener capabilities. At present we believe there are three empirically identified speaker-as-own-listener capabilities—(a) self-talk conversational units, (b) say and do correspondence, and (c) a developmental phenomenon identified by Horne and Lowe (1996) called Naming.

Verbal development requires the joining of the listener and speaker within the same skin that is necessary if one is to be truly verbal (Barnes-Holmes, Barnes-Holmes, and Cullinan, 2000). Skinner (1957) characterized this phenomenon as speaker-as-own listener. One talks to oneself when there is no other audience present, responds to one's own words as a listener and then speaks to the original utterance from the perspective of the speaker. Adults may do this in front of others when they talk to their pets and respond to their pets. Young children engage in self-talk when they play alone. One clear instance of speaker as own listener occurs when children emit self-talk conversational units while engaged in solitary play. Typically developing children readily engage in these speaker as own listener conversational units (Lodhi and Greer, 1989) in certain contexts. This capability appears to form the basis of the kinds of self-editing that occurs in the process of writing and other types of verbal "thinking." Conversational units have been induced or increased by several protocols. The first is the intensive tact protocol that provides extensive tact training on a daily basis (Pistoljevic and Greer, 2006; Schauffler and Greer, 2006). In addition, creating establishing operations for peers to emit conversational units by removing the adults from the context in certain settings has resulted in increases (Donley and Greer, 1993). The use of the yoked contingencies protocols described above show promise for inducing reinforcement effects for the listener (Reilly-Lawson and Walsh, 2007)

Still another instance of the joining of the two capabilities occurs in cases where one says what they are going to do and then one does it (Paniagua and Baer, 1982). This is not simply an instance of "self-management," it is at base an instance of correspondence between the two capabilities. Saying and doing can be taught using procedures similar to those we described in the listener emersion protocol. In this case, reinforcement is contingent upon providing exemplars for saying and doing until say-do correspondence emerges.

Naming is a third type of speaker-as-own-listener capability (Greer, Stolfi et al. 2005; Greer, Stolfi, Pistoljevic, 2007; Lowe, Horne, Harris, and Randle, 2002; Miguel and Petursdottir, in press). In the several studies in which naming has been induced for children missing the capability, the protocol involved multiple exemplar experiences that rapidly rotated listener and speaker responses following the child having heard a tact for, and matched a stimulus with, from one to three sets of 5-stimuli. This protocol has proved effective for children with language delays, typically developing two-year olds, and two-dimensional naming (pictures or abstract symbols) with typically developing six-year olds.

Clearly, there are certain prerequisite verbal capabilities that children need prior to benefiting from the exemplar experiences that have induced naming in children who are missing it. Once it is present other more advanced capabilities become possible, particularly with reference to the joining of naming to print control. Indeed, there may be more advanced naming type capabilities. Maintaining equivalence between one's listener and speaker capabilities may continue throughout ones' life. That is, listener and speaker capabilities remain different but we continuously acquire intercepts between the two.

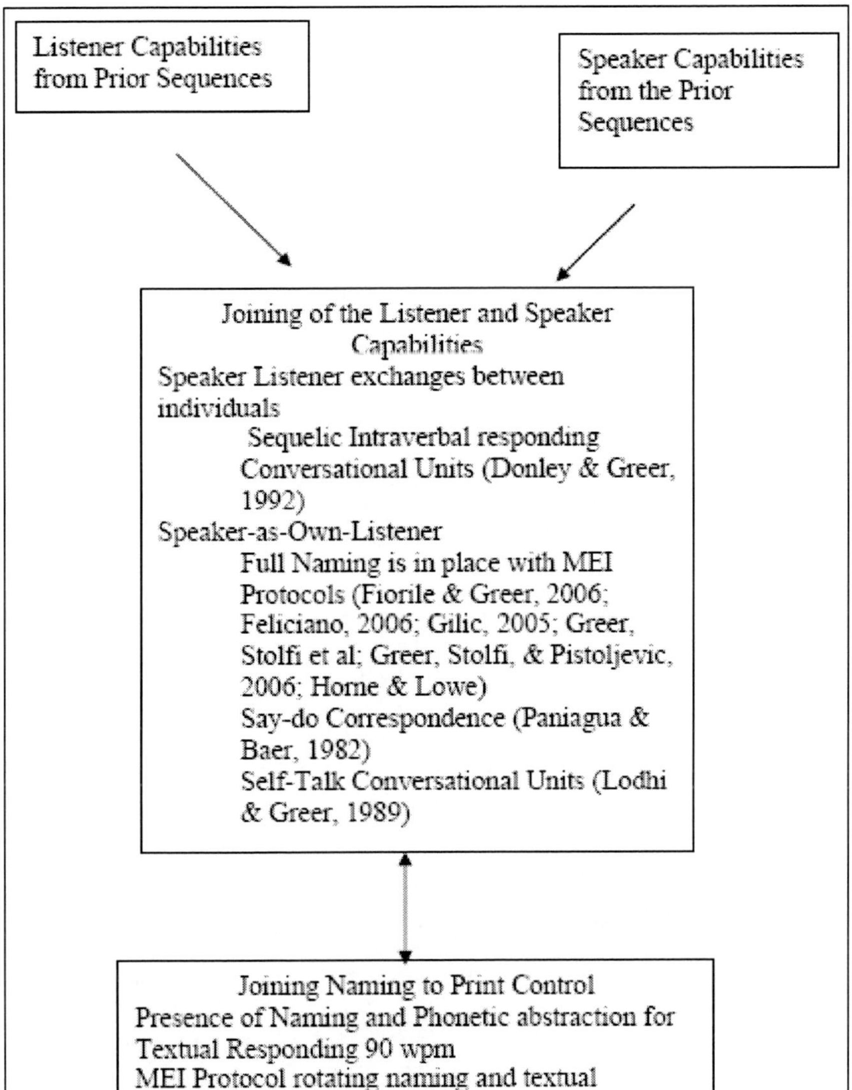

Figure 7.3. Joining the Listener and Speaker for Verbal Episodes with Others and Within the Skin.

When Print Joins the Naming Capability: Reading and Writing

When the child has naming and acquires phonetic reading skills and sounds out an unfamiliar word for the first time if the child has previously acquired a tact for the stimulus (as a function of naming or tact instruction), comprehension is immediate. For example, if a parent points out a blue bunting and the child has Naming the tact and the listener response is available with no further instruction. So, the child hearing that the item is called a blue bunting will be able to respond in the future when asked "What is that?" with the answer "That is a blue bunting" or will be able to tell other individuals in the presence of a blue bunting, "That is a blue bunting." Once the child has phonetic reading skills and textually responses to the printed B-L-U-E B-U-N-T-I-N-G the words are, so to speak, heard (McGuiness, 2004). Once heard, comprehension is immediate. Thus, the exemplar experiences that produce naming lead to reading comprehension at a later stage.

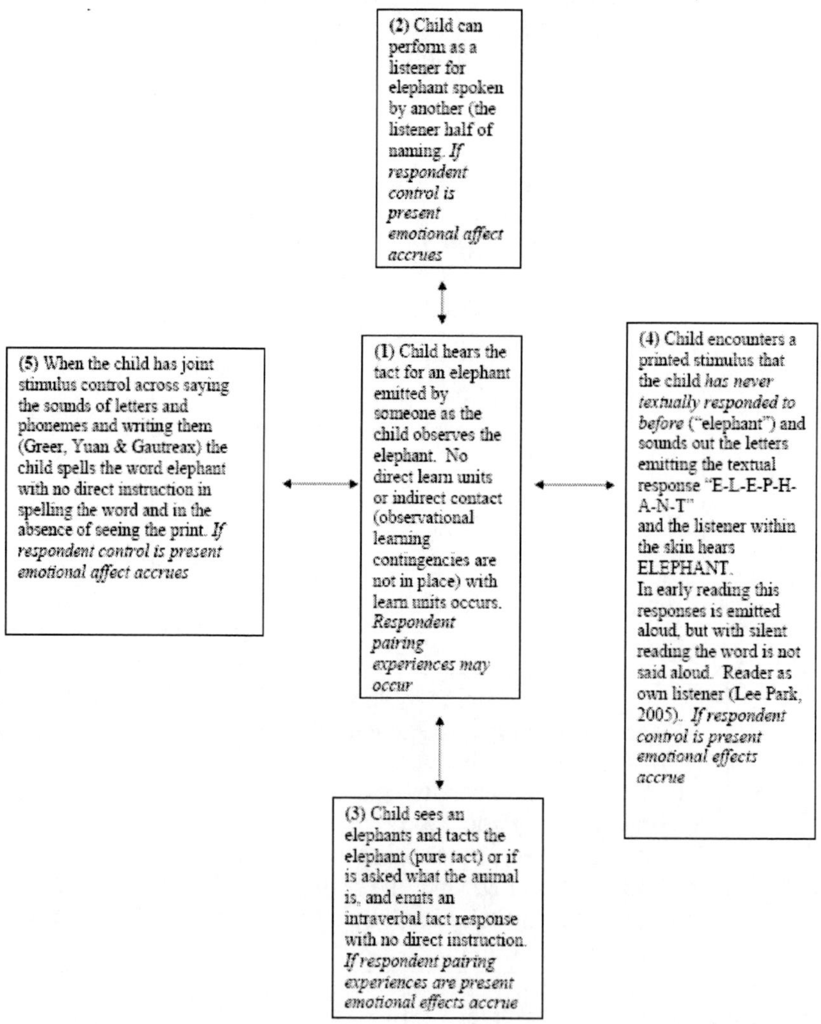

Figure 7.4. Diagram Illustrating the Joining of Print Across Naming, Phonetic Responding, and Joint Stimulus Control Across Saying and Writing: Comprehension as a Higher Order Operant.

Once the responses of saying and writing to the dictated word are present the child not only has reading comprehension but can also write the word. In this case the spoken word results not only in saying the letters for the word but also in writing the letters. Before children have this joint control of the dictated or heard word across saying and writing letters, each needs to be taught separately. Once again multiple exemplar experiences for a subset of stimuli resulted in the emission of untaught responses for novel stimuli (Greer, Yuan et al., 2005). Thus, the exemplar experiences that lead to naming result in the child coming into contact with the experiences those in turn join reading and writing.

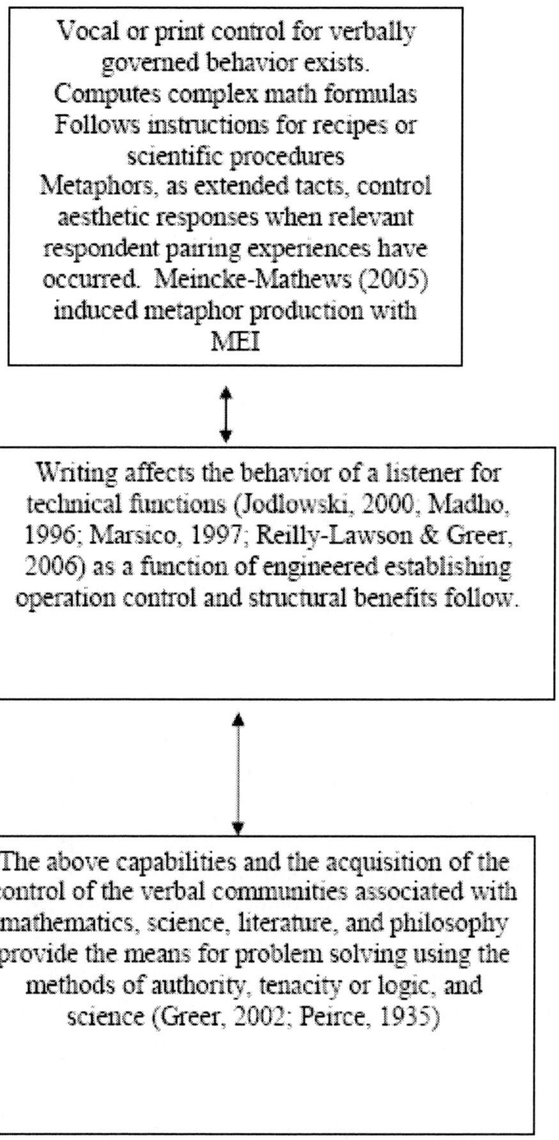

Figure 7.5. Capabilities as the Foundations for More Advanced Complex Verbal or "Cognitive Functions.

Advanced Cognitive or Verbal Capabilities

The joining of print to naming and the resulting relation to writing can then lead to verbally governed behavior of ever increasing complexity. Marsico (1997) showed that once middle school students learned to follow written algorithms they could acquire new repertoires from print stimuli. At a more advanced level Keohane and Greer (2005) identified the verbal stimulus control for scientific decisions. Thus, complex verbally governed behavior builds on the joining of the speaker-as-own-listener within the skin and if the print is isolated as the stimulus the stimulus and response of problem solving is apparent.

The capability of governing the behavior of others with print does not necessarily follow from verbally governed behavior and exemplar experiences across being verbally governed by print and governing others by print requires exemplar experiences (Lee Park, 2005). Without a firm foundation in the verbal cusps that came before, even advanced students will have difficulty moving from responding to printed stimuli to producing print stimuli for others to respond. Responding to math formulas is different from generating formulas unless the necessary exemplars accrue and the prerequisite cusps are present (Gautreaux, Keohane and Greer, 2003).

Once all of these capabilities are present, individuals can draw on the repertoires for all advanced cognitive functions that are verbal in nature. They can use these verbal capabilities in disciplines involving problem-solving repertoires associated with the methods of authority, tenacity (logic) and the methods of science (Peirce, 1935).

Conclusion

One of the interesting outcomes of doing research to identify verbal capabilities, and in turn how to induce them when the child has the necessary prerequisites, is that not only were these useful for working with children who were missing them but they expanded the basic science of verbal behavior. Moreover, concurrent research in stimulus equivalence, Naming and categorization, and Relational Frame Theory in the basic science of behavior was very closely related. Our work added applied validity to their findings and our findings demonstrated the applicability of current basic science work to language functions. The result has been a kind of independent affirmation of higher order operants, relational framing, Naming and categorization, and stimulus equivalence. Our applied work resulted in basic science contributions and the basic science contributions affirmed our direction. For example, Hayes et al. (2001) proposed that multiple exemplar experiences were the source for many types of higher order operants and our work has shown this to be the case in many instances. Sidman believed that stimulus equivalence was useful only if it has an application to explaining language as verbal behavior. While all stimulus equivalence findings do not apply to language, stimulus equivalence is evident in most of our induced higher order verbal operants. We think that other stimulus equivalence findings are probably related to the joining of other emergent observing and producing relations other than language, such as emergent relations in music, dance, and the visual arts. That is, we think that the joining of observing and producing relations by musicians, dancers and artists can result in emergent relations but the reinforcement for these classes of responding differ from the reinforcement of verbal behavior where the listener mediates for the speaker and the speaker mediates for the listener by extending the listener's senses. Horne and Lowe's Naming contribution has shown the utility of Naming to assisting the formation of categorizations, but for us the importance was the fact that Naming was a verbal developmental cusp and the source for research and application of Naming as a dependent variable. Coincidentally, most of our studies on inducing Naming have resulted in novel categorizations. This consensus of findings bodes well for the progress of our science and its usefulness to explaining complex behavior and indeed inducing that behavior when missing.

We outlined the service, research, and demonstration functions of CABAS® schools specifically with reference to our work in verbal development. One of the outcomes of the research and demonstration aspects was the *identification of verbal developmental cusps and capabilities* and *ways to induce them* based on Skinner's verbal behavior theory and research testing the theory's utility for inducing verbal capabilities that were missing in children with language delays (e.g., children with autism spectrum disorders, children from economically disenfranchised communities). Research in stimulus equivalence, relational frame theory, and research experimentally identifying instructional histories that result in productive verbal behavior all contribute to the validity of higher order operant and respondent classes. Taken together this work suggests that no treatments of language in linguistics, anthropology, and neuroscience cannot ignore the contributions of verbal behavior. Most importantly, we now have powerful procedures to induce verbal development capabilities in children; consequently, we can teach children educational objectives that were impossible for them to learn without these. We can save more children with these developmental intervention protocols. As the answers to old questions lead us to new questions we hope to find new procedures that will save even more children.

REFERENCES

Barnes-Holmes, D., Barnes-Holmes, Y., and Cullinan, V. (2001). Relational frame theory and Skinner's *Verbal Behavior. The Behavior Analyst,* 23, 69-84.

Brophy, J.E. (January 1983). If only it were true: A response to Greer. *The Educational Researcher,* 10-13.

Bushel, Jr., D., and Baer, D.M. (1994). Measurably superior instruction means close continual contact with the relevant outcome data. Revolutionary! In R. Gardner et al. (Eds.), *Behavior analysis in education: Focus on measurably superior instruction.* Pacific Groves, CA: Brooks\Cole.

Catania, A.C. (2007). *Learning, interim 4th edition.* Cornwall-on-Hudson, NY: Sloan Publishing.

Chavez-Brown, M. (2005). *The effects of the acquisition of a generalized auditory word match-to-sample repertoire on the echoic repertoire under mand and tact conditions.* (Doctoral dissertation, Columbia University, 2005). Abstract from: UMI Proquest Digital Dissertations [on-line]. Dissertations Abstracts Item: AAT 3159725.

Chavez-Brown, M., and Greer, R.D. (in press). The effect of auditory matching on echoic responding. *The Analysis of Verbal Behavior.*

Decasper, A.J and Spence, M.J. (1987). Prenatal maternal speech influences on newborn's perception of speech sounds. *Infant Behavior and Development,* 2, 133-150.

Dewey, J. (1916). *Democracy and education: An introduction to the philosophy of education.* New York: Macmillan.

Dinsmoor, J.A. (1983). Observing and conditioned reinforcement. *Behavioral and Brain Sciences,* 6, 693-728.

Donahoe, J.W. and Palmer, D.C. (2004). Learning and complex behavior. Richmond, VA: Ledgetop Publishing.

Donley, C.R., and Greer, R.D. (1993). Setting events controlling social verbal exchanges between students with developmental delays. *Journal of Behavioral Education,* 3, 387-401.

Emurian, H. (2004). A programmed-instruction tutoring system for Java: A consideration of learning performance and software self-efficacy. *Computers in Human Behavior,* 20, 423-459.

Emurian, H.H., Hu, X., Wang, J., and Durham, A.G. (2000). Learning Java: A programmed instruction approach using Applets. *Computers in Human Behavior,* 16, 395-422.

Feliciano, G. (2006). *Induction of the listener half of naming in children with little on no speech.* Unpublished Doctoral Dissertation, Columbia Universality.

Fiorile, C.A. and Greer, R.D. (2007). The induction of naming in children with no echoic-to-tact responses as a function of multiple exemplar instruction. *The Analysis of Verbal Behavior*, 23, 71-85.

Gautreaux, G., Keohane, D.D., and Greer, R.D. (2003, July). *Transformation of production and selection functions in geometry as a function of multiple exemplar instruction.* Paper presented at the First Congress of the European Association for Behavior Analysis, Parma, Italy.

Gilic, L. (2005). *Development of naming in two-year-old children.* (Doctoral dissertation, Columbia University, 2005). Abstract from: UMI Proquest Digital Dissertations [on-line]. Dissertations Abstract Item: AAT 3188740.

Greer, R.D. (1998). Comprehensive Application of Behavior Analysis to Schooling (CABAS®). In Howard Sloane (Ed.), *What works in education?* Cambridge, MA: Cambridge Center for Behavioral Studies. (Reprinted in *Behavior and Social Issues,* 1998).

Greer, R.D. (January 1983). Contingencies of the science and technology of teaching and prebehavioristic research practices in education. *Educational Researcher, 12,* pp. 3-9.

Greer, R.D. (January, 1983b). Straightening the nail: A rejoinder. *Educational Researcher*, pp. 13-14.

Greer, R.D. (1980). *Design for music learning.* New York, NY: Teachers College Press.

Greer, R.D. (2002). *Designing teaching strategies: An applied behavior analysis systems approach.* New York: Academic Press.

Greer, R.D. (1994). The measure of a teacher. In R. Gardner III, D. M. Sainato, J. O. Cooper, T. E. Heron, W. L. Heward, J. W. Eschelman, and T. A. Grossi (Eds.), *Behavior analysis in education: Focus on measurably superior instruction* (pp.161-171). Pacific Groves, CA: Brooks/Cole.

Greer, R.D. (2005). Opinion: The two subject matters of behavior analysis and early intervention. *Journal of Early and Intensive Behavioral Interventions, 1 (2), 239-245.* http://www.behavior-analyst-online.org

Greer, R.D. (September 2007). Teaching as a specialization in applied behavior analysis: What we have learned in 26 years of CABAS®. Cambridge Center Newsletter.

Greer, R.D. (1991). Teaching practices to save America's schools: The legacy of B. F. Skinner. *Journal of Behavioral Education,* 1, 159-164.

Greer, R.D., Chavez-Brown, M., Nirgudkar, A.S., Stolfi, L., and Rivera-Valdes, C.L. (2005). Acquisition of fluent listener responses and the educational advancement of young children with autism and severe language delays. *European Journal of Behavior Analysis,* 6, 88-126.

Greer, R.D., and Keohane, D. (2004). A real science and technology of teaching. In D. J. Moran and R. W. Malott, (Eds.*)*, *Evidence-Based Educational Methods* (pp. 23-46). New York: Elsevier/Academic Press.

Greer, R.D., and Keohane, D.D. (2005). The evolution of verbal behavior in children. *Behavioral Development Bulletin,* 1, 31-47. Reprinted in 2006 in the *Journal of Speech and Language Pathology: Applied Behavior Analysis*, Volume 1. http://www.behavior-analyst-today.com

Greer, R.D., Keohane, D.D., and Healy, O. (2002). Quality and applied behavior analysis. *The Behavior Analyst Today,* 3, 120-132. http://www.behavior-analyst-today.org.

Greer, R.D., and McCorkle, N.P. (2003). *CABAS® international curriculum and inventory of repertoires for kindergarten.* Yonkers, NY: CABAS® and The Fred S. Keller School.

Greer, R. D., McCorkle. N.P., and Williams, G. (1989). A sustained analysis of the behaviors of schooling. *Behavioral Residential Treatment,* 4, 113-141.

Greer, R.D., and McDonough, S. (1999). Is the learn unit the fundamental measure of pedagogy? *The Behavior Analyst,* 20, 5-16.

Greer, R.D., and Ross, D.E. (2004). Research in the Induction and Expansion of Complex Verbal Behavior. *Journal of Early Intensive Behavioral Intervention.* 1. 141-165. http://www.behavior-analyst-online.org.

Greer, R.D., and Ross, D.E., (2008). *Verbal behavior analysis: Inducing and expanding complex communication in children severe language delays*. Boston: Allyn and Bacon. (Scheduled for release in May 2007).

Greer, R.D., Singer-Dudek, J, and Gautreaux, G. (2006). Observational learning. *International Journal of Psychology,* 42, 1-14.

Greer, R.D., Stolfi, L., Chavez-Brown, M., and Rivera-Valdez, C. (2005). The emergence of the listener to speaker component of naming in children as a function of multiple exemplar instruction. *The Analysis of Verbal Behavior,* 21,123-134.

Greer, R.D., Stolfi, L., and Pistoljevic, N. (2007). Emergence of Naming in preschoolers: A comparison of multiple and single exemplar instruction. *European Journal of Behavior Analysis*, 8, 119-131.

Greer, R.D., and O'Sullivan, D. (2006). *Preliminary report of Naming for 2-dimensional stimuli in typically developing first graders.* Unpublished Report Columbia University Teachers College.

Greer, R.D. and Yuan, L. (2008). Kids learn to say the darnedest things. *The Analysis of Verbal Behavior*, 24, 103-121.

Greer, R.D., Yuan, L., and Gautreaux, G. (2005). Novel dictation and intraverbal responses as a function of a multiple exemplar instructional history. *The Analysis of Verbal Behavior,* 21, 99-116.

Hart B.M., and Risley, T.R. (1995). *Meaningful Differences in the Everyday Life of America's Children*. Baltimore, MD: Paul Brookes.

Hayes, S., Barnes-Homes, D., and Roche, B. (2001). *Relational frame theory: A Post Skinnerian of human language and cognition.* New York: Kluwer/Academic Plenum.

Hogin, S.E. (1996). *Essential contingencies in correction procedures for increased learning in the context of the learn unit.* (Doctoral dissertation, Columbia University, 1996). Abstract from: UMI Proquest Digital Dissertations [on-line]. Dissertations Abstracts Item: AAT 9631721.

Horne, P.J., and Lowe, C.F. (1996). On the origins of naming and other symbolic behavior. *Journal of the Experimental Analysis of Behavior,* 65, 185-241.

Horne, J., Lowe, C.F., and Randle, V.R.L. (2004). Naming and categorization in young children II: Listener behavior training. *Journal of the Experimental Analysis of Behavior,* 81, 267-288

Ingham, P., and Greer, R.D. (1992). Changes in student and teacher responses in observed and generalized settings as function of supervisor observations of teachers. *Journal of Applied Behavior Analysis,* 25, 153-164.

Jodlowski, S.M. (2000). *The effects of a teacher editor, peer editing, and serving as a peer editor on elementary students' self-editing behavior.* (Doctoral dissertation, Columbia University, 2000). Abstract from: UMI Proquest Digital Dissertations [on-line]. Dissertations Abstracts Item: AAT 9970212.

Keohane, D.D., Greer, R.D., and Ackerman, S.A. (2006a, May). *Effects of teaching sameness across the senses on acquisition of instructional objectives by pre-listeners and listeners and emergent-speakers.* Paper presented as part of a symposium at the annual international Association for Behavior Analysis, Atlanta, Ga.

Keohane, D.D., Greer, R.D., and Ackerman, S.A. (2006b, May). *The effect of conditioning visual tracking on the acquisition of instructional objectives by pre-listeners and pre-speakers.* Paper presented as part of a symposium at the annual international Association for Behavior Analysis, Atlanta, Ga.

Keohane, D.D., Greer, R.D., and Ackerman, S.A. (2006c, May). *Multiple exemplar training across the senses and the capacity for sameness.* Paper presented as part of a symposium at the annual international Association for Behavior Analysis, Atlanta, Ga.

Keohane, D.D., and Greer, R.D. (2005). Teachers' use of verbally governed algorithm and student learning. *International Journal of Behavioral and Consultation Therapy,* 1, (3) 249-259. Available online at <www.behavior_analyst_today.com

Lamarre, J., and Holland, J. (1985). The functional independence of mands and tacts. *Journal of the Experimental Analysis of Behavior,* 43, 5-19.

Lee Park, H.S. (2005). *Multiple exemplar instruction and transformation of stimulus function from auditory-visual matching to visual-visual matching.* (Doctoral dissertation, Columbia University, 2005). Abstract from: UMI Proquest Digital Dissertations [on-line]. Dissertations Abstracts Item: AAT 3174834.

Lodhi, S., and Greer, R.D. (1989). The speaker as listener. *Journal of the Experimental Analysis of Behavior,* 51, 353-360.

Lovaas, O.I. (1977). *The autistic child: Language development through behavior modification.* New York: Irvington Publishers, Inc.

Lovaas, O.I. (1987). Behavioral treatment and normal educational and intellectual functioning in young autistic children. *Journal of Consulting and Clinical Psychology,* 55, 3-9.

Lowe, C.F., Horne, P.J., Harris, D.S., and Randle, V.R.L. (2002). Naming and categorization in young children: Vocal tact training. *Journal of the Experimental Analysis of Behavior,* 78, 527-549.

Luciano, C., Barnes-Holmes, Y., and Barnes-Holmes, D. (2002). Establishing reports of saying and doing and discriminations of say-do relations. *Research in Developmental Disabilities,* 23, 406-421.

Madho, V. (1997). *The effects of the responses of a reader on the writing effectiveness of children with developmental delays*. (Doctoral dissertation, Columbia University, 1997). Abstract from: UMI Proquest Digital Dissertations [on-line]. Dissertations Abstracts Item: AAT9809740.

Marsico, M. J. (1998). *Textual stimulus control of independent math performance and generalization to reading*. (Doctoral dissertation, Columbia University, 1998). Abstract from: UMI Proquest Digital Dissertations [on-line]. Dissertations Abstracts Item: AAT 9822227.

McGuiness, D. (2004). *Early reading instruction: What science really tells us about how to teach reading*. Cambridge, MA: MIT Press.

Meincke-Matthews, K. (2005). *Induction of metaphorical responses in middle school students as a function of multiple exemplar instruction.* (Doctoral dissertation, Columbia University, 2005). Abstract from: UMI Proquest Digital Dissertations [on-line]. Dissertations Abstracts Item: AAT 3174851.

Meltzoff, A.N. (1996). The human infant as an imitative generalist: A 20-year progress report on infant imitation with implications for comparative psychology. In C.M. Heyes and B.G. Galef, Jr. (Eds), *Social Learning in animals* (pp. 347-370). San Diego, CA: Academic Press.

Meltzoff, A.N., and Moore, M.K. (1983). Newborn infants imitate adult facial gestures. *Child Development,* 54, 702-709.

Miguel, C.F. and Petursdottir, A.I. (in press). Naming and frames of coordination. In Y. Barnes-Holmes and R.A Rehfeldt (Eds.), *Derived relational responding: Applications for learners with autism and other developmental disabilities.* Oakland, CA: New Harbinger Publications.

Nuzzolo-Gomez, R., and Greer, R.D. (2004). Emergence of untaught mands or tacts with novel adjective-object pairs as a function of instructional history. *The Analysis of Verbal Behavior,* 24, 30-47.

Paniagua, F. A., and Baer, D. M. (1982). The analysis of correspondence training as a chain reinforceable at any point. *Child Development,* 53, 786-98.

Peirce, C. S. (1935). In C. Hartshorne and P. Weiss (Eds.). *Collected papers of Charles Saunders Peirce.* Cambridge, MA: Harvard University Press.

Petursdottir, A. I., Carr, J. E., and Michaels, J. (2005). Emergence of mands and tacts among preschool children. *The Analysis of Verbal Behavior,* 21, 59-74.

Pinker, S. (1999). *Words and rules*. New York: Perennial.

Pistoljevic, N., and Greer, R.D. (2006). The effects of daily intensive tact instruction on preschool students' emission of pure tacts and mands in non-instructional setting. *Journal of Early and Intensive Behavioral Interventions,* 3.1, 103-120. http://www.behavior-analyst-online.org.

Reilly-Lawson, T. and Greer, R.D. (2007). Teaching the Function of Writing to Middle School Students with Academic Delays. *Journal of Early and Intensive Behavioral Interventions*, 151-169. Available online at http://www.behavior-analyst-online.org

Reilly-Lawson, T., and Walsh, D. (2007). Teaching the social listener reinforcement component of the speaker-listener exchange stage of verbal behavior. Manuscript submitted for publication.

Robinson, A. (1995). *The story of writing: Alphabets, hieroglyphs, and pictograms.* London: Thames and Hudson Ltd.

Rosales-Ruiz, J., and Baer, D.M. (1997). Behavioral cusps: A developmental and pragmatic concept for behavior analysis. *Journal of Applied Behavior Analysis,* 30, 533-544.

Ross, D. E., and Greer, R.D. (2003). Generalized imitation and the mand: Inducing first instances of speech in young children with autism. *Research in Developmental Disabilities,* 24, 58-74.

Schauffler, G., and Greer, R D. (2006). The effects of intensive tact instruction on audience-accurate tacts and conversational units. *Journal of Early and Intensive Behavioral Interventions,* 3.1, *120-132.* http://www.behavior-analyst-online.org

Selinski, J., Greer, R.D., and Lodhi, S. (1991). A functional analysis of the comprehensive application of behavior analysis to schooling. *Journal of Applied Behavior Analysis,* 24, 108-118.

Sidman, M. (1986). Functional analysis of emergent classes. In T. Thompson and M. Zeiler (Eds.), *Analysis and integration of behavioral units* (pp. 213-245). Hillsdale, NJ: Lawrence Erlbaum.

Skinner, B.F. (1968). *A science and technology of teaching.* New York: Appleton, Century, and Crofts.

Skinner, B.F. (1938). *The behavior of organisms: An experimental analysis*. New York: Appleton-Century-Crofts.

Skinner, B.F. (1984). The shame of American education. *The American Psychologist,* 39, 947-954.

Skinner, B. F. (1957, 1992). *Verbal Behavior*. Acton, MA: Copley Publishing Group and the B. F. Skinner Foundation. (Original work published 1957).

Speckman, J. and Greer, R.D. (2009). *Multiple exemplar instruction and the emergence of generative production of suffixes as autoclitic frames*. Manuscript submitted for publication.

Sulzer-Azaroff, B. Drabman, R., Greer, R. D., Hall, R.V., Iwata, B., and O'Leary, S. (Eds.). (1988). *Behavior analysis in education from the Journal of Applied Behavior Analysis, 1968-1987*. Lawrence, KS: Society for the Experimental Analysis of Behavior.

Sundberg, M.L., Michael, J., Partington, J.W., and Sundberg, C.A. (1996). The role of automatic reinforcement in early language acquisition. *The Analysis of Verbal Behavior,* 13, 21-37.

Tsai, H., and Greer, R.D. (2006). Conditioned preference for books and faster acquisition of textual responses by preschool children. *Journal of Early and Intensive Behavioral Interventionsm,*.3.1, 35-60. http://www.behavioranalyst-online.org

Tsiouri, I., and Greer, R.D. (2003). Inducing vocal verbal behavior through rapid motor imitation training in young children with language delays. *Journal of Behavioral Education,* 12, 185-206.

Twyman, J.S. (1996a). *An analysis of functional independence within and between secondary verbal operants*. (Doctoral dissertation, 1998, Columbia University). Abstract from: UMI Proquest Digital Dissertations [on-line]. Dissertations Abstracts Item: AAT 9631793.

Twyman, J.S. (1996b). The functional independence of impure mands and tacts of abstract stimulus properties. *The Analysis of Verbal Behavior,* 13, 1-19.

Vargas, E.A. (1982). Intraverbal behavior: The codic, duplic, and sequelic subtypes. *The Analysis of Verbal Behavior,* 1, 5-7.

Williams, G., and Greer, R.D. (1993). A comparison of verbal-behavior and linguistic communication curricula for training developmentally delayed adolescents to acquire and maintain vocal speech. *Behaviorology,* 1, 31-46.

Yoon, S.Y. (1998). *Effects of an adult's vocal sound paired with a reinforcing event on the subsequent acquisition of mand functions*. (Doctoral dissertation, Columbia University, 1998). Abstract from: UMI Proquest Digital Dissertations [online]. Dissertations Abstracts Item: AAT 9839031.

In: Behavioral Theories and Interventions for Autism
Editor: Phil Reed

ISBN 978-1-60741-165-9
© 2009 Nova Science Publishers, Inc.

Chapter 8

POSITIVE BEHAVIOR SUPPORT: SUPPORTING CHILDREN AND ADULTS WITH AUTISTIC SPECTRUM DISORDERS AND CHALLENGING BEHAVIORS

Ian Grey*[*1], Brian McClean[2], and Niall McCauley[3]
[1]Royal College of Surgeons, Ireland and Medical University of Bahrain, Kingdom of Bahrain
[2]Brothers of Charity Services, Ireland
[3]Health Service Executive, Ireland

INTRODUCTION

In his book *The Ancestor's Tale*, Richard Dawkins describes two distinct species of salamander which do not interbreed, but co-exist at the Southern end of California's central valley. One species dominates the east rim of the valley and the other the west rim. At the north end, however, there is only one species of salamander whose physical traits are a mix of the two species at the other end of the valley. In fact, as you go north along either rim of the valley, each of the species which is so distinct at the south end begins to look more like the other until, at the north end, there is just one homogenous population. There is an obvious parallel with the continuous evolution of Applied Behavior Analysis. Individual mutations are imperceptible, but its practice now is probably utterly unrecognizable from how it was fifty years ago, as different current applications, such as CABAS® and Positive Behavior Support are unrecognizable one from another. Dawkins' genius is to strike a blow against the discontinuous mind. In a world which is supposed to be only black and white, there is no explanation for gray.

Positive Behavior Support may be described as the science of setting events. Of all the variables that co-vary with challenging behavior, it emphasizes those variables which, when removed or ameliorated, may elicit lasting and generalized change in behavior, yielding a net

[*] Please address correspondence to: Dr. Ian Grey Ph.D., D. Clin. Psych. BCBA. Senior Lecturer in Behavioural Sciences, Royal College of Surgeons in Ireland- Medical University of Bahrain, PO Box 15503, Kingdom of Bahrain, e mail: igrey@rcsi-mub.com

increase in the person's quality of life. Interventions are based on the results of functional assessment, which explains behavior based on a descriptive analysis of the factors that are reported or observed to be associated with increases or decreases in the rate of the behavior. To this extent, the methodology employed, called Positive Behavior Support, is derived from Applied Behavior Analysis. However, proponents of Positive Behavior Support argue that it has evolved beyond traditional Applied Behavior Analysis (ABA).

We take as our starting point Horner's (2000) description of the features that characterize Positive Behavior Support. These are (1) behavior support or intervention should not only reduce problem or challenging behaviors but also positively affect the quality of a person's life, (2) a life-span perspective, (3) a concern with ecological validity, (4) an emphasis on stakeholder participation, (5) a consideration of social validity, (6) an emphasis on prevention, (6) flexibility with respect to scientific practices and (7) the use of multiple theoretical perspectives. The question as to whether this exposition of Positive Behavior Support is consistent with the conceptual and practice framework of Applied Behavior Analysis, or has evolved beyond it, is discussed in this chapter.

There has been a clear articulation within the PBS literature that its origins lie within Applied Behavior Analysis, the Normalization/Inclusion Movement and Person Centered Values (Carr et al., 2002) and is probably best viewed as a synthesis of these three areas. The primary goal of PBS is to bring about comprehensive lifestyle change covering dimensions such as social relationships, personal satisfaction, employment, self-determination, recreation and leisure and community integration. Many would argue that focusing on the contexts in which behaviors occur is therefore the primary feature of Positive Behavior Support. The environments of many individuals with developmental disabilities are often deficient at multiple levels. Organizational systems often mitigate against creating and sustaining meaningful change in terms of improving quality of life and reducing problem behaviors. Behavior change is not merely the result of the application of specific techniques to specific challenges (Carr et al., 2002) because the best technology will fail if applied in an unresponsive or disorganized context. This particular emphasis on context leads directly to the other PBS characteristics of multi-component intervention, emphasis on prevention, stakeholder participation, and ecological validity.

To illustrate these characteristics of PBS in practice, the following is a case example of a 13 year old boy with Autistic Spectrum Disorder.

Gary is a charming, energetic 13 year old who has a winning smile and is well loved as the middle brother in a family of three boys. He is thin, healthy and very active. He also has Autistic Spectrum Disorders and severe intellectual disability. He was referred for behavioral intervention after having been suspended from school because of his aggressive behaviors. Gary has hit, kicked, scratched and spat, primarily at his teacher and support staff. These behaviors occur but are less frequent at home, where Gary enjoys familiar routines, freedom of movement and fewer demands. However, he is very active and loud and insistent on snacking regularly.

Six main themes emerged from a functional assessment:

Attention. Gary's ability to rest his attention seems severely compromised. He walks or runs from room to room, and even when he has access to a requested item, such a snack, he may sit for less than a minute before getting up and running to another room.

Organizational abilities. While Gary's gross motor skills are relatively well developed, he can sometimes appear very disorganized. For example, when out walking, he runs on his toes for a few steps, then stops and stoops, as if he is trying to organize his body between inhibiting and disinhibiting responses. Again, when requested to return to classroom, he made several attempts to leave what he is doing, returning to it each time, before finally executing the task requested.

Expressive communication skills. Gary does not use words for communication. He makes his basic needs known by accessing preferred items for himself, and by pointing. Occasionally, he places a hand to his ear, and this is interpreted to mean he may be in pain.

Receptive communication skills. Gary's ability to understand requests in new situations is severely compromised. For example, he made no response when given a verbal prompt to point to a car in front him. He has a picture schedule in his classroom, but appears to require object cues and familiar routines to transition form one activity to another.

Environmental factors. Gary attends school with five other students who have a diagnosis of Autistic Spectrum Disorders, with a teaching staff of five. This means that a total of 11 people share a space that consists of three rooms a hall. The environment can be noisy. Each of the six students follows an individual timetable, with frequent transitions to and from the school. Gary's timetable consists of learning to use pictures to request snacks and to make two way choices, choosing between activities, following verbal requests such as "show me" to select from a visual array, and visual matching and sorting tasks. Each teaching program consists of high rate verbal demand on the part of the instructor.

Antecedents. Based on incident reports for 34 separate incidents of physical aggression in a one month period, it was hypothesized that a majority of incidents occurred at times of unfamiliar situations or transitions.

Consequences. The reactive strategy for responding to Gary's aggressive behavior was to remove the demand and back away. This was followed on most occasions and indeed appeared to be necessary to avoid risk to safety.

As a result of this assessment, it was hypothesized that the function of most of Gary's incidents of aggressive behavior was to communicate "no" or "stop" when he given requests or refusal. This was likely to occur when Gary is over aroused or over-stimulated, when sequences of activity are unpredictable or situations are unfamiliar. A minority of additional incidents occurred without obvious environmental trigger.

A behavior support plan was recommended that involved five main elements

A Low Arousal Environment. Gary moved to an individualized environment. Noise, the frequency of demands, the amount of speech and the loudness of speech were each significantly reduced. In an attempt to explore potential internal sources of stress, Gary had a full medical examination and a food diary. The medical examinations were negative, but the food diary led to a hypothesis of dairy intolerance. Dairy products were removed from his diet. Gary was give free access to healthy, no calorie or low calorie snack.

Rapport Building. Staff were trained in an interaction style protocol of following Gary's lead, naming what he is doing or what he is looking at, waiting for a response from Gary (e.g. a vocalization, a look or a smile) and offering social reinforcement from any request or appropriate social responding. Staff also offered Gary preferred snacks non-contingently, approximately every hour.

Picture Activity Sequencing. When Gary requested an activity using idiosyncratic gestural communication, a picture of that activity was placed on a board. Staff use a "first-then" statement build a two picture activity sequence of "e.g. *first* we will load the dishwasher, *then* we will go for a drive", and a picture of the dishwasher is placed before the picture of the drive on the picture board. Pictures are put away when the activity is completed. Once Gary was using a two picture sequence, a three picture sequence, and then a four picture sequence was introduced.

Reinforcement of Communicating "No". Gary was approached with the pictures in the picture sequence one at a time and the demand was put to him. If he did not respond within 10 seconds, or if he gestured "go away", staff would reinforce his refusal by saying "no" and withdrawing the demand. The demand would then be offered five minutes later

Differential Reinforcement of Low Rates of Behavior. Every time the behavior of spitting was emitted, a token representing a preferred treat was removed. If there was one token left by the end of an activity, an preferred snack (a stick of chewing gum) was exchanged for it. The number of tokens initially presented was systematically reduced.

Interventions were introduced cumulatively. The graph below shows the absolute rate of behavior per week during the first five months of intervention (see Figure 8.1).

Figure 8.1 shows the weekly rate of aggressive behaviors (hitting and hair-pulling) recorded in real time. Interventions were added cumulatively. The graph shows that aggression reduced significantly over the course of intervention, along with the precursor behaviors of hand biting and spitting.

Immediately prior to intervention, Gary's family had reached a point where they were seeking an out of home placement for him. Throughout the intervention, Gary has remained living with his family and attends individualized respite on two nights per week. Gary's family was also involved in the design and directing and monitoring of his day and respite service. Interventions were conducted in naturally occurring settings, not by behavior analysts but by family members and direct care providers. Staff were trained in Positive Behavior Support and designed and re-designed the interventions involved. Particular attention was also paid to the organizational systems needed to implement and sustain the intervention plan across multiple individuals and locations across time.

The main outcome of intervention is net improvement in quality of life, which is reflected in higher levels of engagement with his family, and fewer behaviors at home. Social validity measures indicate that parents regard the changes as highly significant, feel more able to cope with Barry, and can look forward to Gary living at home for the remainder of his teenage years. Gary's brothers report that family life is much less stressful. These included individualized recruitment procedures, staff induction and training in Positive Behavior Support, coaching from intensive support workers and regular team meetings.

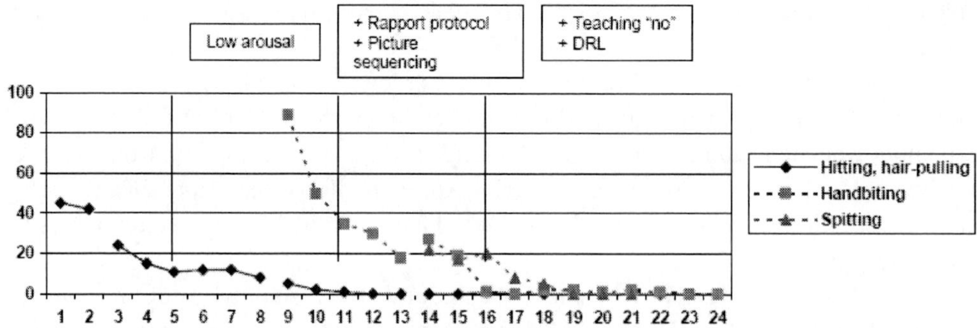

Figure 8.1. Weekly Frequency of Behavior and Cumulative Interventions.

Challenging Behaviors among People with Autistic Spectrum Disorders

The Autistic Spectrum Disorders are pervasive developmental disorders that share a common triad of impairments. These are difficulties with emotional and social understanding; impaired communication and rigidity of thinking or behavior. However, there is very significant heterogeneity of presentation across individuals with the diagnosis. Although many individuals with a diagnosis of autistic spectrum disorders have normal intellectual abilities (so called "high functioning Autistic Spectrum Disorders"), approximately 70% also have a diagnosis of intellectual disability (Baranek et al., 2006). An array of physiological arousal and sensory integration difficulties may accompany the condition. The prevalence of mood instability, psychopathology and particularly anxiety disorders appears strong and appears higher than in the general ID population (Brereton et al, 2007). There is a high co-morbidity of autistic spectrum disorder and both aggressive and self injurious behavior compared with other types of intellectual disability (McClintock 2003; Rojahn et al., 2002; Blancher and McIntyre, 2006). Generally these behaviors are characterized as having a chronic course in Autistic Spectrum Disorders and may be difficult to eliminate or reduce (Murphy, 2005).

Considering the myriad ways in which core features of the disorder (e.g., difficulties with social understanding, impaired expressive ability, rigidity of behavior) can interact with other frequently occurring problems such as sensory integration difficulties (Holden, 2006), it is perhaps not surprising that Autistic Spectrum Disorder is a risk marker for the development of many types of behavioral difficulties. However, research is unclear as to the precise etiology of behavioral difficulties in Autistic Spectrum Disorders or why, for example, many people with diagnosis of Autistic Spectrum Disorders do not present with challenging behavior.

Challenging behaviors such as those described above are frequently a persistent and major cause of isolation and exclusion. In the absence of effective supports people with challenging behaviors can expect exclusion from educational settings, community settings and employment opportunities. Collectively, five themes emerge from the available research regarding Autistic Spectrum Disorders and challenging behaviors: (1) children with Autistic Spectrum Disorders are at significant risk for the development of challenging behaviors (2) in the absence of effective intervention, the trajectory of challenging behaviors is bleak, (3) these behaviors have a detrimental impact on access to and participation in educational, social and community opportunities and a range of quality of life outcomes (e.g. Allen, Lowe, Moore, and Brophy, 2007) (4) these behaviors can have a negative impact beyond the immediate individual to family members, care-givers and professionals (e.g. Feldman, 2007; Hastings and Brown, 2002) and (5) interventions derived from Applied Behavior Analysis have a considerable evidence base in reducing the frequency of challenging behaviors, though their implementation rate can be quite low. What is needed is an intervention or support methodology that has a range of outcomes that is not only effective in reducing behavior but that creates durable behavior change that generalizes across situations, without negative side effects, and which has personal validity (i.e. improves the person quality of life) and social validity (i.e. is positively valued by significant others; LaVigna and Willis, 1995; McClean, Grey, and McCracken, 2007; McGill, 2006)

APPLIED BEHAVIOR ANALYSIS

Applied Behavior Analysis (ABA) is the application of principles of behavior derived from the experimental analysis of behavior, which is based upon the philosophy of radical behaviorism (Skinner, 1953). Its core features of were articulated in the seminal article by Baer and colleagues (1968). They outlined seven key dimensions of ABA which continue to define it and represent the criteria by which behavior analytic work is evaluated (Baer, Wolf, and Risley, 1987). First, ABA is the application of principles of learning to behaviors of social significance. Second, ABA is behavioral, meaning it uses direct measures of participant's behaviors and does not rely on inferential measures of behavior. Third, ABA is analytical meaning that methodologies are selected that allow for experimental demonstrations of functionality consistent with the second criterion. Fourth, ABA is technological meaning that variables are defined operationally and at such a level that they could be readily replicated. Fifth, ABA is conceptually systematic in that it only uses procedures and interpretations of results that are consistent with experimental analysis of behavior and the philosophy of radical behaviorism. Sixth, ABA is effective meaning that it changes the participant's behavior and that these changes are of benefit to them. Finally, ABA is concerned with generality, which means that behavior change should last over time, in different environments, spread to other behaviors not directly treated by the intervention, and continue after intervention.

Since its original application, ABA has shown itself to be effective in reducing the frequency of challenging behavior for individuals with developmental disabilities and Autistic Spectrum Disorders. In summarizing of this body of work, Horner et al., (2002) state that "*the central contributions of this approach to reducing problem behaviors have been the documentation of behavioral mechanisms that describe the relationship between environmental events and the occurrence of specific behaviors and the development of specific strategies for measuring behavior change across time*" (Horner, Carr, Strain, Todd, and Reed, 2002, p. 424-425). The clinical technology that has developed from ABA has been impressive because of its effectiveness in reducing problem behaviors as demonstrated by several hundred single case studies, large outcome studies and meta-reviews (Didden et al, 1997; Campbell, 2003; McClean et al., 2005; Scotti et al., 1991).

These effects have been reported to be independent of location; nature or extent of intellectual disability; gender and age. For example, in a review of interventions to reduce challenging behaviors in school settings for children with Autistic Spectrum Disorders, Machalicek et al. (2007) identified twenty-six studies between 1995 and 2005. Interventions were categorized into one of four categories (1) antecedent manipulations (2) change in instructional content (c) differential reinforcement and (d) self-management techniques. Again, similar findings of effectiveness were reported.

The contribution of ABA has been impressive without doubt. However, it can be argued that ABA has provided only limited access to the full range of environmental events that influence behavior. Early arguments called for a more ecological systems approach to the study of behavior by examining the possible 'side-effects' of behavioral intervention (Willems, 1974) and the inclusion of subjectively measured social validation (Wolf, 1978). Another continuing criticism of ABA relates to the undue emphasis "on the relatively simple and temporally proximate conditions of behavior influence, i.e., the immediate antecedents and consequences for behavior" (Wahler and Fox, 1981, p. 328).

In short, the core argument is that more complex and temporally distant variables or 'setting events' also affect behavior, may have more long term or generalized impact upon behavior, and certainly require investigation.

THE THREE TERM-CONTINGENCY

Most behavioral explanations of challenging behavior rely conceptually on the three term contingency (Skinner, 1953). The rate of behavior, according to this account, is controlled by the consequences occurring after such behaviors and these serve to reinforce or punish the future probability of their occurrence. The person engages in aggressive behavior, for example, in order to elicit attention or to escape from certain tasks or situations. Variation in the rate of delivery of reinforcers helps predict variation in the rate of behavior, such as the behavioral effects observed under various schedules of reinforcement. Behaviors are also under the control of a discriminative stimulus. In other words there is a signal in the environment that reinforcement is available if the behavior is performed, and the probability of behavior increases in response to this stimulus. Functional analysis, or analogue methodology, is the experimental demonstration of one or both forms of control and is perhaps the dominant form of published accounts of contemporary behavioral assessment.

The three term contingency is a useful heuristic for a number of intervention or support strategies. Take for example a behavior maintained by escape from task. Support strategies might include consequence based strategies, such as reinforcing participation or withholding escape (escape extinction), and antecedent-control strategies such as elimination of the task, reducing the difficulty or duration of the task, or improving the availability of preferred activity. The range of support strategies available is wider still when one adopts a behavior constructional perspective. This asks what functionally equivalent behavior could replace the target behavior. Based upon the matching law (Hernstein, 1970), a new behavior will be displayed if it elicits more valuable reinforcement, more reliable reinforcement, or more immediate reinforcement; - or if it requires less effort (cognitive or physical); - than the original target behavior. In the escape-maintained behavior described above, the behavior support plan can include differential reinforcement of socially preferred or non-injurious forms of escape, refusal or requests for help. A person can be offered the same task (discriminative stimulus), but is prompted to lift the red card to communicate "I need a break" and this is reinforced immediately with preferred escape, every time it is reinforced correctly. Teaching consists of fading the physical prompt to lift the red card so that it is being lifted independently, and thinning the frequency and reliability with which the red card leads to escape. Figure 8.2 offers a schematic representation of the three term contingency.

In Figure 8.2 aggressive behavior has been learned as a response to task, and the behavior is rewarded by escape. An intervention plan prompts the person to say "no" or to lift a red card to communicate. If this is more likely to lead to escape, or likely to lead to a higher value escape, or likely to lead to more immediate escape, then the probability saying no or lifting a red card replacing aggressive behavior increases.

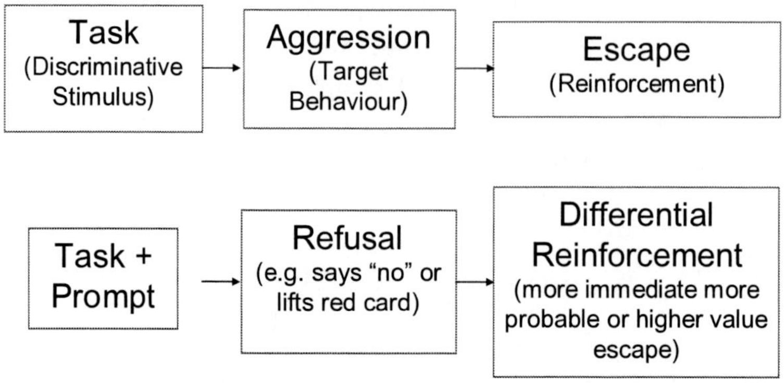

Figure 8.2. Example of three term contingency.

SETTING EVENTS: A FOUR-TERM CONTINGENCY

An ongoing criticism of applied behavior analysis is the primary focus on temporally immediate stimulus events, that is an exclusive reliance on the three term contingency. Such criticisms and arguments for an expansion of the behavioral unit to include more complex relationships have been in existence for almost fifty years. For example, Kantor's interbehavioral psychology (Kantor, 1959), called for an investigation of setting events; - as distinct from stimulus events that were simple, discrete, and immediate (Wahler and Fox, 1981, p. 329). Setting events, by contrast, were conceptualized as more complex conditions such as durational events (i.e., presence or absence of a person) or states of deprivation. Setting events were later expanded to include both those environmental events and the person's responses to them which might subsequently facilitate or inhibit later inter-behavioral relationships. In a classic example, Krantz and Risley (1977) describe a study in a kindergarten class where an antecedent period of vigorous activity set the occasion for reduced attention to the teacher and more disruptive behavior during a subsequent story reading activity. The earlier activity served as a setting event for the reduced attention which occurred at a later point in time. Manipulation of this type of setting event (i.e., providing a rest period antecedent to the story reading session) was as effective as the use of contingency management procedures in the control of inappropriate behavior.

Bijou and Baer (1978) proposed that setting events could include biological variables such as pain, tiredness or menstruation; physical environmental variables such as noise or light; and interpersonal variables such as expectations, presence of other people. Willis and LaVigna (1996) propose a fourth category of programmatic or instructional variables such as task difficulty or variety; choice or predictability.

It is necessary to propose setting events to explain variations in the rate of behavior in the absence of variation in the presentation of antecedents or consequences. Setting events can include personal characteristics, physiological conditions, and environmental factors that establish or exaggerate; abolish or inhibit the probability of behaviors. They include cognitive and communicational abilities, environmental factors such as noise, predictability of activities and of preferred activities, life events, health and medical status. Laraway, Snycerski, Michael and Poling (2003) proposed the term motivating operation as the term for any environmental variable that alters the effectiveness of some object or event as a reinforcer.

While distal antecedents co-vary with behavior in the same way as immediate antecedents do, setting events may also act as super-ordinate variables, providing the necessary conditions for behavior to occur. For example, a task may be the discriminative stimulus for behavior under the condition of a pain, but the same request may not lead to behavior in the absence of pain. Pain thus acts as a motivating operation if it temporarily alters the effectiveness of a stimulus as a reinforcer and evokes behavior likely to produce that reinforcer. Establishing operations may be internal or external, recent or distal. Setting events may also be permanent characteristics of the person or the environment which gives the reinforcer value. For example, one characteristic of Autistic Spectrum Disorders that sets the occasion for challenging behavior is difficulty with verbal memory. An environment which compensates by using visual schedule may increase the predictability of tasks, breaks and changes to routine. In an explanatory model of behavior with setting events, the immediate antecedents may be mere catalysts in a much more long acting behavioral equation.

Few large scale studies on setting events are available. The variables that have been researched are also few in number and largely limited to topics such as otitis media and sleep deprivation (Kennedy and Itkonen, 1993; Kennedy and Meyer, 1996; O'Reilly, 1997). In one study on the relationship between setting events and challenging behavior, McGill, Teer, Rye, and Hughes, (2005) developed an ecological interview with categories that contained, as much as possible, all elements of the "immediate setting containing that person" (Bronfenbenner, 1977, p. 514). Using staff as respondents, the authors reported that the most frequently perceived setting event was mood. Explanatory accounts of behavior using mood are considered tautological by traditional behavior analysts yet they are often considered as a particular type of setting event (e.g. Carr, Magito-McLaughlin, Giacobbe-Grieco, and Smith, 2003). Respondents also rated "doing nothing" as a major category of setting event along with problems in both expressive and receptive communication. Different categories of setting event contributed to different amounts of variance to challenging behaviors. The authors found that although little research attention has been given to the contributions of variables such as client characteristics, staff characteristics, time of year, weather, physical setting, personal and social context; the contribution of these variables to variance in challenging behaviors was approximately 30%.

In an examination of the results of 66 behavioral analyses of functions for challenging behavior, McClean, and Grey (2006) identified that 77% of all challenging behavior was related to escape, a finding similar to existing meta-reviews of the functions of challenging behaviors. Setting events such as confusion, criticism, change of schedule and over-stimulation accounted for the greatest proportion of escape functions. Although the study found no evidence of differential effectiveness of setting event based interventions, setting event interventions were rated by staff as the most effective more frequently than any other component of multi-element behavior interventions.

The limited amount of research in this area may be in substantial part due to the benchmark of experimental manipulation as identified by Smith and Iwata (1997) who state that "the primary goal of research on antecedent variables in behavioral disorders should be the development of research methods that permit experimentally sound analyses of antecedent effects" (p. 369). In effect they call for the demonstration of functional relations through functional analysis to tease apart the complex relations between antecedent, response and consequence relations. Yet, they also conclude that the field of applied behavior analysis has not reached the point where such analyses can effectively inform practice. In a sense, a 'catch-22' situation has evolved where intervention selection may be more readily drawn from well-established consequent operations such as reinforcement and punishment and less from antecedent interventions where the research base is limited. Research of the nature called for by Smith and Iwata (1997) would help in the understanding of behavior disorders yet in its absence the question arises as to what practitioners can do with setting events which relate to features of Autistic Spectrum Disorders. Three common examples of setting event hypotheses will now be considered; arousal, interaction and predictability.

SETTING EVENT HYPOTHESES

The Arousal Hypothesis

In a study using measures of cardiovascular reactivity to environmental stressors, (Goodwin et al., 2006) observed that while children with Autistic Spectrum Disorders showed decreased cardiovascular variance in response to potential stressors in an experimental situation, this was most likely due to high basal heart rates. They identified that all children with Autistic Spectrum Disorders showed a heart rate twenty beats per minute higher than typically developing children. Heightened arousal may enable or exaggerate the effect of a wide range of antecedents, such as task, demand or refusal. It may also play a very important role in constraining the effectiveness of behavioral interventions.

Despite several decades of phenomenological accounts of abnormal sensory processing in children and adults with Autistic Spectrum Disorders, arousal is an area that not attracted as much empirical and intervention attention and certainly little within the field of applied behavior analysis. Measures for assessing autonomic nervous system arousal in routine clinical practice are not well developed and the relationships between it and antecedent stimuli for the occurrence of challenging behaviors poorly developed. In general, two patterns of abnormal sensory processing have been identified: hypo-responsiveness and hyper-responsiveness (Baranek et al., 2006). Hypo-responsiveness is defined as either lack of response or insufficient intensity of response to stimuli (e.g., diminished response to pain, to social stimuli and poor orientation towards novel stimuli). In contrast, hyper-responsiveness is defined as an exaggerated behavioral response to sensory stimuli such as (e.g., covering ears to avoid sounds, avoidance of touch and aversive reaction to lights). Though sensory symptoms are not unique to Autistic Spectrum Disorders, it appears that the rate of these symptoms is higher in children with Autistic Spectrum Disorders than in typically developing children and children with other disabilities. The exact nature of the relationship between sensory abnormalities and core features (Rogers, Hepburn, and Wehner, 2003) remains to be identified as is the relationship between sensory abnormalities and autonomic arousal. Sensory related questions are evident in several of the most frequently used in Autistic Spectrum Disorders assessment instruments including the ADOS, CARS and ADI. There is evidence using parental report that such sensory abnormalities are evident from as early as 24 months and occur at higher rates than in against typically developing children and in others developmentally delayed though with the same mental age. Furthermore, it appears that higher rates of sensory abnormalities are associated with specific diagnoses such as Autistic

Spectrum Disorders and Fragile X syndrome rather than with developmental level (Rogers et al., 2003).

Meta-reviews of challenging behaviors frequently cite escape from aversive stimuli as major functional etiological and maintaining categories for challenging behavior. However, functional analytic methodology (i.e., analogue assessment) has contributed to a dominance of consequence-based interventions. For instance, in the treatment of escape typical consequence-based, interventions include (a) escape extinction, (b) provision of preferred stimuli contingent upon task performance, (c) allowing escape contingent on functionally equivalent socially acceptable behavior and (d) combining escape training with instructional fading. Setting event interventions that may reduce the value of escape from auditory hyper arousal as reinforcement could include reducing the amount of noise, the amount, volume, pace or complexity of verbal language are equally worthy of consideration, but are not studied. Similarly, the hypothesis that over-arousal may be ameliorated by providing short or long breaks from auditory stimuli merits investigation.

The Interaction Hypothesis

A second hypothesis concerning a putative effect of an overarching variable in the challenging behavior of a person with Autistic Spectrum Disorders is the interaction or rapport between the person with Autistic Spectrum Disorders and significant others in the environment. The role of rapport has been highlighted by McLaughlan and Carr (2005) among others, who found evidence of the role of rapport as a setting event to behavior. When rapport was poor, levels of problem behavior were high; when rapport was good, levels of problem behavior were low. The authors evaluated the effectiveness of a multi -element plan designed to improve rapport between the person with disabilities and his or her caregiver. When rapport improved, participants showed a decrease in problem behavior and an increase in task completion in the presence of staff members who had previously been identified as having poor rapport with participants. The primary importance of rapport is recognized noted in most ABA programs, which recommend pairing the instructor with positive reinforcement prior to the presentation of specific requests or demands on the individual.

Joint attention refers to the propensity of a child to engage another's attention to share enjoyment of objects or events. Children display joint attention skills by initiating behaviors to others to pay attention to what they are attending to and by following the line of visual regard and point gestures of a social partner (Mundy and Thorp, 2005). Joint attention represents a critical area in typical development, emerging between the ages of 9 and 15 months. Joint attention skills have been found to be concurrently related to receptive and expressive language skills among typically-developing children. In addition, research indicates that joint attention is important for the development of a host of other, later-emerging, skills, such as more complex expressive language, symbolic play, and theory of mind.

Impairments in the development of joint attention skills are a hallmark of children with Autistic Spectrum Disorders spectrum disorders. While children with Autistic Spectrum Disorders do not differ from typically-developing children in the amount of requesting behaviors, they exhibit far fewer joint attention behaviors (Mundy et al. 1994; Mundy et al. 1996). While children with Autistic Spectrum Disorders consistently used gestural communication to request objects or actions, they rarely attempted to direct adults' attention through the use of gestures (Wetherby and Prizant, 1984). Kasari, Sigman, Mundy, and Yirmiya (1990) have further noted that, even when joint attention is shown, children with Autistic Spectrum Disorders are much less likely than either typically developing or other developmentally delayed children to display positive affect along with joint attention behaviors, so that initial joint attention bids may not be as reinforcing for the parent or others.

This body of research implies that joint attention skills may play a pivotal role in the early development of young children with Autistic Spectrum Disorders. ABA research literature defines pivotal skills as those which, "once strengthened, result in positive changes in other areas of functioning and improvements in subsequent learning" (Jones and Carr, 2004). Evidence for joint attention's role as a pivotal skill is provided by research indicating that there may be a significant interaction between individual differences in joint attention development and later outcome (Charman, 2003; Sigman and Ruskin, 1999). Therefore, it appears especially important to develop interventions to improve joint attention skills in children with Autistic Spectrum Disorders. Some studies have focused on improving the capacity of young children to initiate bids for joint attention. Research in this area has suggested that one effective strategy may be the contingent imitation of children's actions by adults (Dawson and Galpert, 1990; Klinger and Dawson, 1992; Field et al., 2001). Another strategy is to target the behaviors that children use to respond to the joint attention bids of others. This is because responding to joint attention has been found to be related to the development of receptive and expressive language. Ability to engage in joint attention may be critically important for the ability to learn from the environment (naturalistic learning), as opposed to being taught discrete skills in isolation, one of the main bugbears of critics of traditional Applied Behavior Analysis.

A primary criterion for the diagnosis of Autistic Spectrum Disorders is the disconnectedness of the person from the behavior of others. Either the behavior of others is not discriminated by the person, or the person is not reinforced by typical social responses such as praise. The latter may be due to a learning history that has associated social interaction with auditory or tactile over-stimulation, or to a learning history in Autistic Spectrum Disorders in which the social and verbal reinforcement for social responding have become desynchronized from behavior due to specifically slow response times to these forms of stimuli. Pivotal Response Training incorporates a set of specific procedures that may be conceptualized in terms of setting events because they provide contextual variables that enhance the reinforcing value of stimuli. These include allowing a significant amount of choice over the nature of the interaction and materials, reinforcing attempts to respond, and varying tasks frequently. The procedures are more natural because they more closely resemble typical interactions and are utilized in ongoing, natural activities. The potential effectiveness of Pivotal Response Training in establishing and maintaining a repertoire of social behavior may be greatly enhanced if it is implemented by typical peers. In addition, investigating this type of naturalistic procedure is important because of its flexibility and utility not only in the classroom but also on the playground, and in the family. Pivotal Response can use materials in the natural environment (e.g., household objects, toys), and it need not be administered in a rigid, artificial manner. Research attests to the viability of this methodology its capacity to promote generality across stimuli and across collateral behaviors, such as language and attention and social validity (E.g. Murphy, Grey and Honan, 2005; Pearce and Schreibman, 1995).

The Predictability Hypothesis

A third hypothesis regarding settings events and challenging behavior concerns the predictability of events. The lives of many individuals with Autistic Spectrum Disorders are typically characterized by a large degree of uncertainty as to (1) whether and when both preferred and non preferred events will happen and (2) the content and duration of those events. This uncertainty is generated by a mismatch between the reliance on typical environments to provide verbal descriptions about these two domains and characteristics of the individual with Autistic Spectrum Disorders which frequently entail difficulties with attending to, regulating, and understanding auditory input (Hodgdon, 1995). As a result, a broad category of intervention that has developed has been the use of visual activity schedules (Bryan and Gast, 2000). Green et al., (2006) reported that in a sample of 552 parents of children with Autistic Spectrum Disorders, over 43% reported they were currently implementing visual schedules and a further 19% had reported using them in the past. While it has been previously hypothesized that individualized schedules may operate as a form of antecedent intervention to reduce challenging behavior as they limit the impact of various setting events such as unpredictable transitions and stressful activities (O' Reilly et al., 2004), there is a discrepancy between the apparent rates of implementation of such supports and empirical studies supporting their effectiveness in a variety of domains such as challenging behavior and task engagement. This may be at least partly related to two issues, (1) the dominance of consequence based interventions and (2) differences in conceptual underpinning and procedural implementation of schedules.

Few studies have however examined the effects of providing information regarding task sequence, task onset, task duration, task content, and consequences for task performance on rates of escape motivated challenging behavior. All of these dimensions may be regarded as relating to predictability and collectively, studies investigating predictability as a setting event are far fewer in number, and have not kept pace with consequence based interventions.

A number of contemporary lines of research also point to the importance of prediction of an event and challenging behavior. For example, Derrickson et al. (1993) reported that signaling the occurrence of aversive hospital events reduced the frequency of negative behaviors such as crying in a nine month old developmentally delayed infant in between the occurrence of those events. In a school context, Flannery and Horner (1995) evaluated the effects of predictability signals on the rates of escape behaviors for two individuals with moderate to severe intellectual disabilities and Autistic Spectrum Disorders and reported that information on sequence, duration and content of tasks reduced the frequency of aberrant behaviors. Lalli et al. (1994) examined the effects of two daily visual activity schedules (one with textual prompts and one with visual depictions of corresponding events) and reported than frequency of challenging behaviors decreased as compliance with the schedule increased.

Another important aspect of stimuli that predict reinforcement to be considered is not only that reinforcement is coming, but also *when* it is due. Vollmer, Borrero, Lalli, and Daniel (1999) demonstrated that individuals with developmental disabilities and severe challenging behaviors were more likely to exhibit self-control than impulsive choices when longer delays for reinforcement were signaled rather than unsignaled. They also called for further investigation into 'timed' delays.

The above research clearly indicates that 'prediction' has an impact on behavior but it is clear from the available research that schedules are used in several different ways. Firstly, scheduling in some contexts refers to the sequencing of activities in particular ways without visual prompts or without signaling. For example, O'Reilly et al. (2005) assessed the effects of a schedule on the level of task engagement and frequency of challenging behavior in a young boy with Autistic Spectrum Disorders. The schedule was characterized by following brief academic demand sessions with access to play sessions which were non-contingent upon either academic performance or occurrence of challenging behavior. The results indicated that levels of task engagement increased and challenging behavior decreased as a function of the schedule. The use of schedules in this manner may however present some ecological difficulties as the individual may become reliant on a fixed schedule and may not tolerate the frequent changes in schedule that characterize most service settings.

Secondly, schedules are usually used in conjunction with visual supports and represent some of the most common uses of schedules for individuals with Autistic Spectrum Disorders. Such schedules have been reported to be useful in successful transitions (Earles et al., 1998), increasing physical activity (Zimbelman et al., 2007) and skill acquisition across a variety of domains (Kranz, McDuff and McClannahan, 1993). Surprisingly, there is little study of their effects on challenging behavior. Their effect may be due to signaling as they may provide information on when reinforcement will occur, such as the end of a sequence, but research is required. An additional topic that requires focus is their role with respect to more distal events. Anecdotal evidence suggests that the prediction of more distal, low frequency events (can often be highly problematic (e.g., Halloween, birthdays), and preferred activities (e.g., going to the cinema, going to the swimming pool, going home for the weekend) using countdown calendars can alleviate challenging behaviors, but there is little research in this area.

The Assessment of Setting Events

Currently there are three methods for the assessment of setting events; experimental manipulation; direct observation and interview. The most rigorous of these is usually held to be experimental manipulation, which is referred to as *functional analysis*. However, there are at least four sets of problems s associated with this methodology in most applied settings;

Internal validity. Possible sources of artefact in analogue assessment include multiple contingencies in single analogue conditions, adaptation to analogue conditions, carry-over effects, and new learning.

Test – retest reliability. Analogue assessments may be no more objective in their interpretation of test results than descriptive assessments. Martin, Gaffan and Williams (1999) found agreement rates of 35 per cent between analogue assessments conducted just sixteen weeks apart.

Clinical utility. Analogue assessment is only useful for high rate behaviors. In an Irish sample, only 2 per cent of the population of people with challenging behaviors has behaviors that are frequent enough to be subjected to 15-minute analogue assessment conditions (McClean and Walsh, 1995). Other total population surveys of the frequency of challenging behaviors support this finding (e.g. Harris, 1993; Oliver et al., 1987). One of the great ironies of analogue assessment is that interview and observation are usually required prior to analogue assessment in order to generate the hypotheses upon which the experimental conditions are based. The challenge for proponents of analogue assessment is not simply to demonstrate efficacy of interventions based on analogue assessment, but to demonstrate the incremental gain in effectiveness over interventions that are selected from eth results of observation alone.

Ethical concerns. Many services settings do not consider it ethical to sct knowingly the occasion for higher rates of challenging behavior for the purpose of behavior assessment (Rapp, 1994). In these settings naturalistic hypothesis-testing techniques rather than analogue assessments are required.

The challenge for Positive Behavior Support is to develop practical assessment instruments that allow the practitioners to identify relationships between variables related to the occurrence and maintenance of problem behavior and allows them to effectively intervene. Examples of these include the Behavior Assessment Guide (Willis, LaVigna, and Donnellan, 1993); the Functional Assessment Interview (O'Neill et al, 1990); ABC Incident Analysis (Willis and LaVigna, 1993) and the Contextual Analysis Inventory (McAtee, Carr, and Schulte, 2004).

The Intervention Sequence

The primary goal of most behavioral interventions for challenging behavior is to replace the behavior with a more appropriate alternative, and to ensure that the alternative behavior will recruit natural contingencies of reinforcement. Numerous studies have documented that functionally equivalent skills teaching has a significant impact in terms of the reduction of challenging behaviors (Carr and Durand, 1985; Wacker et al., 1990). However several setting event interventions may be necessary to establish or enhance the effectiveness of functionally equivalent skills teaching. A typical intervention sequence is as follows. The first step is the establishment of a low arousal environment. If the child is experiencing over-stimulation or a high degree of stress, efforts to establish rapport or to teach will be less effective. The reinforcement available from any rapport behaviors may not compete effectively with the reinforcement available from escape behaviors for as long as the child experiences high stress. Particularly for dangerous behaviors, the establishment of a low arousal environment will usually involve the control of any idiosyncratic antecedents to the behavior. Once major sources of over-arousal are removed so that the child is not frequently or intensely motivated to engage in escape behavior, the next step is the establishment of rapport and joint attention. If the person associates the presence of an instructor and other contextual features with the possibility of reinforcement, there is a much greater likelihood that the child will orient to an instruction or reinforcement opportunity when presented. The third step in this sequence is to promote predictability using routine activity sequences, transition rituals and visual cues for transitions and activity sequencing. Visual cues can be used to the onset and offset of tasks, progress through tasks or transitions between tasks. The fourth step is the functionally equivalent skills teaching, which precedes the fifth step of using incentive to gain control over behavior because it on the pragmatic (and ethical) grounds that it does not make sense to reward a person for the non performance of challenging behavior until the person has an alternative behavior within the same response class available in his or her behavioral repertoire.

Quality of Life: The Fifth Term

It has been previously mentioned above that a diagnosis of Autistic Spectrum Disorders combined with challenging behavior, can be associated separation from family, less choice and stressful, chaotic environments which place access to meaningful or reinforcing activity or attention at a premium. Improvement in quality of life variables is often promised as an outcome of behavioral interventions, but is seldom measured in published outcome research. Kincaid, Knoster, Harrower, Shannon and Bustamante (2002) specified a number of components to quality of life as the criteria for outcomes of PBS practices. These include (a) emotional well-being (b) interpersonal well-being (c) material well-being (d) personal well-being (e) physical well-being (f) self-determination (g) social inclusion and (h) rights. In one study of quality of life outcomes of positive behavior support with five people with very severe challenging behaviors in community settings, McClean, Grey and McCracken (2007) found significant improvement in the quality of life of three out of the five individuals. Interestingly, scores on the quality of life scores for the two individuals in the study with a diagnosis of Autistic Spectrum Disorders did not change significantly, even though aggressive and self injurious behaviors, respectively, were successfully resolved in both cases.

Increasing the number of times each day that the person experiences choice and preference in daily tasks and activities, preferred foods and preferred possessions have been found to significantly improve behavior (e.g., Malette, 1992), though empirical demonstrations of this are all too rare. Intervention strategies like these could be characterized as setting event strategies, since they alter the establishing operations of behavior. But consider interventions such as increasing family contact in someone who lives away from home, or enabling a person with Autistic Spectrum Disorders to select where and with whom they will live. Could variables such as these play a super-ordinate role to the impact of setting events in explanatory models of individual's challenging behaviors? In other words, if a person with Autistic Spectrum Disorders is well connected with family, has access to meaningful and satisfying activity and is making meaningful choice about the key elements in his or her life, then can the effects of potential setting events such as noise, pain or sleep deprivation be ameliorated? The idea of a super-ordinate role for quality of life variables conflates the values of Person Centered Planning or Social Role Valorization with the methodology of Applied Behavior Analysis as outlined above as a found term contingency.

In Figure 8.3, the role of setting events is included as a fourth term, but quality of life variables are posited as having a super-ordinate role. This leads to the notion of multi-element behavior support plans (LaVigna andWillis, 1995), in which the environment adapted to ameliorate or remove the effect of distal and immediate setting events, skills teaching interventions to provide the person with alternatives to responses for achieving the consequences of behavior, and differential reinforcement strategies designed to maximize the likelihood that non challenging behaviors are selected.

The idea that quality of life variables occupy a super-ordinate role, ameliorating or removing even the impact of setting event themselves is understandably a difficult, though not impossible one to research. However, the notion is at once political as it is scientific. Amanda Baggs, in her video, *In Our Language*, depicts Autistic Spectrum Disorders not as a series of social, communicational and behavioral deficits, but as a constant conversation with her environment.

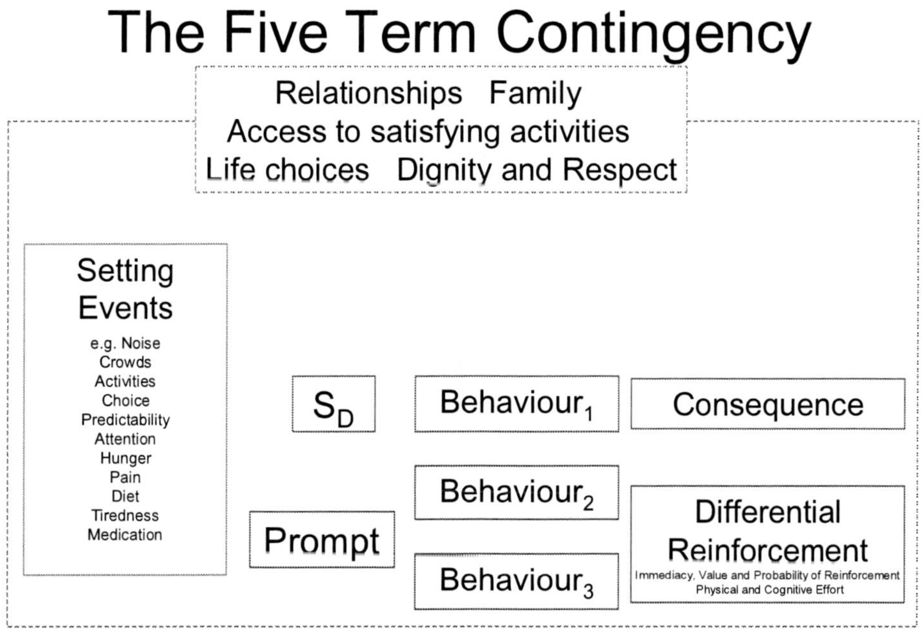

Figure 8.3. The Five Term Contingency.

According to her, the existence or value of different ways of thinking and being in the world determines whether the person with Autistic Spectrum Disorders has any real dignity or rights in the world. The achievement of real dignity and respect for people with Autistic Spectrum Disorders may still appear a far off dream for many with Autistic Spectrum Disorders, and certainly runs contrary to the "treatment" agenda of many advocates of Applied Behavior Analysis, but is the very foundation of the enterprise known as Positive Behavior Support.

Positive Behavior Support and Applied Behavior Analysis

There has been considerable controversy as to whether PBS constitutes a new science (Carr et al., 2002), is merely Applied Behavior Analysis by another name, a service delivery system with philosophical underpinnings (Wacker and Berg, 2002) or even as a delusion of politically minded individuals who have suspended their critical faculties (Mulick and Butter, 2007). There are at least three ways of conceptualizing the relationship between Applied Behavior Analysis and Positive Behavior Support.

Does ABA and PBS Mean the Same Thing?

Positive Behavior Support describes four core practices. Firstly, behavior support should reduce problem behavior and affect how a person lives. Secondly, functional assessment is the foundation for understanding patterns of problem behavior. Thirdly, behavior support should be comprehensive in structure and scope and fourthly the unit of behavioral analysis is expanded beyond the three-term contingency, to setting event variables. These practices echo sharply the original criteria of Baer, Wolf and Risley. However, as Carr et al., (2002) have pointed out, Positive Behavior Support is also characterized by the inclusion of practices from the normalization/inclusion movement and from a concern with person centered values. According to Carr these two conceptions move Positive Behavior Support beyond the original criterion of socially meaningful change into a substantively different conceptual framework (Sailor and Paul, 2004). Positive Behavior Support represents a "melding of values and technology in that the strategies are judged not only with respect to efficacy but also with respect to their ability to enhance personal dignity and opportunities for choice".

Positive Behavior Support differs from Applied Behavior Analysis by encompassing (1) a focus on comprehensive lifestyle change and improvement in quality of life (2) a life-span perspective (3) a concern with ecological validity (4) a focus on stakeholder participation (5) a concern with social validity (5) the use of systems change and multi-component intervention (6) an emphasis on prevention (7) flexibility with respect to scientific practices and (8) the use of multiple-theoretical perspectives. Through this process the person determines the creation of the services they receive rather what the organization may have available. The first six of these aspirations may well be consistent with any modern application of ABA. However, flexibility with regard to scientific practices and the adoption of alternative theoretical perspective would seem to place Positive Behavior Support beyond the definitions of Applied Behavior Analysis. Certainly, putative setting events such as mood or sensory integration difficulties, are not easily measurable, and appear to fall outside the Baer and Wolf definition of behavior analysis. The relationship between challenging behavior and quality of life (as opposed to setting event) intervention is poorly defined as yet, but also may be beyond the remit of a clear behavior analytic framework.

Wraparound services, for example, focus on meeting a person's needs in critical life domain areas such as family, living situation, financial, educational/vocational, social/recreational, behavioral/emotional, psychological, health, legal, cultural and safety (Burns et al, 2000; Eber and Nelson, 1997). Conducting research with these outcomes and implementing interventions with these processes in community settings have induced changes in assessment, intervention practices and the definition of the field. For example, Wolery et al. (2005) examined the content of the Journal of Applied Behavior Analysis (JABA) from its inception in 1968 to 2003. All studies of challenging behaviors from 1968 to 1979 reported using only aversive techniques. Over the entire time-period only 1% examined the effects of providing choices on frequency of challenging behavior and it was not until 1982 that the first articles on replacing challenging behaviors with functional communication training appeared (Carr et al., 1982). Although many of the interventions that are currently cited as examples of Positive Behavior Support are systematically consistent with the principles of Applied Behavior Analysis, almost all interventions described as Applied Behavior Analysis before 1979 are fundamentally inconsistent with the principles of Positive Behavior Support. Self-management and peer modeling appeared as interventions infrequently (2%) and 10% of studies examined environmental arrangements. No article included in the Worley et al analysis included siblings of children with Autistic Spectrum Disorders, only 5% included parents of children and only a further 5% included teachers or other professionals. Ten percent included peers of children with Autistic Spectrum Disorders. Research laboratories, clinics and hospitals accounted for almost a half of all settings and though half were conducted in schools, the majority of school settings were segregated classrooms. By contrast, Clarke and Dunlap (2008) conducted a similar survey of the content of the Journal of Positive Behavior Interventions from 1999 to 2005. They found that two thirds of studies displayed ecological validity, with interventions and measures conducted *in situ* in typical physical, activity and social contexts. By contrast only one fifth of JABA studies occurred in typical contexts in the same time period.

The characteristics of PBS change what are considered appropriate data. If intervention is required at multiple levels then research must also be focused at these various levels and their inter-relationships. For instance, it is a viable hypothesis to speculate that stakeholder participation (e.g., the involvement and collaboration of parents and care-staff) will impact on intervention uptake, outcome and maintenance. Variables such as treatment acceptability and perceived social validity may mediate outcomes and therefore may add to our understanding of the contextual factors affecting uptake. Indeed, recent research does support this (McClean and Grey, 2007). However, such data are more characteristic of the social sciences and is data that typically falls outside the parameters of behavioral theory and practice. Approaches such as ABA have typically focused more on the micro-analysis of environment-behavior relations and investigated macro variables such as relationships between stakeholder participation and outcomes relatively far less. In addition to an expansion in what is considered appropriate data, PBS also draws from other conceptual frameworks beyond operant psychology to include systems theory, social psychology, ecological psychology, environmental psychology and community psychology (Carr et al., 2002).

Social validity relates to the degree of satisfaction associated with a treatment and the feasibility of carrying out a treatment. Social validity has three components (Wolf, 1978) (a) the social importance of treatment goals, (b) the acceptability of treatments relevant to consumers, and (c) the social importance of treatment effects. As such, social validity in itself is likely to be affected by a raft of variables including severity of behavior, intensity of behavior, degree of disruption to local/family routines, culture of both teacher and parents (Machalicek et al., 2007). There is a clear recognition amongst many practitioners that consideration of the contextual fit of an invention plan is a core feature of designing and increasing the likelihood of an effective treatment plan. Schwartz and Baer (1991) have suggested that the real focus of social validity should in fact be to accurately measure when a stakeholder does not like a given intervention as this is likely to be a good predictor of drop-out or non-compliance. The implication of this is that without social validity, there is unlikely to be maintenance of the gains of behavioral intervention, since stakeholders are unlikely to be reinforced by behavior changes that they do not value (McClean and Grey, in press). Although social validity is one of the key criteria by which ABA is defined, it is not measured very often (Kennedy, 2002). Social validity was measured in one third of interventions published in Journal of Positive Behavior Interventions from 1999 to 2005. This compares with three percent of articles published in the Journal of Applied Behavior Analysis for the same period (Clarke and Dunlap, 2007).

These trends suggest significant and emerging separation between the practice of Applied Behavior Analysis and Positive Behavior Support. In Applied Behavior Analysis, there appears to be a continuing bias towards the evaluation of treatment development and the elucidation of basic technological processes rather than factors affecting treatment implementation and evaluation (Carr et., 1999). Applied Behavior Analysis therefore continues to be an expert driven model of service delivery as judged by low use of natural intervention agents, insistence on experimental manipulation of variables; low rates of social validity and more of an interest in basic processes than on the factors affecting implementation and maintenance of behavioral interventions.

Is PBS Loose ABA?

Given that modern ABA may occur within an ethical framework that seeks to improve the quality of life of the person, the only ways in which Positive Behavior Support may deviate from Applied Behavior Analysis are its flexibility with regard to scientific practice and its adoption of multiple theoretical perspective. In this context, is Positive Behavior Support merely a looser, or less scientific, Applied Behavior Analysis. In the same way as, say, a physician may prescribe treatment without subjecting it to double blind trial, perhaps Positive Behavior Support may recommend intervention without the rigours and ethical concerns of an experimental functional analysis? Functional analysis is generally not considered to be a very practical method of assessment in ordinary clinical situations. One survey (Desrochers, Hile and Williams-Mosely, 1997) asked 300 practitioners to rank the degree of usefulness of a number of assessment procedures. ABC analysis and interviews were ranked first and second respectively whereas functional analysis was ranked fifth in terms of usefulness. The concern for advocates of a scientifically pure applied behavior analysis is the prospect of increasing divergence between published examples of Applied Behavior Analysis, and what is used, or allowed, in many everyday service settings.

Critics have argued that the use of the term support is misleading as it lacks specificity (Mulnick and Butter, 2007). Given that the primary goal of PBS is to help an individual change his or her lifestyle in a direction that gives all relevant stakeholders the opportunity to perceive and enjoy an improved quality of life, the case of lack of specificity in ABA may have merit. However, treatment integrity is a separate variable, and as much a challenge to any variety of Applied Behavior Analysis as Positive Behavior Support. Indeed there may be merit in having a looser definition of the conditions or stimuli under which behavioral interventions are introduced. Perhaps the greatest single problem associated with Applied Behavior Analysis is the difficulty achieving generalization and maintenance of it outcomes. Indeed it could be argued that without generalization and maintenance, Applied Behavior Analysis would contribute little of any value to the lives of people with Autistic Spectrum Disorders. “Loose teaching” (Baer, 1999) is a technical terms for teaching conditions in which non-critical antecedent stimuli are varied as much as possible within and across teaching sessions. One of the main reasons why people with autistic spectrum disorders may not generalize learning from one situation to another is that repetitive teaching procedures which inadvertently insert non-critical elements into the teaching procedure, which then become discriminitaive stimuli. Loose teaching varies non-critical elements, such as instructions, tone of voice, setting, so that control of the target behavior is specific to functionally relevant factors. In this way, loose teaching more closely approximates natural learning environments settings in which teaching is opportunistic. Achieving lasting change is a function of the selection of intervention goals that are likely to be significant to, and therefore reinforced by, members of the social system in which the person lives. In addition, though, it requires that teaching methods are less rigorous and precise than some traditions of Applied behavior Analysis would propose.

Is Positive Behavior Support Applied ABA?

According to Horner (2000) Positive Behavior Support "is the application of Behavior Analysis to the social problems created by such behaviors as self-injury, aggression, property destruction, pica, defiance, and disruption. It is an approach that blends values about the rights of people with disabilities with a practical science about how learning and behavior change occur" (p. 97). The emphasis in Positive Behavior Support on altering deficient environments for individuals with developmental disabilities including Autistic Spectrum Disorders can be traced to research which has on the whole identified that the environments that these individuals are place in are generally not conducive to effective learning or a positive quality of life experience. Behavior analysts have long lamented the negative impact of structural, management and staff barriers to the effective uptake of interventions derived from behavior analysis. Growing evidence suggests that when applied in special education and public schools, system wide PBS produces measurable and durable reductions in destructive behaviors and "lasting implementation of empirically supported practices by school personnel" (Liaupsin et al., 2004; p 314.).

However, managing the environment effectively also implies organization in such a way as to prevent the development and maintenance of such problems (Emerson and Gurnalick). In this way, PBS shares an emphasis on placing the environment firmly in the category of intervention. Thus the person is not the locus of the problem but the wider systemic environment that generates the problem. In this area there have been similar calls for an ecological analysis of the ways various systems (e.g., individual, family, neighborhoods, schools, institutions, service organizations and even political structures) interact to confer individual risk for mental problems.

In many countries, the mechanisms for evidence-based development of service delivery for people with intellectual disabilities are not well established. Critical aspects of service provision such as content and point of delivery may be more shaped by issues such as ideology and professional identity than by research evidence. In turn this has serious implications for services which are often less effective than they could do and may even be damaging to personal growth and quality of life. As a consequence, it is the experience of many clients with developmental disabilities including Autistic Spectrum Disorders, that services are more often agency-centered rather than client-centered. While all agencies will espouse positive values such as improved quality of life, such exposition does not translate easily into better practices and better outcomes for people with Autistic Spectrum Disorders.

CONCLUSION

We began this chapter by drawing a parallel between behavioral theory and Darwinian accounts of evolution. It is clear that within a relatively short period of time, Positive Behavior Support has established itself in many human services for developmental disabilities around the world. The selection of Positive Behavior Support may entail that it is better adapted to an ecology that seeks to promote the personal dignity and social role valorization of people with intellectual disabilities. Indeed some have likened the vociferous and unscientific criticisms of Positive Behavior Support (e.g. Mulickk et al., 2005) to an extinction burst, which actually calls on practitioners of Positive Behavior Support to respond not with further ignoring, but with understanding, functional assessment and teaching better survival skills (LaVigna, 2005). We would argue that the acceptance, empowerment and citizenship of people with Autistic Spectrum Disorder is a higher value than the survival of any tool towards that goal, and hope that Applied Behavior Analysis will evolve even beyond the capacity of Positive Behavior Support to realize that goal.

REFERENCES

Allen, D. G., Lowe, K., Moore, K., and Brophy, S. (2007). Predictors, costs and characteristics of out of area placement for people with intellectual disability and challenging behavior. *Journal of Intellectual Disability Research,* 51, 409.

Allik, H., Larsson, J. O., and Smedje, H. (2006). Health-related quality of life in parents of school-age children with asperger syndrome or high-functioning autism. *Health Quality Life Outcomes,* 4, 1.

Baer, D.M. (1999) *How to plan for generalization* (2nd Ed) Austin Texas: Pro-Ed.

Baer, D.M. Wolf, M.M., and Risley, T.R. (1968) Some current dimensions of Applied Behavior Analysis. *Journal of Applied Behavior Analysis,* 10, 405 – 416

Baer, D. M., Wolf, M. M., and Risley, T. R. (1987). Some still-current dimensions of applied behavior analysis. *Journal of Applied Behavior Analysis,* 20, 313-327.

Baranek, G. T., David, F.J., Poe, M.D., Stone, W.L., and Watson, L.R. (2006). Sensory experiences questionnaire: Discriminating sensory features in young children with autism, developmental delays, and typical development. *Journal of Child Psychology and Psychiatry,* 47, 591-601.

Biglan, A. (1995). Translating what we know about the context of antisocial behavior into a lower prevalence of such behavior. *Journal of Applied Behavior Analysis,* 28, 479-492.

Blacher, J., and McIntyre, L.L. (2006). Syndrome specificity and behavioral disorders in young adults with intellectual disability: Cultural differences in family impact. *Journal of Intellectual Disability Research,* 50, 184-198.

Brereton, A.V., Tonge, B.J., and Einfeld, S.L. (2006). Psychopathology in children and adolescents with autism compared to young people with intellectual disability. *Journal of Autism and Developmental Disorders,* 36, 863.

Bryan, L.C., and Gast, D.L. (2000). Teaching on-task and on-schedule behaviors to high-functioning children with autism via picture activity schedules. *Journal of Autism and Developmental Disorders,* 30, 553.

Burns, B.J., Schoenwald, S K., Burchard, J.D., Faw, L., and Santos, A.B. (2000). Comprehensive community-based interventions for youth with severe emotional disorders: Multisystemic therapy and the wraparound process. *Journal of Child and Family Studies,* 9, 283.

Carr, E.G., Dunlap, G., Horner, R.H., Koegel, R.L., Turnbull, A.P., Sailor, W., et al. (2002). Positive behavior support: Evolution of an applied science. *Journal of Positive Behavior Interventions, 4*, 4.

Carr, E.G., and Durand, V. M. (1985). Reducing behavior problems through functional communication training. *Journal of Applied Behavior Analysis,* 18, 111.

Carr, E.G., Horner, R.H., Turnbull, A.P., Marquis, J.G., McLaughlin, D.M., McAtee, M.L., et al. (1999). *Positive behavior support for people with developmental disabilities: A research synthesis*. Washington, DC, US: American Association on Mental Retardation.

Carr, E.G., Ladd, M. V., and Schulte, C.F. (2008a). Validation of the contextual assessment inventory for problem behavior. *Journal of Positive Behavior Interventions,* 10, 91-104.

Carr, E.G., Ladd, M.V., and Schulte, C.F. (2008b). Validation of the contextual assessment inventory for problem behavior. *Journal of Positive Behavior Interventions,* 10, 91.

Carr, E.G., Magito McLaughlin, D., Giacobbe-Grieco, T., and Smith, C.E. (2003). Using mood ratings and mood induction in assessment and intervention for severe problem behavior. *American Journal of Mental Retardation,* 108, 32-55.

Clarke, S., and Dunlap, G. (2008). A descriptive analysis of intervention research published in the journal of positive behavior interventions: 1999 through 2005. *Journal of Positive Behavior Interventions,* 10, 67.

Claude, B. (2006). The autistic child, multiple approaches and divided management. *Soins Psychiatry,* 245, 37-41.

Dawson, G., and Galpert, L. (1990). Mother's use of imitative play for facilitating social responsiveness and toy play in young autistic children. *Development and Psychopathology*, 2, 151-162.

Derrickson, J.G., Neef, N.A., and Cataldo, M.F. (1993). Effects of signaling invasive procedures on a hospitalized infant's affective behaviors. *Journal of Applied Behavior Analysis,* 26, 133.

Desrochers, M.N., Hile, M.G., and Williams-Moseley, T.L. (1997). Survey of functional assessment procedures used with individuals who display mental retardation and severe problem behaviors. *American Journal on Mental Retardation,* 101, 535.

Didden, R., Duker, P.C., and Korzilius, H. (1997a). Meta-analytic study on treatment effectiveness for problem behaviors with individuals who have mental retardation. *American Journal on Mental Retardation,* 101, 387-399.

Didden, R., Duker, P.C., and Korzilius, H. (1997b). Meta-analytic study on treatment effectiveness for problem behaviors with individuals who have mental retardation. *American Journal on Mental Retardation,* 101, 387.

Dubos, R.J. (1959). Medicine as a social science. *Ariz Med,* 16, 668-673.

Eber, L., and Nelson, C.M. (1997). School-based wraparound planning: Integrating services for students with emotional and behavioral needs. *American Journal of Orthopsychiatry,* 67, 385.

Feldman, M., McDonald, L., Serbin, L., Stack, D., Secco, M.L., and Yu, C.T. (2007). Predictors of depressive symptoms in primary caregivers of young children with or at risk for developmental delay. *Journal of Intellectual Disability Research,* 51, 606-619.

Flannery, K.B., O'Neill, R.E., and Horner, R.H. (1995). Including predictability in functional assessment and individual program development. *Education and Treatment of Children,* 18, 499.

Goin-Kochel, R.P., Abbacchi, A., and Constantino, J.N. (2007). Lack of evidence for increased genetic loading for autism among families of affected females: A replication from family history data in two large samples. *Autism,* 11, 279-286.

Goodwin, M.S., Groden, J., Velicer, W.F., Lipsitt, L.P., Baron, M.G., Hofmann, S.G., et al. (2006). Cardiovascular arousal in individuals with autism. *Focus on Autism and Other Developmental Disabilities,* 21, 100-123.

Gouboth, D., Wilder, D. A., and Booher, J. (2007). The effects of signaling stimulus presentation during noncontingent reinforcement. *Journal of Applied Behavior Analysis,* 40, 725.

Green, V.A., Pituch, K.A., Itchon, J., Choi, A., O'Reilly, M., and Sigafoos, J. (2006). Internet survey of treatments used by parents of children with autism. *Research in Developmental Disabilities,* 27, 70.

Greer, F.A., Grey, I.M., and McClean, B. (2006). Coping and positive perceptions in Irish mothers of children with intellectual disabilities. *Journal of Intellectual Disabilities, 10,* 231-248.

Grey, I.M., Honan, R., McClean, B., and Daly, M. (2005). Evaluating the effectiveness of teacher training in applied behavior analysis. *Journal of Intellectual Disabilities,* 9, 209-227.

Harris, P. (1993). The nature and extent of aggressive behavior amongst people with learning difficulties (mental handicap) in a single health district. *Journal of Intellectual Disability Research*, 37, 221-242.

Hastings, R.P. (2002). Do challenging behaviors affect staff psychological well-being? Issues of causality and mechanism. *American Journal of Mental Retardation,* 107, 455-467.

Hastings, R.P., and Brown, T. (2002a). Behavioral knowledge, causal beliefs and self-efficacy as predictors of special educators' emotional reactions to challenging behaviors. *Journal of Intellectual Disability Research,* 46, 144-150.

Hastings, R. P., and Symes, M.D. (2002). Early intensive behavioral intervention for children with autism: Parental therapeutic self-efficacy. *Research in Developmental Disabilities,* 23, 332-341.

Holden, B., and Gitlesen, J.P. (2006). A total population study of challenging behavior in the county of Hedmark, Norway: Prevalence, and risk markers. *Research in Developmental Disabilities,* 27, 456-465.

Horner, R.H. (2000). Positive behavior supports. *Focus on Autism and Other Developmental Disabilities,* 15, 97.

Horner, R.H., and Carr, E.G. (1997). Behavioral support for students with severe disabilities: Functional assessment and comprehensive intervention. *The Journal of Special Education,* 31, 84-109.

Horner, R.H., Carr, E.G., Strain, P.S., Todd, A.W., and Reed, H.K. (2002). Problem behavior interventions for young children with autism: A research synthesis. *Journal of Autism and Developmental Disorders,* 32, 423-446.

Horner, R.H., Dunlap, G., Koegel, R.L., Carr, E.G., Sailor, W., Anderson, J., et al. (2005). Toward a technology of 'nonaversive' behavioral support. *Research and Practice for Persons with Severe Disabilities,* 30, 3-10.

Horner, R.H., Todd, A.W., Lewis-Palmer, T., Irvin, L.K., Sugai, G., and Boland, J.B. (2004). The school-wide evaluation tool (set): A research instrument for assessing school-wide positive behavior support. *Journal of Positive Behavior Interventions,* 6, 3-12.

Jones, E.A., and Carr, E.G. (2004). Joint attention in children with autism: Theory and intervention. *Focus on Autism and Other Developmental Disabilities,* 19, 13-26.

Kasari C, Sigman M, Mundy P, Yirmiya, N., et al. (1990) Affective sharing in the context of joint attention interactions of normal, autistic, and mentally retarded children. *Journal of Autism and Developmental Disorders*, 20, 87-100.

Kennedy, C.H., and Itkonen, T. (1993). Effects of setting events on the problem behavior of students with severe disabilities. *Journal of Applied Behavior Analysis,* 26, 321-327.

Kennedy, C.H., and Meyer, K.A. (1996). Sleep deprivation, allergy symptoms, and negatively reinforced problem behavior. *Journal of Applied Behavior Analysis,* 29, 133-135.

Kincaid, D., Knoster, T., Harrower, J.., Shannon, P., and Bustamante, S. (2002). Measuring the impact of positive behavior support. *Journal of Positive Behavior Interventions,* 4, 109-117.

Klinger, L., and Dawson, G. (1992) Facilitating early social and communicative development in children with autism. In S.F.Warren and J.Reichle (Eds.) *Causes and Effects in Communication and Language Intervention* (pp. 157–186). Baltimore, MD: Paul H.Brookes Publishing.

Knoster, T., Anderson, J., Carr, E.G., Dunlap, G., and Horner, R H. (2003). Emerging challenges and opportunities: Introducing the association for positive behavior support. *Journal of Positive Behavior Interventions,* 5, 183-186.

Kootz, J. P., Marinelli, B., and Cohen, D.J. (1981). Sensory receptor sensitivity in autistic children: Response times to proximal and distal stimulation. *Archives of General Psychiatry,* 38, 271-273.

Kootz, J.P., Marinelli, B., and Cohen, D.J. (1982). Modulation of response to environmental stimulation in autistic children. *Journal of Autism and Developmental Disorders,* 12, 185-193.

Krantz, P. J., and Risley, T.R. (1977). Behavioral ecology in the classroom. In K. D. O'Leary and S. G. O'Leary (Eds.), *Classroom management: The successful use of behavior modification* (2nd Ed., pp. 349-367). New York: Pergamon Press.

Kurtz, P. F., Chin, M. D., Huete, J. M., Tarbox, R. S., O'Connor, J. T., Paclawskyj, T. R., et al. (2003). Functional analysis and treatment of self-injurious behavior in young children a summary of 30 cases. *Journal of Applied Behavior Analysis,* 36, 205-219.

Lalli, J.S., Casey, S., Goh, H., and Merlino, J. (1994). Treatment of escape-maintained aberrant behavior with escape extinction and predictable routines. *Journal of Applied Behavior Analysis,* 27, 705.

Laraway, S., Snycerski, S., Michael, J., and Poling, A. (2003). Motivating operations and terms to describe them: Some further refinements. *Journal of Applied Behavior Analysis,* 36, 407.

LaVigna, G.W. and Willis, T.J. (1995). Challenging behavior: A model for breaking the barriers to social and community integration, *Positive Practices,* 1, 8-16.

Liaupsin, C.J., Jolivette, K., Scott, T.M., Rutherford, R.B., Quinn, M.M., and Mathur, S R. (2004). Schoolwide systems of behavior support: Maximizing student success in schools. In *Handbook of research in emotional and behavioral disorders.* (pp. 487-501). New York, NY, US: Guilford Press.

Lowenthal, R., Campos, M.L., Amorosino, C., Gomila, A., and D'Antino, M.E. (2005). Quality of life in siblings of autistic patients. *Rev Bras Psiquiatr,* 27, 344; author reply 345.

Machalicek, W., O'Reilly, M. F., Beretvas, N., Sigafoos, J., and Lancioni, G.E. (2007). A review of interventions to reduce challenging behavior in school settings for students with autism spectrum disorders. *Research in Autism Spectrum Disorders,* 1, 229.

Magana, S., and Smith, M.J. (2006). Psychological distress and well-being of Latina and non-Latina white mothers of youth and adults with an autism spectrum disorder: Cultural attitudes towards coresidence status. *American Journal of Orthopsychiatry,* 76, 346-357.

Malette, P., Mirenda, P., Kandborg, T., and Jones, P. (1992). Application of a lifestyle development process for persons with severe intellectual disabilities: A case study report. *Journal of the Association for Persons with Severe Handicaps,* 17, 179.

Martin, N.T., Gaffan, E.A., and Williams, T. (1999). Experimental functional analyses for challenging behavior: A study of validity and reliability. *Research in Developmental Disabilities,* 20, 125.

McClean, B., Grey, I.M., and McCracken, M. (2007a). An evaluation of positive behavioral support for people with very severe challenging behaviors in community-based settings. *Journal of Intellectual Disabilities,* 11, 281-301.

McClean, B. and Walsh, P. (1995). Positive programming - an organisational response to challenging behavior. *Positive Practices,* 1, 3-8.

McClintock, K., Hall, S., and Oliver, C. (2003). Risk markers associated with challenging behaviors in people with intellectual disabilities: A meta-analytic study. *Journal of Intellectual Disability Research,* 47, 405-416.

McGill, P., Teer, K., Rye, L., and Hughes, D. (2005). Staff reports of setting events associated with challenging behavior. *Behavior Modification,* 29, 599-615.

McLaughlin, D.M., and Carr, E.G. (2005a). Quality of rapport as a setting event for problem behavior: Assessment and intervention. *Journal of Positive Behavior Interventions,* 7, 68-91.

McLaughlin, D.M., and Carr, E.G. (2005b). Quality of rapport as a setting event for problem behavior: Assessment and intervention. *Journal of Positive Behavior Interventions,* 7, 68.

Mirenda, P L., and Donnellan, A.M. (1986). Effects of adult interaction style on conversational behavior in students with severe communication problems. *Language, Speech, and Hearing Services in Schools,* 17, 126-141.

Mugno, D., Ruta, L., D'Arrigo, V.G., and Mazzone, L. (2007). Impairment of quality of life in parents of children and adolescents with pervasive developmental disorder. *Health Quality Life Outcomes,* 5, 22.

Mundy, P. and Thorp, D. (2006). The neural basis of early joint-attention behavior. In T. Charman and W. Stone (Eds.), *Social communication development in autism spectrum Disorders*, (pp. 296-336). New York, NY: Guilford Publications.

Mundy, P., Sigman, M., Kasari, C., and Sigman, M. (1994). Joint attention, developmental level, and symptom presentation in autism. *Development and Psychopathology*, 6, 389-401.

Murphy, G.H., Beadle-Brown, J., Wing, L., Gould, J., Shah, A., and Holmes, N. (2005). Chronicity of challenging behaviors in people with severe intellectual disabilities and/or autism: A total population sample. *Journal of Autism and Developmental Disorders,* 35, 405-418.

Mulick, J.A., Butter, E.M., Jacobson, J.W., Foxx, R.M., and Mulick, J. A. (2005). Positive behavior support: A paternalistic utopian delusion. In *Controversial therapies for developmental disabilities: Fad, fashion and science in professional practice.* (pp. 385). Mahwah, NJ, US: Lawrence Erlbaum Associates Publishers.

Oliver, C., Murphy, G. and Corbett, J.A. (1987). Self-injurious behavior in people with mental handicap: a total population study. *Journal of Mental Deficiency Research,* 31, 147-162.

O'Reilly M, F., Sigafoos, J., Lancioni, G., Rispoli, M., Lang, R., Chan, J., et al. (2007). Manipulating the behavior-altering effect of the motivating operation: Examination of the influence on challenging behavior during leisure activities. *Research in Developmental Disabilities.*

O'Reilly, M.F. (1997). Functional analysis of episodic self-injury correlated with recurrent otitis media. *Journal of Applied Behavior Analysis,* 30, 165-167.

Orsmond, G.I., Seltzer, M.M., Greenberg, J.S., and Krauss, M.W. (2006). Mother-child relationship quality among adolescents and adults with autism. *American Journal of Mental Retardation,* 111, 121-137.

Pierce, K., and Schreibman, L. (1995). Increasing Complex Behaviors in children with autism: Effects of Peer-Implemented Pivotal Response Training. *Journal of Applied Behavior Analysis,* 28, 285-295.

Prizant, B.M., Wetherby, A.M., Volkmar, F.R., Paul, R., Klin, A., and Cohen, D. (2005). Critical issues in enhancing communication abilities for persons with autism spectrum disorders. In *Handbook of autism and pervasive developmental disorders, vol. 2: Assessment, interventions, and policy (3rd ed.).* (pp. 925-945). Hoboken, NJ, US: John Wiley and Sons Inc.

Reinke, W.M., Herman, K.C., and Tucker, C.M. (2006). Building and sustaining communities that prevent mental disorders: Lessons from the field of special education. *Psychology in the Schools,* 43, 313-329.

Reiter, S., and Vitani, T. (2007). Inclusion of pupils with autism: The effect of an intervention program on the regular pupils' burnout, attitudes and quality of mediation. *Autism,* 11, 321-333.

Renty, J.O., and Roeyers, H. (2006). Quality of life in high-functioning adults with autism spectrum disorder: The predictive value of disability and support characteristics. *Autism,* 10, 511-524.

Repp, A.C. (1994). Comments on functional analysis procedures for school-based behavior problems. *Journal of Applied Behavior Analysis,* 27, 409-412.

Rogers, S.J., Hepburn, S., and Wehner, E. (2003). Parent reports of sensory symptoms in toddlers with autism and those with other developmental disorders. *Journal of Autism and Developmental Disorders, 33,* 631-642.

Rojahn, J., Matson, J.L., Naglieri, J.A., and Mayville, E. (2004). Relationships between psychiatric conditions and behavior problems among adults with mental retardation. *American Journal on Mental Retardation,* 109, 21.

Sailor, W., and Paul, J. L. (2004). Framing positive behavior support in the ongoing discourse concerning the politics of knowledge. *Journal of Positive Behavior Interventions,* 6, 37-49.

Schumann, C.M., Bauman, M.D., Machado, C.J., Amaral, D.G., Moldin, S.O., and Rubenstein, J.L.R. (2006). The social brain, amygdala, and autism. In *Understanding autism: From basic neuroscience to treatment.* (pp. 227-253). Boca Raton, FL, US: CRC Press.

Schwartz, I.S., and Baer, D.M. (1991). Social validity assessments: Is current practice state of the art? *Journal of Applied Behavior Analysis,* 24, 189.

Scott, T.M., and Barrett, S.B. (2004). Using staff and student time engaged in disciplinary procedures to evaluate the impact of school-wide pbs. *Journal of Positive Behavior Interventions,* 6, 21-27.

Scott, T.M., Liaupsin, C., Nelson, C.M., and McLntyre, J. (2005). Team-based functional behavior assessment as a proactive public school process: A descriptive analysis of current barriers. *Journal of Behavioral Education,* 14, 57-71.

Scott, T.M., McLntyre, J., Liaupsin, C., Nelson, C.M., Conroy, M., and Payne, L.D. (2005b). An examination of the relation between functional behavior assessment and selected intervention strategies with school-based teams. *Journal of Positive Behavior Interventions,* 7, 205-215.

Scotti, J.R., Evans, I.M., Meyer, L.H., and Walker, P. (1991a). A meta-analysis of intervention research with problem behavior: Treatment validity and standards of practice. *American Journal on Mental Retardation,* 96, 233-256.

Scotti, J.R., Evans, I.M., Meyer, L.H., and Walker, P. (1991b). A meta-analysis of intervention research with problem behavior: Treatment validity and standards of practice. *American Journal on Mental Retardation,* 96, 233.

Sen, E., and Yurtsever, S. (2007). Difficulties experienced by families with disabled children. *J Spec Pediatr Nurs,* 12, 238-252.

Sigman, M., and Ruskin, E. (1999). *Change and continuity in the social competence of children with Autism, Down syndrome, and developmental delays*. Monograph of the Society for Research in Child Development. London, England: Blackwell.

Smith, R.G., and Iwata, B.A. (1997). Antecedent influences on behavior disorders. *Journal of Applied Behavior Analysis,* 30, 343.

Sugai, G. (2003). Commentary: Establishing efficient and durable systems of school-based support. *School Psychology Review,* 32, 530-535.

Sugai, G., and Horner, R. (2002). The evolution of discipline practices: School-wide positive behavior supports. *Child and Family Behavior Therapy,* 24, 23-50.

Sugai, G., Horner, R.H., Dunlap, G., Hieneman, M., Lewis, T.J., Nelson, C.M., et al. (2000). Applying positive behavior support and functional behavioral assessment in schools. *Journal of Positive Behavior Interventions,* 2, 131-143.

Vollmer, T.R., Borrero, J.C., Lalli, J.S., and Daniel, D. (1999). Evaluating self-control and impulsivity in children with severe behavior disorders. *Journal of Applied Behavior Analysis,* 32, 451.

Wacker, D.P., and Berg, W.K. (2002). PBS as a service delivery system. *Journal of Positive Behavior Interventions,* 4, 25.

Wacker, D.P., Steege, M.W., Northup, J., and Sasso, G.M. (1990). A component analysis of functional communication training across three topographies of severe behavior problems. *Journal of Applied Behavior Analysis,* 23, 417.

Wahler, R.G., and Fox, J.J. (1981). Setting events in applied behavior analysis: Toward a conceptual and methodological expansion. *Journal of Applied Behavior Analysis,* 14, 327.

Wetherby, A., and Prizant, B.M. (1999) Enhancing Language and Communication Development in Autism: Assessment and Intervention Guidelines. In D.B. Zager (Ed.) *Autism: Identification, Education and Treatment 2nd Edition*. London: Lawrence Erlbaum.

Willis, T.J., and LaVigna, G.W. (1993). *ABC Incident Analysis*. Los Angeles: Institute of Applied Behavior Analysis

Willis, T.J., and LaVigna, G.W. (1996) Behavior Assessment: An overview. *Positive Practices*, 1, 1-16.

Willis, T.J., LaVigna, G.W., and Donnellan, A.M. (1993). *The Behavior Assessment Guide*. Los Angeles: Institute of Applied Behavior Analysis.

Wolery, M., Barton, E.E., and Hine, J.F. (2005). Evolution of applied behavior analysis in the treatment of individuals with autism. *Exceptionality,* 13, 11.

Zahn, T.P., Rumsey, J.M., and Van Kammen, D. . (1987). Autonomic nervous system activity in autistic, schizophrenic, and normal men: Effects of stimulus significance. *Journal of Abnormal Psychology,* 96, 135-144.

Zimbelman, M., Paschal, A., Hawley, S.R., Molgaard, C.A., and St.Romain, T. (2007). Addressing physical inactivity among developmentally disabled students through visual schedules and social stories. *Research in Developmental Disabilities,* 28, 386.

PART 3: FAMILY, PROFESSIONAL AND TRAINING ISSUES

In: Behavioral Theories and Interventions for Autism
Editor: Phil Reed
ISBN 978-1-60741-165-9
© 2009 Nova Science Publishers, Inc.

Chapter 9

A Dynamic Transactional Model of Parent-Child Interactions in Autistic Spectrum Disorders

Lisa A. Osborne*
Swansea University, U.K.

Recent work has identified a number of important theoretical reasons for examining the relationships between parenting stress, parenting behaviors, and child behavior problems in Autistic Spectrum Disorder (ASD) samples. These reasons revolve around ascertaining whether these three family-centered parent-child elements interact with, or impact on, one another, and, if so, how, and what the nature, and degree, of such influences would be. The results of these examinations may also have practical implications for the development of future teaching interventions for ASD, especially regarding parent training, counseling, and support.

A review of the existing literature for families of children with ASD suggests a relationship between parenting stress and child behavior problems (Blacher and McIntyre, 2006; Donenberg and Baker, 1993; Floyd and Gallagher, 1997; Lecavalier, Leone, and Wiltz, 2006), but Osborne and Reed (2009b) identified a large range of questions that remained unanswered by this literature. For example, in relation to the association between patenting stress and child behaviors, there was a clear need to determine: firstly, whether parenting stress is most strongly associated with the severity of the ASD, or with the severity of the child behavior problems; secondly, the temporal directionality of any such parent-child interactions; and thirdly, whether high parenting stress levels impact negatively on child outcomes during, and following, teaching interventions for children with ASD.

A further area in need of research is whether parenting stress impacts on parenting behaviors, and the types of parenting behaviors that are influential for subsequent child behavior problems in the context of ASD. For example, it is unknown whether any association between parenting behaviors and subsequent child behavior problems is a direct

* Correspondence regarding this chapter should be sent to: Lisa A. Osborne, Department of Psychology, Swansea University, Singleton Park, Swansea, SA2 8PP, U.K.

one, or a by-product resulting from these two behavioral elements being impacted upon by additional factors, such as parenting stress.

An additional area of investigation lacking in the current literature revolves around how, and from where, parenting stress levels initially emerge, and whether parents' contact with, and communication experiences of, professionals leading up to, and during, the diagnostic process is of particular significance in the generation of such parenting stress in the context of ASD. Furthermore, the additional, and related, influences of both the initial emergence and parental noticing of problems with the child, and of the ASD diagnosis concerning the child, on the parents' levels of stress were in need of investigation.

On the basis of these questions, a series of studies were conducted in order to provide some clarification of, and even answers for, these related areas of enquiry. Furthermore, it was hoped that an empirically-based model of the interrelationships between all of these family elements could be developed, on the basis of any findings that had emerged, and that this model may contribute to inform theory, aid practice, and promote further development of previous ideas and notions in this, somewhat, neglected field in the context of ASD. This chapter provides a summary of these recent findings, and a new model for parent-child interactions emerging from these results.

FINDINGS

Osborne, McHugh, Saunders, and Reed (2008a) presented the results from a community-based study, which examined the influences of early teaching interventions on sixty-five young children who had been diagnosed with ASD. In addition, this study explored the dynamics between the time-intensity of the early teaching interventions (hours per week), and the levels of parenting stress measured prior to intervention, on the child outcomes nine to ten months after the interventions had first commenced. The intellectual, educational, and adaptive behavioral and social, functioning of the children were all measured. The children in this study were divided into four groups, based on both the levels of time-intensity of their interventions, and on their parents' levels of stress. The study found that there were gains in the intellectual, educational, and adaptive behavioral and social, functioning of the children over the nine to ten month period of assessment, and that there was a positive relationship between the time-intensity of the early teaching interventions and the child outcome gains. It was noted also that high levels of parenting stress counteracted the overall effectiveness of the early teaching interventions. Children whose parents reported higher levels of stress made fewer outcome gains, even when engaged in higher time-intensity interventions, than the children whose parents reported lower levels of stress (see Figure 9.1).

Findings of a similar detrimental relationship between high levels of stress reported by parents, and the development of subsequent child behavior problems, were obtained in the pair of studies reported by Osborne and Reed (2009a). This study presented the results from two longitudinal studies, involving a total of one hundred and thirty-seven children, and examined the interaction between stress in parents and the behavior problems of children with ASD. Study 1 focused on the effects of these family dynamics in very young children, while Study 2 employed a wider range of child ages. Both of these studies assessed levels of stress in parents, and child behavior problems, at two points in time separated by about ten months.

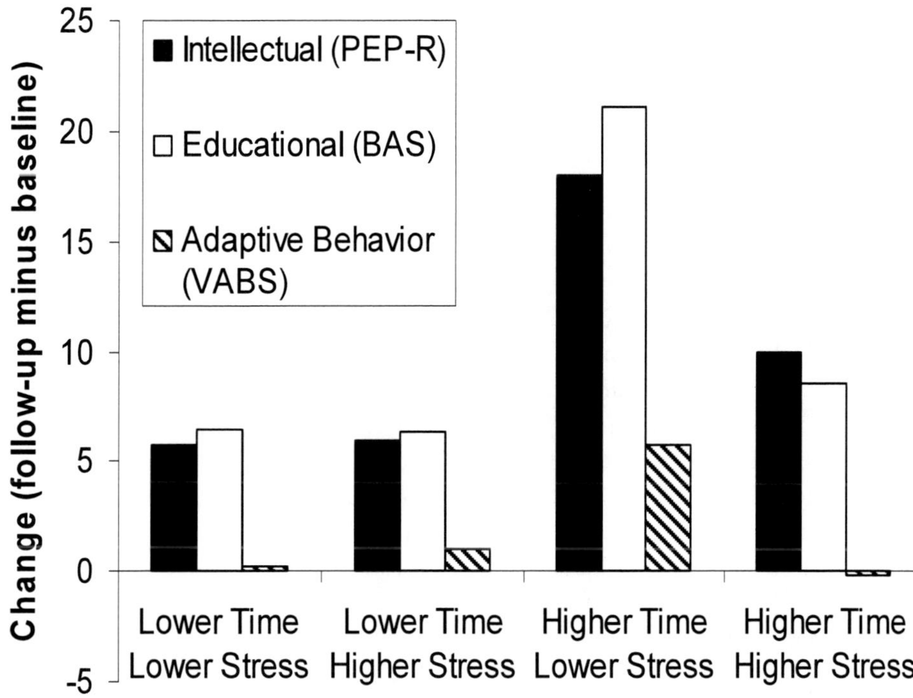

Figure 9.1. Change scores (follow-up minus baseline) for child measures from Osborne et al. (2008a).

Both studies noted that, in general, higher levels of self-reported stress in parents were strongly associated with higher reported levels of child behavior problems, even when other factors, such as the severity of the child's ASD, and the child's intellectual functioning, were controlled for. However, Study 1 found that, when the children were very young (2:6 to 4:0 years old), their severity of ASD was related most strongly to levels of stress in parents. In addition, both Study 1 and Study 2 found that stress levels in parents at baseline were a stronger predictor of child behavior problems at follow-up, than the reverse relationship. Thus, children with ASD, of all ages, whose parents initially reported higher levels of stress, displayed more behavior problems about ten months later, than did those children whose parents initially reported lower levels of stress.

Two further studies (Osborne and Reed, 2009c; Osborne, McHugh, Saunders, and Reed, 2008b) explored potential mechanisms, and influences, whereby high parenting stress may have a negative impact on child outcomes and child behavior problems, specifically via the possible impact of parenting stress on parenting behaviors. Osborne and Reed (2009c) examined the relationships between parenting stress and parenting behaviors in one hundred and thirty-eight parents of children of various ages with ASD, over a period of nine to ten months. Apart from the parents' communication with their child being attenuated, relative to that of parents of typically developing children, which might be expected, there were no obvious major areas of parenting weakness in this sample. Parenting stress was found to closely interact with the parenting behaviors of involvement, communication, and limit setting over the time period of this study. For the parents of the older children (i.e. those children aged above four years), parenting stress and the parenting behaviors of communication, and limit setting, interwove bidirectionally to improve, or exacerbate, each other. However, in the sub-set of the parents of the younger children (i.e. those children aged below four years), the interaction between parenting stress and parenting behaviors was not bidirectional, but was unidirectional; higher initial levels of parenting stress were found to result in less subsequent involvement, and poorer communication, with the child. In contrast, within this sub-set of parents, good initial parenting skills in limit setting resulted in subsequently lower levels of parenting stress. These findings suggest that the relationship between parenting stress and parenting behaviors evolves, that is, develops, and alters, over time.

The relationships noted by Osborne and Reed (2009c) could enhance understanding, and form the basis of a possible explanation, concerning the impact of parenting stress on child behavior problems, and outcomes, as mediated by parenting behaviors. The research reported by Osborne et al. (2008b) explored the relationships between parenting behaviors (which are impacted upon by parenting stress), in parents of children with ASD, and subsequent child behavior problems. The sample deployed by Osborne et al. (2008b) consisted of seventy-two children with ASD (aged from five to sixteen years old), and their parents, who were assessed over a period of nine to ten months. The results of this study noted a relationship between parenting behaviors and subsequent child behavior problems, but only for the parenting behavior of limit setting. It was found that, the better the limit setting abilities of the parents at baseline, the fewer the child behavior problems reported at follow-up nine to ten months later. Importantly, the parenting behavior of limit setting was found to mediate the relationship between parenting stress and subsequent child behavior problems.

Two further studies (Osborne and Reed, 2008; Osborne, McHugh, Saunders, and Reed, 2008c) sought to investigate potential sources of early stress in parents of children with ASD, as parenting stress appears to trigger changes in parenting behaviors that lead to subsequent child behavior problems. One obvious source of initial stress for parents of children with ASD is the experience of seeking, and obtaining, a diagnosis of ASD for their child, and their contact and communication with professionals involved in this diagnostic process. In order to gain the views of parents concerning their perceptions, and experiences, of the process of getting a diagnosis of ASD for their child, Osborne and Reed (2008) presented the findings from fifteen focus groups, conducted across a range of locations in South East England. These focus groups were split into separate sets of parents of pre-school, primary-aged, and secondary-aged, children who had received an ASD diagnosis. The analyses of these focus groups showed that, at the time of diagnosis, most of the parents involved in this study wished for a quicker and easier process. In particular, they would have preferred the procedure to have had a more coherent structure and content. They also requested greater professional training regarding ASD, especially concerning the level of information about ASD that some professionals possess, and the interpersonal skills of some professionals. The idea of general information sheets that could be provided to parents, at the time of diagnosis, was suggested, and agreed to be of value, especially in order to combat negative information obtained from other sources.

The final study mentioned above (Osborne et al., 2008c) investigated the impact of an ASD diagnosis for children on the levels of parenting stress in their parents. The parents of eighty-five children with ASD (aged from three to sixteen years) completed measures of their parenting stress, and gave a brief history of their child and their child's diagnosis. The children were assessed for their severity of ASD, and for their adaptive behavioral functioning. The results revealed that the severity of a child's ASD predicted that their parents would first notice a problem at an earlier stage in that child's development. The speed at which parents first noticed a problem with their child, rather than their child's severity of ASD, predicted obtaining an earlier diagnosis of ASD (see Figure 9.2 for a schematic representation of the results).

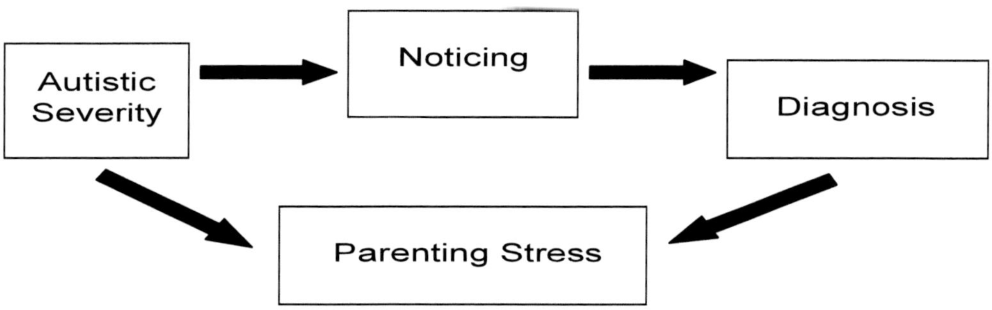

Figure 9.2. A schematic representation of the interactions between autistic severity, parents' first noticing a problem with their child, receiving a diagnosis, and parenting stress.

While the severity of a child's ASD was related directly to parenting stress, a somewhat surprising finding to emerge from this study was that an earlier diagnosis may be detrimental to levels of parenting stress. While parenting stress declined over time from the point at which the parents had first noticed a problem with their child, it failed to change by any significant degree, once the diagnosis of ASD had been received. Given this possible contra-indication for early diagnosis of ASD, this finding warrants some caution, and further investigation, in this area.

A Dynamic Transactional Model of Parent-Child Interactions

The results from the six empirical studies, summarized above, in addition to the context of the previous background literature (see Osborne and Reed, 2009b, for a review), are graphically crystallized and depicted in an empirically-based model shown in Figure 9.3. The model presents the relationships between the various elements of parent and child behaviors and interactions involved in parenting a child with ASD.

The model presented in Figure 9.3 is particularly complex, involving multiple elements, and their interactions, which alter over time, and which are triggered by different stimuli at different points in the child's development, and in the parent's experience of that development. It should be noted that "parent-child interactions" refer only to the relationships between those elements represented in Figure 9.3; namely, those between a child's ASD severity, parenting stress, parenting behaviors, and child behavior problems. The two terms used to describe the model, "dynamic" and "transactional", are explained and discussed below, and act to place this model within a behavioral framework.

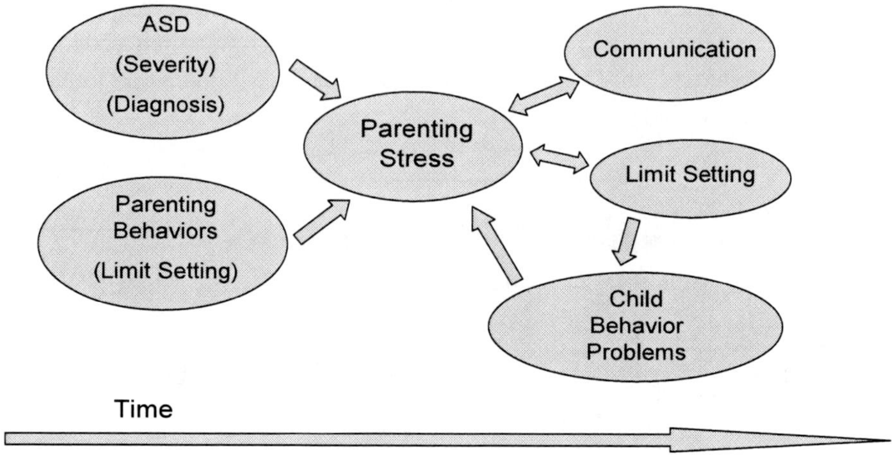

Figure 9.3. A dynamic transactional model.

Dynamic Model

This model has been termed "dynamic" in order to indicate the movement, change, and flux of the relationships presented. That is, what is true for the younger children with ASD and their parents, is not necessarily true for the older children with ASD and their parents, and *vice versa*. In some sense, this model, therefore, could be classed as a 'developmental' model; one that seeks to encapsulate and depict the alterations in the processes, and the changes in parent-child interactional behaviors, that occur as the child grows older. However, although this model may be viewed as 'developmental', in this sense, it should not be taken to imply that this is a model concerning 'developmental maturation'. This model does not present a picture of set developments within a child, based purely on changes that come about as a result of innate catalysts, such as are often postulated in typical 'stage' models of development (see Brainerd, 1978, for a comprehensive critique of such 'stage' models). These models, typically characterized for example by Piagetian theories (Piaget, 1954), are often postulated in the area of ASD (e.g., Frith and Frith, 2003), and are related to the age of a child, such as Theory of Mind accounts of ASD (e.g., Baron-Cohen, Leslie, and Frith, 1985; Leslie, 1991).

Rather, what is intended by this model is to display a representation of complex mechanisms, and interactive components, that are triggered by environmental and experiential events, which are compatible with a behavioral interpretation. That is, the interactions that occur, and that drive the model, will depend on the behaviors, and events, that are most salient at a particular time in the development of a child. Parent and child behaviors feed into each other, and particular relationships between these behaviors will build up to influential capacities over time, creating different patterns of triggering at different points in time.

Transactional Model

This model has been termed "transactional" in order to encompass the various multiple bidirectional interactions involved between the many elements present. Models that are composed entirely, or largely, of one-way interactions could be termed 'unidirectional'. There are some examples of such models in the developmental area. For instance, the model presented by Keogh, Garnier, Bernheime, and Gallimore (2000; see Figure 9.4) could be referred to as a 'child-driven' unidirectional model, in that a child's competences determine and produce accommodation for those abilities, or deficits, by the family, but influence does not act in the reverse direction.

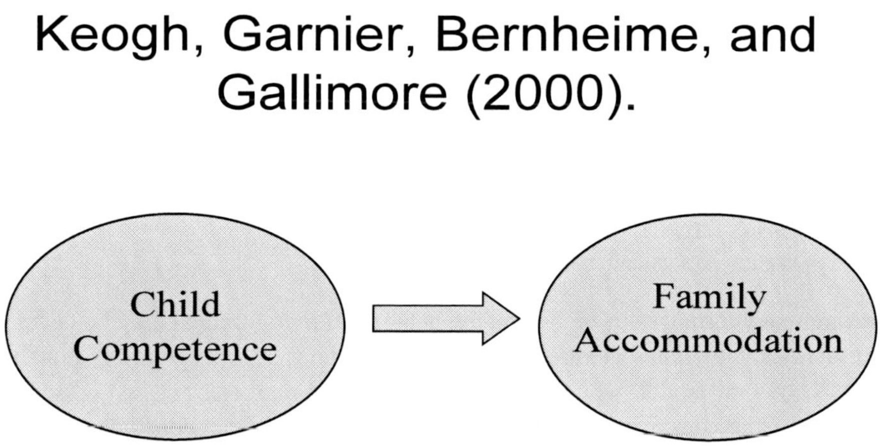

Figure 9.4. A simple unidirectional model.

A somewhat more complicated, and triangular, model is the theoretical model of parent-child relationships for learning disabilities, presented by Hastings (2002; see also Deater-Deckard, 1998; see Figure 9.5). This model shows three elements impacting upon each other, in a linear fashion. According to Hastings' model (2002), child behavior problems impact on parental stress, which, in turn, impacts on parenting behavior, which, in turn, impacts on child behavior problems. Thus, the direct effect of each element upon the next element in line is one way, and so is unidirectional, and, if this model were not 'triangular' in structure, then it could not be said to be transactional in any sense. Thus, although in Hastings' (2002) model, one element does impact on another directly (e.g., parental stress impacts directly on parenting behavior), the reverse relationship between these elements is not direct, but, rather, this reverse relationship is mediated. For example, the relationship between two elements (e.g., the impact of parenting behavior on parental stress) is always mediated by a third element (e.g., child behavior problems). In this sense, this model could be termed a 'mediated transactional' model.

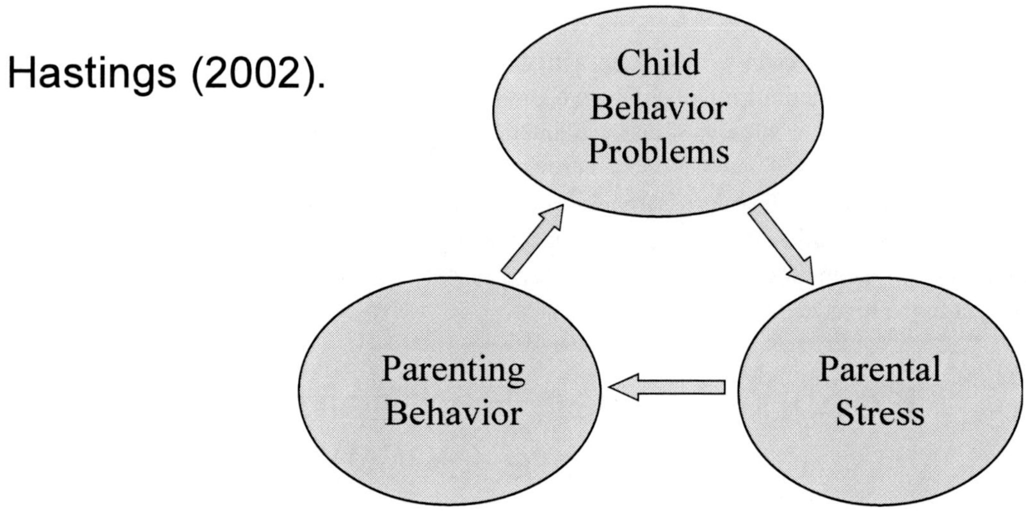

Figure 9.5. A mediated transactional model.

There are many instances of models in the behavioral literature that may be deemed to be 'fully transactional' in their structure. For example, in the field of marketing, Foxall (1999) proposed a behavioral model, whereby the behavior of the marketer acts as a discriminative stimulus (Sd) for the consumer, and the subsequent behavior of the consumer acts as an Sd for the marketer's subsequent behavior. These two behaviors could be said to 'interlock', and to be 'fully transactional' (see Figure 9.6).

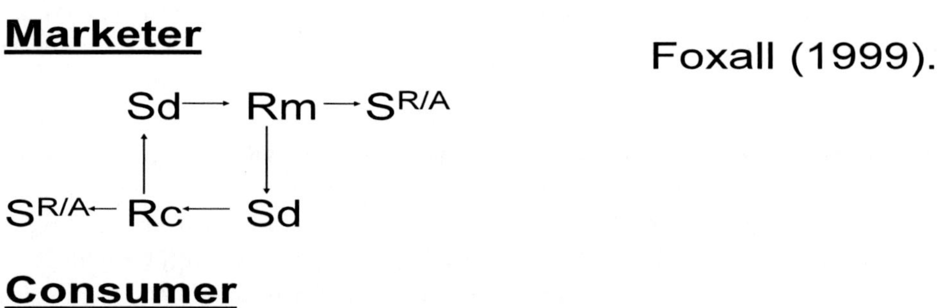

Figure 9.6. A fully transactional model.

In the field of educational interventions that have been widely used for children with ASD, the concept of the 'learn unit' also could be said to be 'fully transactional'. The behavior of the teacher acts as an Sd for the behavior of the child, and the child's subsequent behavior acts as an Sd for the teacher's subsequent behavior, and so on (see Greer, 2002; Keohane, Greer, and Ackerman, 2007).

The Model for Younger Children

In order to untangle some of the complexities of the current model, presented in Figure 9.3, it is necessary to break the model down into two separate parts, based on the different ages of the children represented on the timeline of this model. By breaking down this model into two separate parts (for younger and older children with ASD), it may be easier to see how, and when, different processes 'kick in' in order to determine, or trigger, behaviors. This present section examines the interactions between the elements for younger children (below the age of four years), when the initial signs, and early problems, of ASD are first becoming apparent to the parents, and when diagnosis is usually sought and obtained. This part of the model is represented in Figure 9.7.

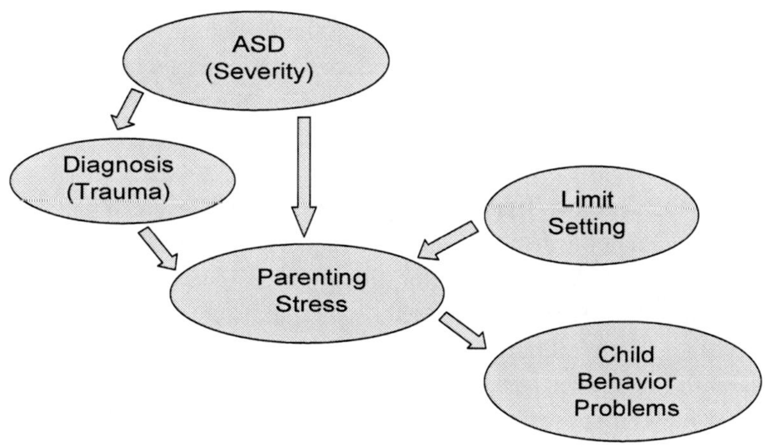

Figure 9.7. Model part for younger children and their parents.

The key elements, at this stage of the timeline of the model, are the severity of the child's ASD, the process of seeking and obtaining a diagnosis, the parents' ability to limit set for their child, and the levels of parenting stress. At this stage, it appears that the severity of the child's ASD has an impact, both directly and indirectly, on the levels of parenting stress. Osborne and Reed (2009a) noted that, for younger children (between 2:6 and 4:0 years old), there was a strong direct relationship between the severity levels of the ASD and the levels of parenting stress. This relationship was stronger, at those young ages, than that between the levels of child behavior problems and parenting stress. Although there has been some debate about the relative strengths of these relationships (see Osborne and Reed, 2009b), this finding does correspond to several other reports that have sampled very young children, and which have found the level of ASD to be a very strong predictor, at such young ages, of parenting stress (Duarte, Bordin, Yazigi, and Mooney, 2005; Eisenhower, Baker, and Blacher, 2005).

Many reasons could be postulated for this finding; for instance, when a child is very young, child behavior problems (e.g., externalized behaviors) may not be particularly salient or troublesome for a parent, as the child is smaller, less strong, and so aggressive behaviors are easier to restrain. As a child grows older, larger, and stronger, such behaviors become more difficult to manage and control, and the relationship between child behavior problems (e.g., aggressive and externalizing behaviors) and parenting stress will become more closely bonded. However, when a child is very young, those behaviors that are more integrally associated with the core problems of ASD (e.g., weak social interaction, poor eye contact, etc.) will be more immediate, and salient, concerns for parents.

As noted by Osborne et al. (2008c), these ASD-related behaviors often alert parents initially to notice a problem with their child, and prompt parents to seek help and advice, and to obtain a diagnosis concerning these problems. While the levels of parenting stress appear to reduce from the point at which parents first notice a problem, the point of diagnosis, itself, is strongly correlated with future levels of parenting stress, and this traumatic event appears to 'set', or 'crystallize', these levels of parenting stress. Previous studies also have reported a relationship between obtaining a diagnosis of ASD, and levels of stress in parents (e.g., Schuntermann, 2002). This may be due to the difficulties involved in obtaining a diagnosis, and due to experiences of contact and communication with professionals involved in the diagnostic process and system, as suggested by the results reported by Osborne and Reed (2008; see also Brogan and Knussen, 2003; Evans, Stoddart, Condon, Freeman, Grizzell, and Muller, 2001; Goin-Kochel, Mackintosh, and Myers, 2006).

Thus, there are two factors that appear to increase levels of parenting stress in the parents of younger children (often just recently diagnosed) with ASD: the severity of the ASD, and the diagnosis of ASD. A third factor, that of the parents' skills in limit setting for their child, was also shown by Osborne and Reed (2009c) to be connected with levels of parenting stress. The better a parent's limit setting behaviors, the lower their subsequent levels of parenting stress were found to be, and, of course, the worse their abilities to limit set for their child, the higher were their subsequent levels of parenting stress. Although not previously noted in an ASD sample, there is some additional evidence for this relationship in the general population (Kotchick, Dorsey, and Heller, 2005; Meyers and Miller, 2004).

These factors all contribute to the initial production, and continual generation, of parenting stress. In turn, this factor of parenting stress was associated with more exacerbated child behavior problems (see Osborne and Reed, 2009a). For this younger age group, it is not yet determined whether this relationship is a direct one, or whether it is mediated through parenting behaviors, as the sample used by Osborne et al. (2008b) did not include very young children. However, it is established that child behavior problems become more strongly associated with parenting stress as children grow older. This relationship becomes stronger over time than that between a child's ASD severity and parenting stress (see Osborne and Reed, 2009a). This finding is consistent also with that noted in the literature for slightly older children of around four years and above (see Blacher and McIntyre, 2006; Lecavalier, Leone, and Wiltz, 2006), and Lecavalier et al. (2006) have previously noted a bidirectional relationship between parenting stress and child behavior problems for such a sample.

The Model for Older Children

The part of the model that deals with children with ASD as they get older (i.e. above four years old), and their parents, is a little less complicated than the part of the model that applies to younger children. Firstly, this is because the initial powerful effects of undergoing the diagnostic process, and obtaining such an ASD diagnosis (see Osborne and Reed, 2008), although not necessarily dissipated over time (see Osborne et al., 2008c), are no longer present and ongoing in the environment of the child and parents. Secondly, it should be noted that the effects of the core ASD behaviors do not exert a major influence on parenting variables, such as parenting stress and parenting behaviors, at this point in a child's development (Blacher and McIntyre, 2006; Donenberg and Baker, 1993; Floyd and Gallagher, 1997; Lecavalier et al., 2006; Osborne and Reed, 2009a). Rather, the key behaviors of the child that are important, at this stage, are their behavior problems, such as externalizing, anti-social, and aggressive, behaviors, for the reasons discussed above. Thus, the major components of the part of the model for older children are parenting stress, parenting behaviors (communication and limit setting), and child behavior problems. The relationships between these components for older children are seen in Figure 9.8.

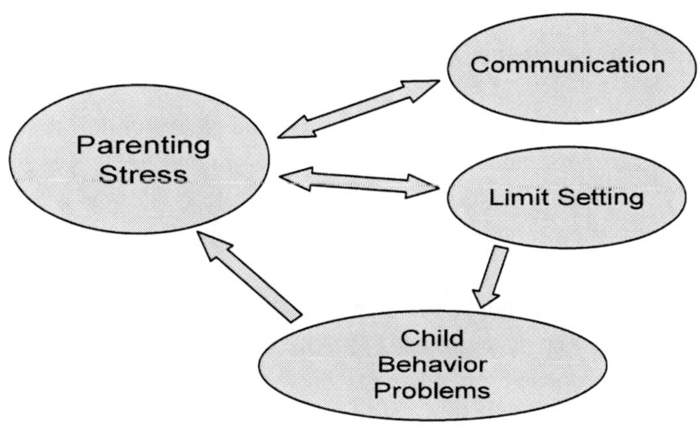

Figure 9.8. Model part for older children and their parents.

The evidence obtained in the studies described in this chapter suggests that the relationships between these three elements are straightforward. As noted by Osborne and Reed (2009c), the levels of parenting stress impact upon the types of parenting behaviors that are utilized. In particular, high levels of parenting stress are associated with subsequently lower abilities to communicate with, and limit set for, a child with ASD. Also, it was noted by Osborne and Reed (2009c) that the reverse relationships were relatively strong. That is, parental levels of communication, and limit setting skills, are related to subsequent parenting stress: the better these parenting skills, the lower the subsequent parenting stress.

Such findings have not previously been reported in an ASD sample, but there is evidence from the general population of broad links between parenting stress and parenting behaviors that supports this current model (Kotchick et al., 2005; Meyers and Miller, 2004).

Osborne et al. (2009c) noted that there was a relationship between parental limit setting for a child with ASD and subsequent behavior problems displayed by that child. However, there were found to be no relationships between other forms of parenting behaviors measured in the study and subsequent child behavior problems. Moreover, the limit setting behavior of parents was found to be the variable that mediated the relationship between parenting stress and child behavior problems. Of course, the fact that the parenting behavior of communication did not impact on subsequent child behavior problems could reflect the specifics of this sample of children with ASD, and for whom communication may not be a prime concern. This finding may not necessarily generalize to samples that are more able linguistically.

Implications and Practical Applications

The findings of this series of studies, and the resulting empirically-based model presented and outlined in this chapter, have a number of theoretical implications, and possible practical applications, that merit brief discussion.

Relationship to Other Models of Parenting

There have been numerous models of parenting, and parent-child interactions, relating to various conditions, disorders, and disabilities (e.g., Hastings, 2002; Keogh et al., 2000), as well as to typically developing children and their parents (e.g., Deater-Deckard, 1998). There are probably too many such models to list and review here, but some of the more pertinent models are worth brief mention.

A difference between the model presented in this chapter and many of the previous models (e.g., Hastings, 2002; Keogh et al., 2000) is that these previous models tend to be unidirectional in their proposed interchanges between the elements therein, whereas, the currently proposed model is much more 'fully transactional', in that it postulates a mutual bidirectional exchange between many of the elements involved. Moreover, many of the previous models cannot be said to be truly 'developmental' in nature, as they do not propose that these exchanges modify as a child grows older. Rather, they tend to propose a static situation with regard to the manners in which the various components relate to one another. The current model attempts to accommodate, and describe, developmental changes by reference to the most environmentally salient events, and states, that fuel and propel the interchanges between the components at particular times in a child's development.

These theoretical differences were discussed above, however, there are also empirical reasons presented in this chapter that separate the current model from most previous models. In particular, previous models tend to suggest that it is the child's behavior problems that trigger parenting stress (e.g., Deater-Deckard, 1998; Hastings, 2002), or that lead to family accommodation concerning those child competencies, or behavioral problems and deficits (e.g., Keogh et al., 2000). The parenting stress, in many of these models, then impacts on parents' ability to parent. That parenting stress impacts on the ability to parent is also part of the current model, at least for older children (see Osborne and Reed, 2009a), and has been noted in the general literature (Kotchick et al., 2005; Meyers and Miller, 2004). However, the current series of studies found very little evidence that it is the child behavior problems that impact on parenting stress, but, rather, it found a large amount of evidence that the impact was in the opposite direction (Osborne et al., 2008a; Osborne and Reed, 2009a), and perhaps mediated through parenting behaviors (Osborne et al., 2008b).

For instance, one link in Hastings' (2002) theoretical model (i.e. child behavior problems impacting on parental stress) would imply that temporal precedence is from child behavior problems to parental stress. If this hypothesis of causal directionality were true, then the relationship between child behavior problems at a baseline measurement and parental stress at a follow-up measurement would be stronger than the relationship between parental stress at baseline and child behavior problems at follow-up. However, Osborne and Reed (2009a) found that the relationship between child behavior problems at baseline and parenting stress at follow-up was not statistically significant, and was weaker than the relationship between parenting stress at baseline and child behavior problems at follow-up. This latter relationship was statistically significant. Hence, regarding this link in Hastings' (2002) theoretical model, it would appear that the temporal directionality, as indicated by the data reported by Osborne and Reed (2009a; see also Osborne et al., 2008a), runs in opposition to that put forward in Hastings' (2002) model, as well as in other similar models (e.g., Deater-Deckard, 1998; Keogh et al., 2000).

This contrary evidence relates only to that link in Hastings' (2002) model between child behavior problems and parental stress. This model was offered as a theoretical account for learning disabilities, as a whole, and was not intended specifically for ASD. Nevertheless, it has served as a useful device for focusing attention on the specifics of the complex interactions between parenting stress levels, parenting behaviors, and child behavior problems, when applied to ASD. Furthermore, Hastings (2002) suggested that two tests were necessary in order to substantiate this model. Firstly, that the relationship between child behavior problems and parental stress had to be demonstrated as non-spurious to rule out the possibility of other factors, or confounds, having an influence on parental stress. Secondly, that temporal precedence needed to be established for any suggestion of causal directionality to be supported. In claiming that these two aspects needed examination, Hastings (2002) proposed rigorous criteria against which to substantiate his model, and, indeed, any future models.

Hence, the current model proposed here, which places more emphasis upon the impacts of parents' behaviors on their child's behaviors, than the other way around, represents something of a return to the earlier behavioral models, for example, as suggested by Ferster (1961). This change in conception may help to mark a turning of the tide in terms of the ways in which disorders, such as ASD, are being approached (see also Drash and Tudor, 2004, for a similar argument), and this sea change is due to pivotal and prominent work within the behavioral field (e.g., Lovaas, 1987; Greer, 2002), which has placed the emphasis on environmental, rather than within-child, factors.

Developing Interventions

In terms of the practical implications of these current findings for the treatment of ASD, it may be noted that focusing purely on the impact of any intervention on the child neglects the important role that parents play in the management of their child's problems. There is increasing research on the effects of ASD on family functioning (e.g., Eisenhower et al., 2005; Hastings and Brown, 2002; Hastings and Johnson, 2001; Mash and Johnston, 1983), and growing amounts of research on the influences of the family and parents on the child with ASD (see Blacher, Neece, and Paczkowski, 2005, for a review), especially concerning their effects on the child's behavior problems, and outcomes following intervention (e.g., Lecavalier et al., 2006; Robbins et al., 1991). For example, Osborne et al. (2008a) highlighted, in the context of early teaching intervention programs, the influence of parenting stress on child outcomes. Thus, the results outlined in this chapter may have implications for, and be consistent with, the development of interventions for parents, in order to enhance their behavioral strategies, to more effectively deal with their extreme parenting stress levels.

There are many interventions now targeted at the parent, rather than the child. However, the results of the current research help to identify the specific aspects that such interventions should target. The present findings, especially from Osborne et al. (2008b), suggest that intervention programs that focus on providing parents with enhanced behavior management skills (e.g., Harris, Handlemann, Arnold, and Gordon, 2000; Lovaas and Smith, 2003) will have benefits for both the parent and the child. In particular, those programs that aid the parent to limit set more effectively may help to reduce subsequent child behavior problems, and also to reduce parenting stress. Moreover, reductions in parenting stress, as a consequence of better limit setting skills, may subsequently feed into promoting other successful parenting behaviors, such as involvement and communication, which high parenting stress otherwise attenuate (see Osborne and Reed, 2009c).

However, it is clear that interventions should focus also on the reduction of parenting stress at their commencement, as this may allow development of better parenting behaviors and skills subsequently. Numerous intervention programs target parents of children with ASD, and note improvements in the children's behaviors and functioning as a result of parents' reductions in stress and increases in their coping abilities (e.g., Harris et al., 2000; Lovaas and Smith, 2003; see Blacher, Neece, and Paczkowski, 2005, for a review).

In addressing the issues and problems resulting from having a child with ASD, the importance of the parent cannot be underestimated. As noted above, in the context of developing interventions, the importance of involving the parents with the interventions given to the child has been recognized (e.g., Schuntermann, 2002; Stoddart, 1999). However, the parental and family influences that contribute to the effectiveness of interventions should continue to be documented and assessed, to gain a more complete picture of the influencing factors on child behavior problems, and on child outcomes (see Harris, 1984; 1994; Harris et al., 2000; Lovaas and Smith, 2003; Robinson and Anderson, 1983).

It is of essential importance to highlight the ethical implications embedded in this area of parenting and ASD, and to emphasize that the re-focus on the parents' role in managing ASD, and in promoting intervention outcomes, should not be misunderstood and taken to imply that the parent is being held responsible, or blamed, for the original development of the child's ASD. This is not a return to any view that suggests that such responsibility, or blame, is attributed to the parent. It is not intended to heap further burdens upon parents who are already struggling with their child's problems, but, rather, to point to ways in which parents may be helped and supported to manage the problems of their child. "*Blame is for God and little children*"; as this Dalton Trumbo quote implies, it is neither relevant, nor meaningful, to use such terms as "blame", and to apportion it is not helpful or constructive (see also B.F. Skinner's *Beyond Freedom and Dignity* for a similar analysis).

The various theories regarding the possible causes of ASD, like most other theories, are greatly influenced by the times in which they are postulated. These theories, and especially those that relate to the impact of parental care, are often conceived in the first place as a result of their political, social, and economic contexts (e.g., see the debate regarding the post-war political agenda that helped to promote and encourage the notion of maternal deprivation, Bowlby, 1951). Theories come in waves, and each wave seems to react to, or against, whatever has preceded it. Depending on the requirements of the time in question, certain theories will be favored more than others, and, as public, political, and scientific opinions change, some theories will fall out of favor and be replaced by others. The social climate determines what is 'in', and what is 'out', but this will fluctuate, and is never constant. Hence, many theories of ASD are agenda-driven and agenda-laden, and these alter over time to fulfill the requirements, or fit the needs, of their socio-political times. The current model views parental factors as one of potentially many factors that influence the behaviors of a child with ASD, and not as the 'cause' of the ASD.

On the other hand, certain 'within-child' causal theories of ASD may diminish feelings of guilt in parents, reduce panic, and alleviate blame. However, although rendering 'more digestible' the causal theories of ASD, and readily reducing some of the certain anguish and anxiety of parents, such 'within-child' views will not, on their own, offer any real assistance in practical terms, in managing the inherent problems of having a child with ASD. Such causal theories may inform, educate, and comfort parents, families, and the public in general, but they cannot help in practical ways to manage behaviors that are deemed inappropriate, anti-social, and even damaging. Nor can 'within-child' causal theories actively promote other behaviors that are regarded as appropriate. In contrast, if identification can be made of some child problems resulting from parenting stress and parenting behaviors, then this knowledge will aid both the child and the parents. To aid and support parents to help their children is not to blame those parents!

Diagnostic Practice

There are also implications for diagnostic practice, and the role that the process of diagnosis may play in generating parenting stress. The impact of the diagnosis on parenting stress was studied by Osborne et al. (2008c), and parents' perceptions of the diagnostic process were documented by Osborne and Reed (2008). These results suggest that the period of diagnosis may be critical in producing, and setting, parenting stress levels, and that high parenting stress has a subsequent negative impact on child outcomes and behaviors.

While there is increasing pressure to provide early diagnosis of ASD, there is a lack of evidence relating to the impact of early diagnosis on parents. Osborne et al. (2008c) suggested that early diagnosis may not necessarily be helpful to parents if they already experience high levels of parenting stress. This creates a tension, as it is often assumed that intervention for ASD is more effective if offered early, rather than remedially later (Lovaas, 1987), and such suggestions produce pressure for earlier diagnosis of these conditions. However, as mentioned by Osborne et al. (2008c), the diagnosis of mental problems can have unexpected effects (see Bentall, 1990, for a discussion relating to 'labeling' and schizophrenia).

In cases of ASD, the impact of a diagnosis can often be seen in parents (Osborne et al., 2008c), and this impact, in turn, will affect the children. Thus, although an early diagnosis of ASD may facilitate access to services, and enhance treatment prognosis for the child, the diagnosis of ASD can contribute to the production of extreme levels of stress in parents. These high levels of stress in parents have been shown to have detrimental impacts on children in terms of treatment outcomes (e.g., Osborne et al., 2008a; Robbins et al., 1991), and behavior problems (e.g., Lecavalier et al., 2006; Osborne and Reed, 2009a). Thus, parents play a pivotal role in the prospects for the child with ASD, but these parents suffer from extreme levels of stress, which can be heightened by the diagnostic process, and which have, in turn, a negative impact on the prospective outcomes for the child with ASD.

As shown in the results reported by Osborne and Reed (2008), many of the early stressors experienced by such parents revolve around communication and contact with professionals during the critical period of time in which a diagnosis of ASD is sought and obtained. Such contact often comes prior to engagement in treatment programs, and, if this contact has been stressful or aversive, it may well lead to less success in the subsequent treatment. Hence, as high parenting stress can inhibit the effectiveness of such treatments, the communication experiences of parents with professionals during the diagnostic process may be of particular importance.

Given this situation, there is a very clear need to provide further empirical evidence regarding the impacts of diagnosis on parents, and how this process could be made less stressful for parents whose children are undergoing such a diagnosis. One way forward may be to uncouple diagnosis (or a Statement of Special Needs) from accessing help, support, and intervention for children with ASD. Of course, if ASD is not regarded as a unitary disorder, but, rather, as a set of conditions, composed of a collection of behaviors, then help can be directed at those specific behaviors, as and when needed, rather than at a disorder as a whole. Such a philosophy underlies much of the applied behavioral interventions for ASD, and has recently been suggested as a policy to be adopted by the Welsh Assembly Government (Welsh Assembly Government's *The Autistic Spectrum Disorder Strategic Action Plan for Wales*, 2007).

Poverty and Economic Deprivation

If ASD is approached as a collection of behavioral difficulties, rather than as a disorder *per se*, it could be argued that ASD can be seen to share some similarities with a number of other problem areas. The practical implications that can be derived from adopting this approach, and from the current model of parent-child interactions, could then be generalized to some of these other areas of concern. One such area, which is of long-term and continuing significance, is that of economic deprivation and poverty, and its immediate and lasting impacts on children. Comparing the natures, and the approaches to alleviating the effects, of ASD and poverty may lead to possibly enhanced mutual informing and understanding. There are three points that could be made in this regard.

Firstly, it would not be sensible to suggest that poverty and economic deprivation present a single, or unique, profile of difficulties for the children who experience them. Neither could it be said that there is one single cause of poverty. Nevertheless, attempts are often made to counteract the various serious impacts of poverty on children who experience such economic deprivation problems, and such attempts are often made governmental priorities. Similarly, as argued above, it should not be thought necessary to provide evidence for a single cause of ASD, and, indeed, such a search may be fruitless. Despite this, numerous interventions have been developed for ASD. In both cases, a search for a single cause may be distracting from the search for remedies for the effects of the problems.

Secondly, there have been numerous initiatives aimed at helping children in poverty, or in areas of economic deprivation, to overcome the often debilitating effects of such deprived conditions on their learning and behaviors. Many of these initiatives are aimed at younger children, and can be called 'early interventions' (e.g., Head Start, Sure Start, etc.). The links to early teaching interventions for ASD (e.g., Lovaas, 1987) are obvious, and have, importantly, not gone unnoticed by prominent researchers and investigators in the field of ASD. In a recent interview, Greer ("*The Unorthodox Behaviorist*", 2007) makes a clear link between the effects of ASD and the impacts of poor, deprived, environments, especially in terms of their influences on language acquisition and development:

> "…they may have had thousands fewer language interactions than their peers. Other research shows that the teacher then speaks to them less than to the other kids, because she doesn't know how to deal with them, and then the kid misbehaves to get attention. By fourth grade, he's in special ed, and by 14, she's pregnant, and it's a generational repeat. And it's absolutely about poverty, not race. There were plenty of black families in the higher-income group that Hart and Risley studied and plenty of whites in the welfare group." (Greer, 2007.)

If this is the case, then early teaching interventions could be applied to aid the development of economically deprived children, of which, of course, there have been numerous examples. However, few of these examples, such as Head Start or Sure Start, have the strong empirical investigative foundations, and developed knowledge regarding their effectiveness, that many of the behavioral teaching interventions for ASD possess. Given this, the attempts to alleviate, and reverse, the effects of poverty could benefit greatly from the field of behavioral interventions for ASD.

Thirdly, this argument is mainly based on similarities in the effects of economically deprived environments, and of ASD, on language acquisition and development. However, the similarities may go much further than this, and may well involve the area of parenting practices. In fact, much of the evidence that helps to support the current model of parent-child interactions in ASD comes from studies of parenting in economically deprived families and neighborhoods. For instance, there have been some investigations of the effects of parenting stress on parenting behaviors in economically deprived populations. Rodgers (1993; 1998) found that parenting stress directly, and indirectly, affected parenting behaviors in mothers of young children in a Head Start program. Likewise, Kotchick et al. (2005; see also Meyers and Miller, 2004), in a longitudinal study of low-income, urban-dwelling, single mothers, noted that higher levels of neighborhood stress had relationships with greater psychological distress, and with detrimental effects on psychological functioning, in these mothers. This subsequently went with less engagement in positive parenting practices, and resulted in poorer parenting over time. Similarly, Ehrensaft, Wasserman, Verdelli, Greenwald, Miller, and Davies (2003) examined the long-term effects of maternal anti-social behaviors and parenting practices on behavior problems in boys at risk of developing anti-social behaviors. They found that lower levels of maternal involvement and monitoring, and higher levels of conflict between the mothers and sons, contributed to worse subsequent child behavior problems seen one year later. This overall pattern of results from economically deprived families reflects the pattern of results found in the current investigation of ASD. Thus, it is clear that there are real opportunities and fruitful possibilities to be had from a cross-fertilization, and mutual informing, of these two disparate areas.

Limitations and Future Research

As with all research, there are areas that should be acknowledged as limitations to the generality of the results, and which may inform any ongoing or future work in the field. These limitations are discussed below, and relate to participant selection, assessment of various behaviors of the participants, and the need to explore additional areas of behavior. Many of these general limitations are characteristic of all 'real world' research, and, to some extent, community-based research needs to be pragmatic in its approach, and to acknowledge the difficulties in controlling all possible variables.

Participant Selection

There are a couple of limitations to the empirical work reported in this chapter that should be mentioned with respect to the selection, and possible characteristics, of the participants involved. These limitations may affect the generality of the extrapolation of these current findings to other samples. Firstly, of course, caution needs to be exercised when extrapolating from any particular sample to the whole population of parents of children with ASD. In all of the present studies conducted by Osborne and colleagues, the samples of parents and their children studied were always volunteers. It may be that parents of children with ASD who volunteer for such research studies display different characteristics to those who do not volunteer. Consequently, the findings may be somewhat biased. However, self-selection of participants is a recognized limitation, and an acknowledged difficulty, of all such community-based studies, and this problem is not specific to this particular research. Such participant self-selection would have been the case in the vast majority, if not all, of the studies cited in this chapter. Moreover, it is not clear how this limitation could be overcome, short of coercion. Such studies depend on the voluntary participation of those involved, and participants cannot be forced to take part against their wishes. To the extent that all studies in this area have this same constraint, the findings reviewed in the current chapter are perfectly generalizable to other studies in the field.

The second participant-related issue regarding possible characteristics that might have implications for the generality of these findings, and which future research could address, is that of the impacts of the demographic characteristics (e.g., age, ethnicity, marital status, religion, socio-economic status, etc.) of the parents involved. Unfortunately, few measures of these variables were taken in the current studies, and there is no way, with sufficient accuracy, to identify precisely the social or economic background, for example, of each individual participant.

It is not known precisely how demographic factors, such as these mentioned above, may impact on the current results. Although parents' age, ethnicity, marital status, religion, and socio-economic status appear to have little impact on the probability of having a child with ASD (Ritvo, Cantwell, Johnson, Clements, Benbrook, Slagel, Kelly, and Ritz, 1971), Dumas and Wekerle (1995) looked at differences between high and low socio-economically disadvantaged families, and they found that, in the high disadvantaged group, there was a relationship between stress and parenting, but this relationship was not found in the less disadvantaged families. It is highly likely that parents from higher socio-economic backgrounds may have access to greater levels of support, in that they may be able to afford to 'buy in' help, perhaps in the form of home interventions, perhaps with greater access to day care, professional support, respite, and facilities, such as private special nurseries. In addition, such parents may be in a position to provide greater amounts of educational materials for their child (e.g., books, puzzles, toys, computers, and even extra rooms in the family home in which to hold home-based interventions, etc.). Thus, while there is little direct evidence bearing on this demographic issue that would allow assessment of its impacts, the discussion in this chapter would imply that poverty and economic deprivation are associated with greater parental stress, and can act as a break on the developmental progress of a child.

Measures of Parenting Behaviors

One of the central themes of this current chapter, and of the empirically-based model that arises from the work reported here, concerns parenting behaviors. As such, it is important to be able to assess such parenting behaviors accurately and objectively. It should be noted that the measure of parenting behaviors used in many studies reported here (e.g., the Parent-Child Relationship Inventory, PCRI) is a self-report measure. On the one hand, the PCRI is a well-standardized, reliable, validated, and widely used measure. On the other hand, it has to be acknowledged that such a measure suffers from two potential problems. Firstly, it does produce a measure of parents' self-reported perceptions of their own parenting abilities, rather than a direct measure of these behaviors. Secondly, although well-standardized for the general population, it has had limited use with the ASD population. Thus, further research that employs a range of additional measures of these parenting behaviors would help to corroborate, and systematically replicate, the current findings.

The degree to which the PCRI could be shown to correlate with other measures of parenting behaviors for this ASD sample would be an important finding. It may be that parental perceptions of their own behaviors, and those of their child, are affected by factors, such as the high levels of parenting stress that they experience. For instance, Fong (1991) noted that highly stressed mothers reported more threatening appraisals, based on video-taped scenes of adolescents with ASD engaged in everyday activities, than did low stress mothers. This might imply, simply, that highly stressed parents rate the same behaviors differently to low stress parents (albeit sometimes more accurately linked to child behaviors, see Kasari and Sigman, 1997). However, the parenting reactions of the highly stressed mothers, studied by Fong (1991), based on their assessments, were subsequently different to those of the low stress mothers; the former having more negatively emotional responses. Such differences in their subsequent reactions (i.e. in their parenting behaviors and interactions with their children) to their appraisals may lead to differences in their perceptions, and reporting, of their own parenting behaviors.

A study in which the PCRI were to be used alongside direct observation and rating of parenting behaviors would also add to the evidence concerning the validity of the PCRI for this sample. Moreover, direct observation of the parenting of children with ASD could help to corroborate the findings reported in this chapter. Although, it should be mentioned that this latter, more direct, approach would severely limit the sample size, relative to the method employed in most of the research conducted to date. Moreover, a direct observational approach would not appear to be highly feasible, or viable, given the range of parenting behaviors, and the time course of the study needed, and such an approach would be highly intrusive and invasive for the parents and families involved. Indeed, the invasiveness of such a direct and intrusive observational procedure may well lead to changes in the parenting behaviors being observed, as parents may show some reactivity to the process of being observed while parenting their children.

Role of Coping Strategies

One area of parenting that was not discussed in the current chapter was that of coping, namely, the strategies employed in order to deal with and counteract parenting stress, and adopted to handle stressful parenting situations. Neither the parents' abilities to cope with the high levels of parenting stress that they reported, nor their coping strategies, were examined in this chapter. Both of these aspects, of course, could have moderated the effects of parenting stress. This is clearly an area that could be investigated in subsequent work, and the impacts of parents' coping strategies and abilities could be incorporated in to the model of parent-child interactions postulated in this chapter.

Certainly, in models that examine the effects of stress, both degrees of coping ability and different strategies of coping are often thought of as important moderators, and/or mediators, of the effects of stress. For example, there has been work using the Double ABCX model for parents of children with ASD (Bristol, 1987), which suggests that coping strategies impact on the behaviors that stressful situations will produce. Some models of parenting incorporate coping strategies into their descriptions of the parenting process (e.g., Kurtz and Derevensky, 1994; Lazarus, 1991), and, in an extension to the basic theoretical model presented by Hastings (2002), parental coping with stress was added as a factor, although very limited evidence was presented in support of this addition of coping.

In terms of what is known about the coping strategies used by parents of children with ASD, research indicates that parents deploy a variety of coping strategies to deal with their child's ASD, including support from family and friends (Marcus, 1977), the use of service providers (DeMeyer, 1979), and religion (Gray, 1994). Hastings, Kovshoff, Brown, Ward, Degli Espinosa, and Remington (2005) documented four coping dimensions: active avoidance coping, problem-focused coping, positive coping, and religious/denial coping, and they suggested that reliance on 'avoidance' coping is detrimental, and should be decreased, if possible, and that increasing the use of 'positive' coping strategies may be beneficial.

However, the results from two other studies suggest that this advice may not be entirely appropriate, or, at least, may be over simplistic. Gray (2006) noted that parental coping strategies change over time. As time passes, fewer parents cope via reliance on service providers, family support, social withdrawal, and individualism, and more parents cope via religious faith, and other emotion-focused strategies. These results support other research on parental coping that indicates the benefits of more emotion-focused coping strategies. For example, Waddington and Reed (2009) noted greater intellectual, and educational, gains for children with severe ASD, whose parents used passive reappraisal coping strategies, rather than active or confrontive coping strategies.

This work on parent coping ties in with intervention studies that have shown that teaching parents 'mindful parenting' reduced aggression, non-compliance, and self-injury in their children, and promoted parental satisfaction with their parenting skills, as well as with their parent-child interactions (Singh, Lancioni, Winton, Fisher, Wahler, McAleavey, Singh, and Sabaawi, 2006).

A related area that may warrant some study in this ASD context is that of Acceptance and Commitment Therapy (ACT; Hayes, 1994; Hayes, Strosahl, and Wilson, 1999). ACT was originated, in part, to help people who suffer chronic levels of distress, which have debilitating effects on their functioning across many aspects of their lives. Traditional threads of Psychotherapy were designed to decrease the intensity, and frequency, of aversive affect and cognition, and ACT was developed as an alternative to these more traditional approaches. Rather than attempting, directly, to decrease such aversive feelings, emotions, and thoughts, ACT focuses on increasing behavioral effectiveness, regardless of the presence of unpleasant feelings and thoughts. Given the persistent high levels of stress in parents of children with ASD, and, given the apparent improvements for children associated with parental passive reappraisal coping strategies, ACT, in this context, may be beneficial, and is certainly worthy of future investigation in relation to possibly aiding this population.

SUMMARY

In summary, the research reported in this chapter examined relationships between parenting stress, parenting behaviors, and child behavior problems in ASD. An empirically-based model of parent-child interactions was developed, which may contribute to inform theory, and aid practice, in this neglected area of ASD research, especially regarding teaching interventions, and parent support.

REFERENCES

Baron-Cohen, S., Leslie, A. M., and Frith, U. (1985). Does the autistic child have a 'theory of mind'? *Cognition*, 21, 37-46.

Bentall, R.P. (1990). *Reconstructing schizophrenia*. London: Routledge.

Blacher, J., and McIntyre, L.L. (2006). Syndrome specificity and behavioural disorders in young adults with intellectual disability: Cultural differences in family impact. *Journal of intellectual and Developmental Disabilities*, 50, 184-198.

Blacher, J., Neece, C.L., and Paczkowski, E. (2005). Families and intellectual disability. *Current Opinion in Psychiatry*, 18, 507-513.

Blader, J.C. (2006). Which family factors predict children's externalizing behaviors following discharge from psychiatric inpatient treatment? *Journal of Child Psychology and Psychiatry*, 47, 1133-1142.

Bowlby, J. (1951). Maternal care and mental health. *Bulletin of the World Health Organization*, 3, 355-533.

Boyd, B.A. (2002). Examining the Relationship between Stress and Lack of Social Support in Mothers of Children with Autism. *Focus on Autism and Other Developmental Disabilities,* 17, *208-215.*

Brainerd, C.J. (1978). The stage question in cognitive-developmental theory. *The Behavioral and Brain Science*, 12, 173–213.

Bristol, M. M. (1987). Mothers of children with autism or communication disorders: Successful adaptation and the Double ABCX Model. *Journal of Autism and Developmental Disorders,* 17, 469-486.

Brogan, C.A., and Knussen, C. (2003). The disclosure of a diagnosis of an autism spectrum disorder. *Autism*, 7, 31-46.

Deater-Deckard, K. (1998). Parenting stress and child adjustment: Some old hypotheses and new questions. *Clinical Psychology: Science and Practice*, 5, 314-332.

DeMeyer, M.K. (1979). *Parents and children in autism*. Washington, DC.: V.H. Winston and Sons.

Donenberg, G., and Baker, B. L. (1993). The impact of young children with externalizing behaviors on their families. *Journal of Abnormal Child Psychology*, 21, 179-197.

Drash, P. W., and Tudor, R. M. (2004). An analysis of autism as a contingency-shaped disorder. *The Analysis of Verbal Behavior,* 20, 55-62.

Dumas, J.E., and Wekerle, C. (1995). Maternal reports of child behavior problems and personal distress as predictors of dysfunctional parenting. *Development and Psychopathology*, 7, 465-479.

Durate, C.S., Bordin, I.A., Yazigi, L., and and Mooney, J. (2005). Factors associated with stress in mothers of children with autism. *Autism*, 9, 416-427.

Ehrensaft, M.K., Wasserman, G.A., Verdelli, L., Greenwald, S., Miller, L.S., and Davies, M. (2003). Maternal antisocial behavior, parenting practices, and behavior problems in boys at risk for antisocial behavior. *Journal of Child and Family Studies*, 12, 27-40.

Eisenhower, A.S., Baker, B.L., and Blacher, J. (2005). Preschool children with intellectual disability: Syndrome specificity, behaviour problems, and maternal well-being. Journal of Intellectual Disability Research, 49, 657-671.

Evans, M., Stoddart, H., Condon, L., Freeman, E., Grizzell, M., and Mullen, R. (2001). Parents' perspectives on the MMR immunisation: a focus group study. *British Journal of General Practice*, 51, 904-910.

Ferster, C.B. (1961). Positive reinforcement and behavioral deficits of autistic children. *Child Development*, 32, 437-456.

Floyd, F. J., and Gallagher, E. M. (1997). Parental stress, care demands, and use of support services for school-age children with disabilities and behavior problems. *Family Relations*, 46, 359-371.

Fong, P.L. (1991). Cognitive appraisals in high- and low-stress mothers of adolescents with autism. *Journal of Consulting and Clinical Psychology*, 59, 471-474.

Foxall, G. R. (1999). The marketing firm. *Journal of Economic Psychology, 20.*

Frith, U., and Frith, C.D. (2003). Development and neurophysiology of mentalizing. *Philosophical Transactions of the Royal Society London – Series B: Biological Sciences*, 358, 459-473.

Goin-Kochel, R.P., Mackintosh, V.H., and Myers, B.J. (2006). How many doctors does it take to make an autism spectrum diagnosis. *Autism*, 5, 439-451.

Gray, D.E. (1994). Coping with autism: Stresses and strategies. *Sociology of Health and Illness*, 16, 275-300.

Gray, D.E. (2006). Coping over time: the parents of children with autism. *Journal of Intellectual Disability Research*, 50, 970-976.

Greer, R.D. (2002). *Designing teaching strategies: An applied behavior analysis systems approach*. London: Elsevier.

Greer, R.D. (2007). *The Unorthodox Behaviorist*. Teachers College, Columbia University. Press Room Article, published: *06/04/2007*.

Harris, S.L. (1984). The family of the autistic child: A behavioral-systems view. *Clinical Psychology Review*, 4, 227-239.

Harris, S.L. (1994). Treatment of family problems in autism. In E. Schopler and G.B. Mesibov (Eds.), *Behavioral issues in autism* (pp. 161-175). New York, NY: Plenum Press.

Harris, S.L., Handleman, J.S., Arnold, M.S., and Gordon, R.F. (2000). The Douglass Developmental Disabilities Center: Two models of service delivery. In J.S.Handleman and S.L.Harris (Eds.), *Preschool Education Programs for Children with Autism (2nd ed.)*, (pp. 233–260). Austin, TX: Pro-Ed.

Hastings, R. P. (2002). Parental stress and behaviour problems of children with developmental disability. *Journal of Intellectual and Developmental Disability*, 27, 149-160.

Hastings, R.P., and Brown, T. (2002). Behavior problems of children with autism, parental self-efficacy, and mental health. *American Journal on Mental Retardation*, 107, 222-232.

Hastings, R. P. and Johnson, E. (2001). Stress in UK families conducting intensive home-based behavioral intervention for their young child with autism. *Journal of Autism and Developmental Disorders*, 31, 327-336.

Hastings, R.P., Kovshoff, H., Brown, T., Ward, N.J., Espinosa, F.D., and Remington, B. (2005). Coping strategies in mothers and fathers of preschool and school age children with autism. *Autism*, 9, 377-391.

Hayes, S.C. (1994). *Acceptance and change: Content and context in psychotherapy*. Reno: Context Press.

Hayes, S.C., Strosahl, K., and Wilson, K.G. (1999). *Acceptance and Commitment Therapy: An experimental approach to behavior change*. New York: Guilford Press.

Holroyd, J., and McArthur, D. (1976). Mental retardation and stress on the parents: A contrast between Down's syndrome and childhood autism. *American Journal of Mental Deficiency*, 80, 431-436.

Jackson, A.P. (2000). Maternal self-efficacy and children's influence on stress and parenting among single black mothers in poverty. *Journal of Family Issues*, 21, 3-16.

Jackson, A.P., and Huang, C.C. (2000). Parenting stress and behavior among single mothers of preschoolers: The mediating role of self-efficacy. *Journal of Social Service Research*, 26, 29-42.

Kasari, C., and Sigman, M. (1997). Linking parental perceptions to interactions in young children with autism. *Journal of Autism and Developmental Disorders*, 27, 39-57.

Keohane, D.D., Greer, R.D., and Ackerman, S. (2007). Conditioned observation for visual stimuli and rate of learning. *Paper presented at the third conference of the International Association for Behavior Analysis, Beijing, China.*

Keogh, B.K., Garnier, H.E., Bernheimer, L.P., and Gallimore, R. (2000). Models of child family interactions for children with developmental delays: child-driven or transactional? *American Journal of Mental Retardation*, 105, 32-46.

Konstantareas, M.M. and Homatidis, S. (1989). Assessing child symptom severity and stress in parents of autistic children. *Journal of Child Psychology and Psychiatry,* 30, 459-470.

Kotchick, B.A., Dorsey, S., and Heller, L. (2005). Predictors of parenting among African American single mothers: Personal and contextual factors. *Journal of Marriage and Family*, 67, 448-460.

Kurtz, L., and Derenvensky, J. L. (1994). Adolescent motherhood: An application of the stress and coping model to child rearing attitudes and practices. *Canadian Journal of Community Mental Health*, 13, 5–24.

Lazarus, R. (1991). *Emotions and adaptations*. New York: Oxford University Press.

Lecavalier, L., Leone, S., and Wiltz, J. (2006). The impact of behaviour problems on caregiver stress in young people with autism spectrum disorders. *Journal of Intellectual Disability Research*, 50, 172-183.

Lovaas, O.I. (1987). Behavioral treatment and normal educational functioning in young autistic children. *Journal of Consulting and Clinical Psychology*, 55, 3-9.

Lovaas, O. I., and Smith, T. (2003). Early and intensive behavioral intervention in autism. In E. Kazdin and J. R. Weisz (Eds.), *Evidence-based psychotherapies for children and adolescents* (pp. 325-340). New York: Guilford.

Marcus L. (1977). Patterns of coping in families of psychotic children. *American Journal of Orthopsychiatry,* 47, 383-399.

Mash, E.J., and Johnston, C. (1983). Parental perceptions of child behavior problems, parenting self-esteem, and mothers' reported stress in younger and older hyperactive and normal children. *Journal of Consulting and Clinical Psychology*, 51, 86-99.

Meyers, S.A., and Miller, C. (2004). Direct, mediated, moderated, and cumulative relations between neighborhood characteristics and adolescent outcomes. *Adolescence*, 39, 121-144.

Osborne, L.A., McHugh, L., Saunders, J., and Reed, P. (2008a). Parenting stress reduces the effectiveness of early teaching interventions for Autistic Spectrum Conditions. *Journal of Autism and Developmental Disorders*, 38, 1092-1103.

Osborne, L.A., McHugh, L., Saunders, J., and Reed, P. (2008b). The effect of parenting behaviors on subsequent child behavior problems in Autistic Spectrum Conditions. *Research in Autism Spectrum Disorders*, 2, 249-263.

Osborne, L.A., McHugh, L., Saunders, J., and Reed, P. (2008c). A possible contra indication for early diagnosis of Autistic Spectrum Conditions: Impact on parenting stress. *Research in Autism Spectrum Disorders.*

Osborne, L.A., and Reed, P. (2008). Parents' perceptions of communication with professionals during the diagnosis of autism. *Autism*, 12, 259-274.

Osborne, L.A., and Reed, P. (2009a). The relationship between parental stress and behavior problems of children with autistic spectrum disorders receiving teaching interventions. *Exceptional Children.*

Osborne, L.A., and Reed, P. (2009b). The role of the family in Autistic Spectrum Conditions: Theory and Practical Implications. Under review

Osborne, L.A., and Reed, P. (2009c). Stress and perceived parenting behaviors in parents of children with Autistic Spectrum Conditions. Under review

Piaget, J. (1954). *Intelligence and affectivity: Their relationship during child development.* Palo Alto, CA: Annual Review, Inc.

Ritvo, E.R. Cantwell, D., Johnson, E., Clements, M., Benbrook, F., Slagle, S., Kelly, P., and Ritz, M. (1971). Social class factors in autism. *Journal of Autism and Childhood Schizophrenia*, 1, 297-310.

Robbins, F.R., Dunlap, G., and Plienis, A.J. (1991). Family characteristics, family training, and the progress of young children with autism. *Journal of Early Intervention*, 15, 173-184.

Robinson, E.A., and Anderson, L.L. (1983). Family adjustment, parental attitudes, and social desirability. *Journal of Abnormal Child Psychology*, 11, 247-256.

Rodgers, A.Y. (1993). The assessment of variables related to the parenting behaviour of mothers with young children. *Children and Youth Services Review*, 15, 385-402.

Rodgers, A.Y. (1998). Multiple sources of stress and parenting behavior. *Children and Youth Services Review*, 20, 525-546. Cambridge: Cambridge University Press.

Schuntermann, P. (2002). Pervasive developmental disorder and parental adaptation: Previewing and reviewing atypical development with parents in child psychiatric consultation. *Harvard Review of Psychiatry*, 10, 16-27.

Singh, N.N., Lancioni, G.E., Winton, A.S.W., Fisher, B.C., Wahler, R.G., McAleavey, K., Singh, J., and Sabaawi, M. (2006). Mindful parenting decreases aggression, noncompliance, and self-injury in children with autism. *Journal of Emotional and Behavioral Disorders,* 14, 169-177.

Stoddart, K.P. (1999). Adolescents with Asperger syndrome: Three case studies of individual and family therapy. *Autism,* 3, 255-271.

Waddington, E.M., and Reed, P. (2009). Comparison of the affects of mainstream and special school placements on outcomes in children with ASD: An archive-based analysis. *Submitted for publication.*

Welsh Assembly Government (2007). *The Autistic Spectrum Disorder Strategic Action Plan for Wales*. Welsh Assembly Government.

In: Behavioral Theories and Interventions for Autism
Editor: Phil Reed
ISBN 978-1-60741-165-9
© 2009 Nova Science Publishers, Inc.

Chapter 10

TEACHING PARENTS TO USE APPLIED BEHAVIOR ANALYSIS WITH THEIR CHILD WITH AN AUTISTIC SPECTRUM DISORDER

Kate E. Fiske and Sandra L. Harris*
Rutgers, The State University of New Jersey, USA

The field of Applied Behavior Analysis (ABA) has a long-standing tradition of inviting parents to be partners in the process of change for their children with autism. Early research showed that many parents were fully capable of collaborating in the process of implementing ABA programs in the home and community. Based on those findings, teaching mothers and fathers the fundamental skills necessary to implement ABA instructional programs became standard practice in many settings. This partnership between parents and professionals is especially important when addressing the needs of children on the autism spectrum, as many of them have considerable difficulty generalizing skills learned in one setting to different places, persons or activities. In spite of their potential to be superb ABA partners, parents and other family members face a number of challenges in raising a child with an autism spectrum disorder. These challenges may impact their ability to work effectively at implementing ABA programs.

The present chapter first reviews the research on methods of teaching ABA to parents of children with autism spectrum disorders. We will review both the initial work demonstrating that parents could have a valued role in implementing primarily discrete trial instruction and more recent studies addressing their role in the latest naturalistic methods of instruction. When we use the term "discrete trial" we are referring to a very structured method of teaching in which a task is presented to the child (e.g., "touch your nose"), the child is given time to respond, and the teacher reacts to the child's response. The reaction may be in the form of positive reinforcement (e.g., stating, "Good job, you touched your nose") or in the form of corrective feedback (e.g., stating, "This is touching your nose" while guiding the child's hand to his nose). When we use the term "naturalistic," we are referring to methods that, while

* Please address correspondence to: Sandra L. Harris, Ph.D., Professor Emerita and the Executive Director of the Douglass Developmental Disabilities Center, Rutgers, The State University of New Jersey, New Brunswick, New Jersey, USA, e-mail: sharris@rci.rutgers.edu

based on the principles of ABA, closely resemble the ways in which children and adults typically interact in less structured settings. Naturalistic teaching is well-planned and has clear goals that are evident to the teacher/parent even when an outside observer might not immediately recognize the underlying principles.

Research indicates that both discrete trial and naturalistic teaching methods are highly effective and that each has its place in instruction for individuals with autism (e.g., Farmer-Dougan, 1994; Lovaas, Koegel, Simmons, and Long, 1973; McGee, Krantz, and McClannahan, 1985, 1986; Smith, 1993. Many clinicians indicate that discrete trial instruction may be best utilized to teach skills that require much repetition and for which there is low motivation (e.g., Sundberg and Partington, 1998, 1999), while naturalistic teaching may be best utilized to teach skills that require initiation. A combination of both teaching methods may maximize a child's skill acquisition and generalization (McGee, Krantz, and McClannahan, 1985; Smith, McAdam, and Napolitano, 2007). In addition to examining parent training using each of these approaches, we will also look briefly at the small body of research on teaching the basics of ABA to siblings of children on the autism spectrum.

In addition to exploring the effectiveness of parents as teachers, we will describe how parental stress changes with various challenges posed by the child on the autism spectrum and consider what little is know about how these stressful events influence a parent's ability to carry out home- and community-based ABA programs. Similarly, we will examine how cultural factors may influence parental reactions to their child's developmental disorder and consider how these factors may influence the involvement of parents in ABA teaching. Finally, we will point to some areas where more data-based knowledge would be of considerable value.

PARENTS AS TEACHERS: A BRIEF HISTORY

The engagement of parents in their child's treatment is not unique to ABA. Typically, non-ABA parent training has less empirical support than do ABA methods and, in many cases, non-ABA parent training has placed less emphasis on making parents experts in the teaching methods and more on helping them understand autism and the assumptions of the various approaches. However, the behavioral—but not ABA-based—Treatment and Education of Autistic and Related Communication-Handicapped Children (TEACCH) program teaches parents how to implement TEACCH methods (e.g., Olley, Robbins, Morelli-Robbins, 1993). Similarly, the Early Bird Program run by the National Autistic Society in Great Britain reports on their website about significant changes in parenting skills and feelings following parent training in their treatment methods (http://www.nas.org.uk/-nas/jsp/polopoly.jsp?d=10). It is important to recognize that a variety of treatment approaches have recognized the valuable role that parents can play.

Notably, however, the most extensive and research-based parent training practices have been done from an ABA perspective. Before we look at that work, it is interesting to examine briefly some earlier efforts to involve parents in the treatment of their child. One of the best known case studies was that of Little Hans, a young boy with a horse phobia whom Sigmund Freud treated in the 1800s. Freud (1959) enrolled Hans' father as his son's therapist in what was reported as a successful intervention. More recently, some client-centered therapists—building on the initial work of Carl Rogers (1951)—taught parents the reflective and interpersonally sensitive skills that are part of the client-centered approach (e.g., Guerney, 1969) and enrolled them as co-therapists in treating their own children.

In spite of the interest of these early efforts, not until behavior therapists began to engage parents in the change process was a persuasive body of research developed documenting that behavioral interventions carried out by parents could significantly alter problem behaviors and enhance skill acquisition of children. In the 1930s, Weber (1936) taught parents to use behavioral procedures to reduce their children's fears and O. H. Mowrer and W. M. Mowrer (1938) trained parents to address their child's bedwetting problems.

In the 1960s, behaviorally-based parent training began to gain more general attention from practitioners. At a meeting of the American Psychological Association in 1965, Pumroy described a procedure for teaching parents what was know then as "behavior modification" for their child. The work increased in frequency and sophistication in the years that followed (e.g., Lindsley, 1966; Patterson and Brodsky, 1966; Patterson, McNeal, Hawkins, and Phelps, 1967). By the 1970s, a sufficient body of work justified two major reviews, one by Berkowitz and Graziano (1972) and another by O'Dell (1974).

Much of the early work on parent training focused on teaching parents to intervene behaviorally with relatively common problems such as bedwetting (e.g., Azrin, Hontos, and Basalel-Azrin, 1979) and oppositional behavior (Wahler and Fox, 1980). By the 1970s, however, a growing appreciation of the power of teaching parents to use "operant conditioning" to meet the needs of children with autism and mental retardation had emerged (e.g., Harris and Romanczyk, 1976; R. L. Koegel, Glahn and Nieminen, 1978; Kozloff, 1973).

PARENTS AS TEACHERS: THE EARLY RESEARCH

A compelling early paper by Lovaas, Koegel, Simmons and Long (1973) reported that, no matter how effective the behavioral treatment a child might receive in a specialized institutional setting, the youngster was at significant risk of regression when returned to a less supportive setting such as a state institution without trained staff, or a home where the parents were not skilled in the use of behavioral teaching methods. These findings underscored the importance of training parents in behavioral methods to ensure that the children would receive treatment in the natural environment. Without preparing both caregivers and children for the shift from one setting to another, it was close to impossible for behavior change to be maintained. Training of staff members and parents, as well as gradual fading of cues to prepare the child for the novel setting, were essential if the child were to retain learned behaviors and acquire new ones. Eric Schopler and his colleagues at the TEACCH program in North Carolina had come to a similar conclusion and were among the first to include systematic parent training as part of their program of intervention for children with autism (1978).

As the report by Lovaas et al. (1973) became known to professionals using behavioral methods to serve children with autism, and as these clinical researchers saw for themselves the consequences that followed when a strong link between school or center based treatment and home was not established, they developed an interest in looking empirically at the role parents could play in the education and treatment of their child on the autism spectrum. Several different groups, as well a number of individual investigators, were involved in this seminal research. A review of a sample of this work follows.

Koegel, Schreibman et al.

One major body of early work was conducted by Robert Koegel, Laura Schreibman and their colleagues in California (e.g., Koegel, Schreibman, Britten, Burke and O'Neill, 1982; Koegel, Schreibman, Johnson, O'Neill, and Dunlap, 1984). In one study, they compared the relative benefits of 25 to 50 hours of parent training in ABA with 225 hours of child-focused ABA treatment in an outpatient clinic (Koegel et al., 1982). They also systematically analyzed the acquisition of ABA teaching skills by parents and subsequent adaptive skill acquisition by their children (e.g., Koegel, Glahn and Nieminen, 1978). These researchers found that children whose parents participated in training made more progress 3 months after training ended than did children who received clinic treatment. The parents who participated in behavioral training also reported that they engaged in more leisure time activity at follow-up than did those parents whose children were enrolled in the out-patient clinic. Of note, children who received clinic-based instruction received 4 ½ hours of instruction a week by a skilled therapist, and the parents who received training provided an unknown number of hours a week for their children. Based on what we have learned since about the crucial role of hours of instruction, it may well be that the small number of weekly clinic hours, no matter how skillfully provided, was insufficient to have much impact on the clinic treated children. We can speculate that some of the parents who had been trained devoted much more extensive time to their children than was provided for clinic children.

Regardless of this limitation, this interesting initial work set the stage for many years of fine research on the inclusion of parent training in the treatment of people with autism. In recent years their work has focused on naturalistic ABA teaching methods (e.g., Koegel and Koegel, 2005; Ingersoll and Schreibman, 2006). Some of this work is discussed below in conjunction with recent naturalistic approaches to educating children on the autism spectrum and in the section on teaching ABA methods to siblings.

Howlin et al.

Another important body of research was developed in England by Patricia Howlin and her colleagues (e.g., Hemsley et al., 1978; Howlin, 1981a, 1981b; Howlin, Marchant, Rutter, Berger, Hersov and Yule, 1973). These investigators focused on how parents might enhance the use of speech and language by their child with autism. They conducted a home-based study of parent training with the families of 16 boys with autism between the ages of 3 and 11 years with nonverbal IQs of 60 of higher. Two matched control groups were used to compare changes over 6 months and at a later follow-up. Howlin (1981b) reported that the boys in the treatment condition demonstrated significant benefits from their parents' use of behavioral interventions to stimulate speech. The later follow-up, however, indicated a significant relation between continued benefits of treatment and the child's functioning level at the start of treatment. Holmes et al. (1982) note that many parents reported major challenges in being able to sustain their teaching effort over time.

Harris et al.

A third stream of the early research on parent training was done by Harris and her colleagues at the Douglass Developmental Disabilities Center of Rutgers, The State University of New Jersey. These studies, all done in small training groups of 5 or 6 couples, showed gains in parents' teaching skills (e.g., Weitz, 1982), and improvement in children's speech and language skills, as well as gains in appropriate behavior (e.g., Harris, 1983; Harris, Wolchik and Milch, 1982; Harris, Wolchik and Weitz, 1981).

While immediate skill acquisition by parents and behavior change by children is important in treatment, the follow-up data for this research suggest considerable variability in the long-term outcome of parent training courses. Harris (1986) reported on a 4- to 7-year follow-up of 42 families who participated in one of a series of intensive 10-week parent training courses between 1977 and 1981. Among the 30 parents who responded to a questionnaire (approximately 75% of the original sample), Harris (1986) found a significant positive correlation between child IQ at intake as estimated by the *Developmental Profile* (Alpern and Boll, 1972) and parental report of child skill level at follow-up. Children who had more speech at intake had higher skill levels at follow-up and those children who exhibited echolalia at intake had higher follow-up language ratings than those who were not echolalic at intake. In a second follow-up study with this same population of families, Harris (1987) reported that 86% of parents had used behavioral skills in the week prior to their self-report, and 54% said they still used behavioral methods to teach new skills to their child. More than half no longer collected data on teaching programs. She also found that parents whose children were enrolled in ABA programs were much more likely to have continued using ABA teaching methods than were those parents whose children entered generic special education classrooms.

The General Impact of Parent Training

Among the most important findings from the early work on parent training was the demonstration that parents could learn the ABA skills needed to modify such varied behavior as speech and language (Harris, 1983; Howlin, 1981a, 1981b), eating problems (e.g., Stimbert, Minor and McCoy, 1977), rituals, crying, whining and noncompliance (Moore and Bailey, 1973; Nordquist and Wahler, 1973) and self-injury (Harris and Romanczyk, 1976). Some studies taught parents the specific skills they needed to address a particular problem behavior (e.g., Harris and Romanczyk, 1976; Holmes et al., 1982) and others used a broader curriculum, including both skill acquisition and behavior management, to allow parents to intervene in an array of settings (e.g. Baker, Heifetz, and Murphy, 1980; Heifetz, 1977; Howlin, 1981a, 1981b; Koegel et al., 1982). Parent training that focuses on a single behavior problem or new skill may have more limited utility for parents than does an approach that teaches an array of skills and problem solving strategies. Because the needs of parents and families change over time as the child grows and develops, training in the broader curriculum may help them adapt their treatment approach using general principles of behavior change. Notably, however, the work of Harris (1987) suggests that parents often require on-going support in developing interventions if they are to remain effective in their role as teachers.

The early studies on teaching parents an array of skills often focused much of the parent training curriculum on the use of discrete trial instruction (Koegel, Russo and Rincover, 1977). Early work at the Douglass Developmental Disabilities Center taught parents to use a variety of methods within a discrete trial format, including how to establish attending, teach imitation, shape behavior, deliver reinforcement, and program for generalization and maintenance. The research showed that parents became more skillful in these methods over time and that they used the skills with their children who, in turn, demonstrated improved behavior (e.g., Harris, Wolchik and Milch, 1982; Harris, Wolchik and Weitz, 1981; Weitz, 1982). Howlin's (1981a, 1981b) research reported similar findings on training parents to stimulate child speech using ABA methods. Both individual (e.g., Tymchuk, 1979) and group (e.g., Harris, 1983) instruction of parents were found to be effective contexts for teaching parents new skills to use with their children on the autism spectrum and/or with mental retardation.

The benefits of parent training for children with autism are so well documented that recent studies have compared a parent training intervention with intensive clinic directed intervention. For example, Smith, Groen, and Wynn (2000) compared the benefits of intensive ABA treatment for an average of 24.52 hours a week with parent training for preschool-aged children. Parents whose children were assigned randomly to the parent training condition participated in 5 hours a week of training in ABA over 3 to 9 months. Smith et al. (2000) found children in the intensive treatment group made greater gains in IQ scores, visual-spatial abilities, language, and academic work than did the children whose parents were trained to use ABA. The two groups did not, however, differ on standardized tests of the children's level of adaptive functioning or the presence of behavior problems following intervention.

More recently, Sallows and Graupner (2005) compared preschool-aged children who were randomly assigned either to an intensive ABA program or to a parent-directed program. Children in the intensive treatment group received a mean of 39 hours a week of treatment in Year 1 and 37 hours in Year 2. Parents in the parent-directed group were allowed to choose the number of hours of treatment they wished to provide for their child, and this group was expected to provide the less intensive treatment. In Year 1, however, they implemented a mean of 32 hours per week and in Year 2, they implemented 31 hours of instruction per week. In this case, where more consultation was provided to the parent directed group than in the Smith et al. (2000) study, the parent-directed children performed just about as well as the clinic-directed group. In addition to documenting the potential power of early intervention, these two studies highlight the need for intensive support and consultation when the parents assume the primary responsibility for the treatment of their child with autism. In those cases where a school, center, or experienced consultant takes the primary role in intervention provision and parents provide supplementary instruction, parents may not require the number of hours of support and supervision that are essential for effective intervention when they take the lead role in instruction. Whether children are being treated in the home or school, however, parents are vulnerable to considerable stress because of the challenges inherent in raising a child with a serious developmental challenge. We discuss some of these sources of stress later in the chapter.

EARLY USE OF NATURALISTIC METHODS

The roots of naturalistic teaching methods, as well as highly structured teaching had their start in the early era of parent training. As we noted above, naturalistic teaching, while thoughtfully planned and based on the principles of ABA, is less structured in approach than is discrete trial instruction, and is very attuned to the shifting interests of the child. An early example of naturalistic teaching is found in the work of Hart and Risley (1980) who introduced the concept of incidental teaching to enhance speech among educationally disadvantaged young children. This method was quickly demonstrated to be effective for teaching learners on the autism spectrum to use speech during meal preparation (McGee, Krantz, Mason and McClannahan, 1983; McGee, Krantz and McClannahan, 1985).

In her initial parent training research, Harris (1983) included what she termed "informal teaching," during which parents were asked to play with their child and interact verbally throughout the day. As they did so, they were taught to apply basic concepts such as keeping speech simple, labeling items and activities, repeating back to the child things he or she said, making simple expansions of the child's speech, and rewarding speech attempts with attention and other reinforcements. Parents were also encouraged to create circumstances that required the child to use communication skills to obtain desired items that were out of reach or could not be accomplished by the child alone (Sosne, Handleman and Harris, 1979). This informal teaching was intended to extend the structured discrete trial language instruction into the natural environment and support the meaningful and generalized use of speech. Similar successful work had been done that blended formal and informal instruction for parents of children with Down Syndrome (Salzberg and Villani, 1983) and language delay (MacDonald, Blott, Gordon, Spiegel and Hartmann, 1974).

Taken as whole, the early research on parent training demonstrated that parents could be effective teachers for their child on the autism spectrum, but that a number of issues required continuing research including the refinement of naturalistic teaching methods and strategies to ensure generalization and maintenance of newly acquired skills by both children and parents (Harris, Alessandri, and Gill, 1991). The initial research also highlighted the importance of taking into account the impact on the family of raising a child with autism and how this experience influenced family members' ability to persist in implementing home-based work with their child (e.g., Harris, 1986, 1987; Holmes et al., 1982). The impact of this unique parental role on the stress and coping of parents of children with autism is discussed later in this chapter.

NATURALISTIC PARENT TRAINING

Much of the recent research on parent training has focused on the use of naturalistic teaching strategies in the home setting. While sharing the advantage of increasing quantity and availability of instruction with other methods of teaching (Koegel, Symon, and Koegel,

2002), naturalistic teaching responds to the criticism that training in other methods, such as discrete trial teaching, can be both time-consuming and poorly maintained by parents (Laski, Charlop, and Schreibman, 1988; Holmes et al., 1982). As has been discussed, early research in naturalistic teaching strategies demonstrated positive results. Laski, Charlop, and Schreibman (1988), for instance, trained parents to implement the natural language paradigm (NLP) with their children with autism in the home setting. The procedure was designed to increase child motivation through the use of turn-taking and shared control over choice in activities, to increase responding through the delivery of natural reinforcement for all verbal attempts, and to increase generalization through loose structure and multiple exemplars. Parents were taught to use these strategies via video modeling and in vivo teaching. Training resulted in an increase in parent requests for verbalizations from their child in generalization settings and, more importantly, in increases in child verbal responsiveness.

Most research in the use of naturalistic teaching strategies with parents of children with autism is focused on the use of pivotal response training (PRT). Proponents of PRT maintain that optimal gains in skill acquisition can be attained by focusing on what are termed "pivotal skills," or skills that, once acquired, will result in collateral gains in other areas (Koegel, Koegel, and Schreibman, 1991; Koegel, Symon, and Koegel, 2002). These pivotal behaviors are motivation and responsivity to multiple cues. That is, researchers suggest that a child who demonstrates increased motivation and ability to respond to multiple cues in the environment simultaneously will show collateral improvements in areas such as verbal communication, adaptive behavior, and academic performance. Parent training in PRT has been used to improve both generalization and maintenance of the skills taught using these techniques.

One of the advantages of parent training in PRT is that the model for training has been well developed. Parents are trained in a variety of techniques critical to the implementation of PRT. For instance, parents are trained to deliver clear instructions to their child, to intersperse maintenance tasks with tasks not yet learned, to provide multiple cues in instruction (e.g., "give me the *red* ball" rather than "give me the ball"), to share control of the activity with the child, and to provide clear, immediate, natural reinforcement contingent upon correct responses or attempts (e.g., handing the child the ball when he says or attempts to say the word "ball"; Koegel, Koegel, and Schreibman, 1991). Training for parents includes the use of a PRT training manual which details the above techniques, viewing of video models of PRT instruction with opportunities for discussion, as well as direct modeling and in vivo training with feedback for the parents in the context of everyday activities (e.g., meals, playground, etc.). The training model also allows for measurement of generalization and maintenance through the analysis of video samples of parents implementing the techniques in the context of family routines (e.g., family dinner) over time (Koegel, Koegel, and Schreibman, 1991).

This parent training model has been used to successfully train parents in PRT, resulting in improvements in parent skills and child behavior. Koegel, Symon, and Koegel (2002) report on the use of the training model to train parents living in areas geographically distant from the training center. The above training model was provided in an individualized format to five families of children with autism. The 25 hours of training took place over the course of one week. Analysis of video samples of family routines in the home setting before and after training show increased parent use of PRT in the home setting, as well as increased verbal production from the children following training. In analysis of the videos, parents were also observed to demonstrate increased positive affect in interactions with their child following

PRT training. These promising results were maintained for as long as 1 year following training (Koegel, Symon, and Koegel, 2002).

Research indicates that PRT may result not only in collateral effects on the target children, but also in collateral effects among the parents. Koegel, Bimbela, and Schreibman (1996) demonstrated that parents of children with autism were more likely to demonstrate positive affect while interacting with their child at dinner following PRT training than were those parents who received training in teaching individual target behaviors (ITB). Teaching individual target behaviors required parents to run adult-structured teaching sessions with their child in which they reinforced their children for correct or successive approximations of target skills using edible reinforcement and praise. In contrast, PRT was child-directed and utilized natural reinforcement of correct responses and attempts of skills. In response to the findings, researchers postulated that PRT allowed parents to generalize teaching strategies to dinner more readily than parents who had been instructed in ITB, resulting in decreased stress and increased positive affect during this time (Koegel, Bimbela, and Schreibman, 1996).

The success of PRT during family routines has been noted by many and indicates that parent training that is compatible with family routines may result in greater parent and child skill acquisition, generalization, and maintenance than does less compatible training. The use of training that fits well into family context is termed "contextual" training, and relies on the integration of interventions in the preexisting family structure. Moes and Frea (2000) indicate that prescriptive interventions that are not altered to fit the family structure are less likely to be maintained than contextual interventions. To contextualize an intervention, professionals must assess the abilities and needs of family members who will implement the intervention, the daily routines and activities taking place during times when the intervention will be implemented, competing demands on and responsibilities of family members, available resources for the family members, and the desired interaction patterns of the family members (Moes and Frea, 2000).

An example of contextualized intervention in the home was demonstrated by Moes and Frea (2002) in training parents of their child with autism to implement functional communication training (FCT) to decrease disruptive behavior. Families were first asked to conduct daily functional communication training sessions as prescribed by the consultants, without taking family context into account. Following this phase, the consultants assessed the family's beliefs, needs, and desires as described above and altered the FCT procedure accordingly. The adjustments resulted in naturalistic teaching procedures in which FCT was integrated into daily routines such as play sessions with siblings and at dinner. Decreases in disruptions no longer remained the only goal of the interventions; goals also included increased support for parents, including emotional support, from various family members during daily routines. While prescriptive FCT resulted in only minimal decreases in disruptive behavior, contextualized FCT resulted in near-zero levels of disruptive behavior in all children in generalization settings and at a 2-month follow-up. In addition, parents reported that contextualized FCT would be much more sustainable in their family than would the traditional FCT package. This finding was especially prominent among mothers of children with autism, which is notable given that mothers were the sole providers of the prescribed FCT sessions (Moes and Frea, 2002).

Recently, researchers have begun to examine the use of parenting programs, such as the Stepping Stones Triple P (SSTP), in the treatment of individuals with autism (Sanders, Mazzucchelli, and Studman, 2004; Sanders, Plant, and McHale, 2002). SSTP teaches parenting strategies based on behavior and behavior analytic principles to parents of children with developmental disabilities, and is an adaptation of the original Triple P-Positive Parenting Program, which was initially developed to address the concerns of families of children with behavioral problems (Sanders, Markie-Dadds, Tully, and Bor, 2000; Sanders, Mazzucchelli, and Studman, 2004). The program is structured to address parent concerns at a number of levels, from basic parent management skills to the skills that are required to manage multiple behavior problems. Notably, SSTP is designed to be implemented within the family context, and at its most intensive level addresses not only child concerns but also family problems such as relationship conflict, depression, and adapting to having a child with a disability (Sanders, Mazzucchelli, and Studman, 2004).

In SSTP, parents are taught a variety of skills—all within the context of daily family activities and routines—including addressing the function of problem behavior, managing behavior, teaching skills to their child that may reduce problem behavior, and problem solving for future challenges (Sanders, Mazzucchelli, and Studman, 2004). The body of evidence among families of autism, while emerging, suggests that the contextualized approach is deemed acceptable and usable by parents (Whittingham, Sofronoff, and Sheffield, 2006). Early research with individuals with autism suggests that this contextual approach to parent training reduces parent report of difficult child behavior and increases parents' sense of efficacy (Sanders, Plant, and McHale, 2002). While additional research on the use of parent training programs like SSTP is necessary to fully assess the impact on families of children with autism, they do highlight the potential importance of contextualizing treatment to promote parent skill acquisition and generalization.

Research in naturalistic teaching strategies indicates positive results of parent training in these techniques. Not only do naturalistic approaches such as NLP, PRT, and contextualized interventions result in increases in appropriate behavior among children with autism when implemented by parents, but they also facilitate impressive generalization and maintenance of parent teaching skills and child behavior. The incorporation of naturalistic teaching strategies into daily routines improves parents' ability to generalize the skills to new settings and sustain the teaching strategies over time. The use of the strategies is easily integrated into the family structure, allowing all members of the family to become involved in the teaching process. We shall now consider the siblings' role in instruction of the child with an autism spectrum disorder.

The Role of Siblings

Brothers and sisters of children with autism can be valuable allies in supporting the process of change. In an early study, Colletti and Harris (1977) used an ABAB reversal design to demonstrate that a 10-year-old girl could teach her 9-year-old sister with autism to string beads by using clear directions and edible reinforcement. A study of the role of siblings as "teachers" by Schreibman, O'Neill and Koegel (1983) was successful in teaching siblings to help their brother or sister with autism complete academic work. In a study with an older sibling, Lobato and Tlaker (1985) trained a 21-year-old sister to teach her 13-year-old brother essential self-help skills. Similarly, Swenson-Pierce, Kohl and Egel (1987) effectively trained siblings to teach domestic skills to their sibling with mental retardation. All of these early sibling studies involved having the children interact during highly structured tasks such as stringing beads, simple academic activities and basic self-help routines. Thus, while they were useful demonstrations of the extent to which a broad range of people could teach fundamental skills to individuals with autism and/or mental retardation, they did not address instruction in more typical sibling interactions, including—most importantly—play.

For the most part, parents help us learn self-help and academic skills and our siblings are our partners at playtime (Wulff, 1985). Being able to play with their sibling is a fond wish of most brothers and sisters of a child with autism and they are often frustrated by their inability to engage their sibling in childhood fun. In recognition of this problem, several studies have demonstrated the feasibility of increasing playful behavior among siblings. In an early study, Powell, Salzburg, Rule, and Itzkowitz (1983) showed that parents could facilitate cooperative play for their mentally retarded child and a typically developing sibling. These parents used social praise and prompts to encourage the interactions but did not teach any special behavioral skills to the typically developing child. In a study with children with autism, Coe, Matson, Craigie and Gossen (1991) indicated that the siblings of two children on the autism spectrum could learn to use prompting and reinforcement techniques in a play setting.

El-Ghoroury and Romanczyk (1999) compared the play of parents and siblings with a child with autism. Among their findings were that parents tried harder to engage the child with autism in play than they did their typical child, and the harder the child with autism was to engage, the harder the parents tried to make the connection. The siblings, in contrast, made less effort to help their brother or sister on the spectrum compensate for skill deficits than did the parents. There was, however, some evidence that children with autism had an interest in interacting with their typically developing sibling. These findings highlight the importance of teaching both the child with autism and the typical sibling skills with which to engage one another in playful activities.

Celiberti and Harris (1993) systemically taught children the ABA skills needed to gain their brother or sister's attention: Give a clear, simple instruction; give their sibling time to follow the direction; and use a variety of requests during the play time. The siblings also learned to give social praise and to use prompts when necessary. The typically developing siblings were girls ranging in age from 7 to 10 years old and their siblings with autism—two boys and one girl—were preschool-aged. All three couplets showed measurable gains in play interaction during the training period and these changes were impressively maintained at a 16-week follow-up. Undergraduates naïve to the purposes of the study watched videos of the children pre- and post-training, and indicated that all children exhibited positive changes in play. In brief, they looked like they were having fun!

Children with autism can also learn the skills they need to play with their brother or sister. Belchic and Harris (1994) showed that when preschool-aged children with autism were taught to initiate social interactions with a peer at school, they were able to generalize this skill to a sibling at home. Thus, siblings can learn to play and interact with one another via instruction given to either child. In addition, these same skills can be valuable for peers to master when they learn and play along side of a child with autism in an inclusive educational setting.

PARENT STRESS OVER TIME

As we have suggested, the professional involved in training parents must be aware of the impact of stress on parents' ability to take on the role of teacher for the child with autism. The unique stresses of raising a child with autism—seeking appropriate services, advocating for the child, intensive care for the child in the home—may make the additional challenge of parent training seem overwhelming to the parent. Additionally, the stress may interfere with even the best-trained parent's implementation of behavioral techniques. Despite these concerns, parent training may also have therapeutic effects for the parent and, transitively, the child. These effects will be reviewed here.

Stress is defined as an individual's response to life strains, demanding events, or crises. Stress is manifested in physiological and psychological patterns that can either be in immediate response to the event or delayed (Rabkin and Streuning, 1976). Parents of children with autism experience a greater level of stress than do parents of typically developing children, and even experience more stress than do parents of children with other disabilities such as Down Syndrome and mental retardation (Donovan, 1988) or parents of children with fatal or chronic illnesses (Bouma and Schweitzer, 1990).

The higher level of stress among parents of children with autism may be attributed to the lack of effective communication with their child, the maladaptive behavior frequently exhibited by these children, as well as the absence, in many cases, of a positive affective relationship with their child (Donovan, 1988; Olsson and Hwang, 2001). The increased stress may contribute to greater rates of depression among mothers of children with autism (Olsson and Hwang, 2001) and increased anxiety among fathers (Hastings and Brown, 2002). Stress and decreased mental health may make parents reluctant or unable to participate in parent training or implement teaching strategies in the home environment.

Parent stress is a phenomenon that will shift over time and be affected by multiple factors. Child transitions may serve as a significant stressor for parents, and professionals should be aware that parents may be especially susceptible to stress during such times. For instance, researchers have postulated that transitions into adolescence and adulthood may result in increases in parental stress as parents are forced to consider new treatment options, to plan for the new stage of their child's life, and to face the pervasiveness and long-term effects of their child's disorder (Donovan, 1988; Hanline, 1991; Scorgie, Wilgosh, and McDonald, 1998; Wikler, 1986). While reactions to initial diagnosis are obviously stressful, laced with feelings of sorrow, guilt, blame, resentment, and disbelief (Midence and O'Neill, 1999), these experiences can be triggered by successive events in the child's life that remind the parent of the child's diagnosis and of "what could have been." These events may include when a younger sibling developmentally surpasses the child with autism, the affected child's entry into school, medical crises (Hanline, 1991), increases in the child's maladaptive behavior (Baker et al., 2003; Mansell and Morris, 2004), and consideration of residential placements (Baker and Blacher, 2002; Hanline, 1991).

Despite the pervasiveness of parent stress among families of children with autism, a number of factors increase parents' resiliency in managing their child with autism. For example, parents may experience less stress if they have higher education, greater financial resources, more effective problem-solving skills, stronger faith (Kwai-Sang and Li-Tsang, 1999), more optimism (Baker, Blacher, and Olsson, 2005), and a greater sense of control, commitment, and acceptance of challenge (Weiss, 2002). The reported best predictor of coping success among parents of children with autism is the quality of the parents' marital relationship (Kwai-Sang and Li-Tsang, 1999).

An additional factor that increases parents' ability to cope with stress and stave off depression and anxiety is social support (Boyd, 2002; Hanline, 1991; Gill and Harris, 1991; Hastings and Johnson, 2001; Weiss, 2002). Social support can take many forms, including friends, parent support groups, educators, and—of particular relevance here—parent training. Bristol, Gallagher, and Holt (1993) reported that parents who received training in teaching their child with autism through the TEACCH program reported a greater decrease in stress than did parents who did not receive training. Tonge et al. (2006) conducted a randomized, group-comparison study in which parents of children with autism were either assigned to a manual-based parent education and counseling intervention or a manual-based parent education and behavior management intervention. The parents assigned to the behavior management condition received action-based educational and skills training in identifying features of autism, behavioral management strategies, methods of improving social interaction and communication, teaching new skills, managing parental stress, and understanding family responses to autism. Skills were taught via workbooks, video modeling, in vivo practice, homework, and feedback. To control for the effects of therapist attention and support, the second group of parents received the same educational training through discussion only, and did not receive skills training or homework. Emphasis was instead placed on non-directive discussion and counseling with the parents.

Tonge et al. (2006) reported that, while both treatments were effective in improving parents' mental health, parents who received the behavior management intervention experienced greater alleviation of mental health symptoms such as anxiety, insomnia, somatic symptoms and family dysfunction at 6-month follow-up than did those who had received counseling. These findings, taken with Bristol et al.'s (1993) earlier findings, indicate that parent training may be beneficial in reducing parent stress and mental health risks over time. Parent training may increase parents' sense of self-efficacy, which has been demonstrated to protect mothers from stress-related disorders such as depression and anxiety (Hastings and Brown, 2002).

These results suggest that, while parent stress may make parent training more challenging for the professional, persistence in training efforts may serve to benefit the parent immensely. Parent training may counteract this stress by improving parents' ability to manage their child's behavior and transitively improving the child's skills. While naturally occurring transitions and events may trigger increases in parent stress, the parents' ability to effectively manage and improve their child's behavior may inhibit the ultimate level of stress experienced by the parent, as well as have a protective effect for parents' mental health.

The Impact of Cultural Factors

Parents of varying cultural, ethnic, racial and socioeconomic status bring differing views to their understanding of their child on the autism spectrum and their own role as teachers for their child. We use the term "culture" broadly here to include the effects of ethnicity, race, and socioeconomic status on one's values. For example, one can grow up in a culture of poverty that—regardless of nationality—will significantly influence one's values and beliefs and make one different than the more affluent members of one's own nation. The professional engaged in parent training should be alert to these cultural differences and able to adapt the methods to the many different families he or she encounters. Regardless of our own specific cultural assumptions, the more we understand and respect how people with other assumptions view their lives, the more likely we are to help them be effective in working with their child on the autism spectrum. We have little data on the specifics of how one's cultural assumptions impact one's ability to learn and implement ABA parent training methods with individuals on the autism spectrum, so it is important in this discussion to consider what we know from research with other populations and also what we know about cultural values more broadly.

North America and much of Western Europe have become an increasingly diverse in the past two decades (e.g., Hanson, Lynch and Wayman, 1999) and this has resulted in increased demands on professionals from cultural majority backgrounds to broaden their own perspective on the differences that exist among us. This heightened cultural heterogeneity appears to be arising as ease of travel and technological advances, including the internet, have led to many more encounters across cultural lines.

Respect for the differences among us is important in and of itself. Professionals serving families should strive to understand others' cultural assumptions if they are to adapt interventions to meet a family's needs. For example, Heller, Markwardt, Rowitz, and Farber (1994), in comparing Hispanic and non-Hispanic white families that were raising a child with moderate to profound mental retardation, found that the groups resembled one another in terms of use of informal supports and out-of-home placements. The families of Hispanic background, however, had greater difficulty obtaining services than did the non-Hispanic families. Additionally, the Hispanic families viewed raising their child with mental retardation as less burdensome than did the non-Hispanic families.

Both Hispanic (Heller at al, 1994) and Orthodox Jewish families (Leyser, 1994) report a reliance on their religious traditions as an important source of support in raising a child with a disability. Religious faith can have an impact on parents' readiness to take an active stance in addressing their child's needs. Several studies have shown that when parents believe that God will provide for their child and/or that the disability is God's will, parents may have a more passive stance toward addressing changes in their child's behavior. In many other cases, however, parents report that their faith in God gives them the strength they need to actively meet their child's needs (e.g., Freidrich and Friedrich, 1981; Shapiro and Tittle, 1986).

Several studies have highlighted parents' lack of fluency in the dominant culture's language as a barrier in using professional services. This has been found true for Hispanic (Prieto-Bayard and Baker, 1986; Shapiro and Simonsen, 1994) and Chinese speaking parents (Smith and Ryan, 1987) in the United States. Families from other backgrounds who are not fluent in English may likely have the same problem with locating and using services in English speaking countries.

Lau (2006) has written at length about making cultural adaptations to evidence-based treatments (EBT) using parent training as her exemplar of this process. She points out the paucity of data about the benefits of any EBT for minority communities and turns to Parent Management Training (PMT) for specific examples of the impact of culture on treatment. Although the populations of parents and children who have participated in this research are facing different problems than are the families of children with autism, it is worth noting that immigrant and minority families are less likely to enter these parent training programs (e.g., Cunningham et al., 2000) and more likely to drop out of training (e.g., Holden, Lavigne, and Cameron, 1990) than are Caucasian families. Lau (2006) points to the sensitivity of cultural issues involved in asking parents to change their methods of raising their children. She notes that some research supports the value of recruiting and retaining parents in treatment by using training materials that reflect the family's culture and offering services in settings that are comfortable for participants, such as their local church or other community based settings. This is followed by the caveat, however, that even with these adaptations treatment outcomes are roughly equivalent to standard versions (Lau, 2006). She concludes that these more superficial changes do not target the cultural differences in a way that has a major benefit for families. She then cites examples of PMT programs that have effectively targeted the specific needs of Black and Hispanic families by modifying the content in a culturally meaningful way and argues that as these targeted interventions are developed, they may well inform work being done to serve the cultural majority community as well. Research on teaching ABA methods to parents of children with autism requires a similar focus on incorporating parent training into the cultural values and traditions of participants. That work remains to be done.

Where Are We Headed?

While research on training parents of children with ASD to implement ABA strategies in the home setting has resulted in a solid research base on the utility of including parents in a child's education, gaps in the current body of knowledge prompt continued investigation in this area. Areas that warrant additional attention include the development of effective methods of integrating parent training into our current educational models, increasing parent adherence to instructional methods, the further assessment of the reciprocal effects of parent stress on parent training outcome, and continued study of the impact of family structure and culture on the successful implementation of parent training in the home setting.

Though research suggests that parent training may be critical in enhancing the generalization and maintenance of skill development among children with autism, many programs for the treatment of autism still approach parent training as an afterthought, rather than as a staple of the teaching model. Investigations into barriers to implementing parent training programs in schools will aid in the development of structured parent training programs and their integration in these programs. Ingersoll and Dvortscak (2006) indicate that the obstacles of dissemination and training of parents may impede such development, and offer a model for incorporating parent training into a preexisting educational program for children with autism. The authors acknowledging that teachers of children with autism have little time to devote to training parents in addition to the time they spend teaching, and that few teachers know how to teach skills to adults. Accordingly, the authors describe a parent training protocol in which teachers in classrooms for children with autism (1) were instructed in how to train parents in the use of developmental and naturalistic behavioral strategies in working with their children and (2) trained parents during group instruction during school hours and during individualized sessions in the evenings. The authors reported high teacher and parent satisfaction with the model. Though effects on parents' teaching skills were not assessed for the purposes of the study, teachers provided anecdotal reports that both parents' teaching skills and children's communication skills improved in response to the training.

This study takes a first step toward detailing a model in which parent training is integrated into a child's educational curriculum. Such integration requires attention to school and teacher resources. Ingersoll and Dvortscak admit that even the 50 hours required of each teacher to implement the above procedure may be excessive and interfere with continued use of the program. Additional models of incorporating parent training into pre-existing educational programs should be investigated.

Ingersoll and Dvortscak also report, however, that only 56% of parents recruited for the program participated in the entire program. The low rate of participation was cited by teachers as a primary impediment to the success of the program. In addition to assessing models of incorporating parent training into educational programs, research should investigate barriers to parent participation in these programs and suggest methods that such programs might use to facilitate parent participation. Obstacles such as child care during parent training and the location of training may impede participation. The provision of child care during training and conducting training in the home setting may result in higher participation and, in the case of the latter, may also increase generalization of skills to the home setting (Ingersoll and Dvortscak, 2006).

An additional impediment to parent participation, as cited earlier, may be levels of stress among parents of children with autism. Research should further investigate the events that may trigger increased levels of stress among parents (e.g., transitions) to better prepare professionals in providing support and training parents during these difficult times. Parent training may actually provide a protective effect for parents with regard to stress and mental health problems (Bristol et al., 1993; Tonge et al., 2006), but further study is required in this area to identify which parent training methods and models might be most effective in maximizing this effect. For example, Koegel, Bimbela, and Schreibman (1996) noted that positive parent affect—a possible indicator of low parent stress—was higher among parents who received training in PRT rather than ITB. While replication and extension of this research is required, these initial findings indicate that parent stress may be most mitigated by naturalistic teaching strategies that are easily incorporated into daily family routines.

Relatedly, substantial research is required to better assess the integration of parent training into families of different cultures. As noted earlier, cultural approaches to child rearing and the understanding of autism may alter the way in which parent training can be incorporated into a family structure. The use of contextualized interventions will be paramount in this endeavor. Additional investigation of the methods by which common interventions can be contextually adapted to fit cultural and familial beliefs, attitudes, and goals may vastly improve our understanding of how best to implement parent training in households of different cultures and structures.

Parent training has evolved over the years to assert its utility in the instruction of children with autism using ABA methods. From early research in discrete trial training to the most recent research in naturalistic teaching methods, parent training has consistently resulted in improvements in parents' instructional skills and child behavior. The contextualized integration of parent training into a family's daily life results in training models that are highly sustainable and facilitate improved generalization of skill acquisition for both parents and children. Future research on the impact of parent stress, culture, and context on the implementation of parent training, as well as on the most effective means of incorporating parent training into a child's educational placement, will serve to further enlighten the field of ABA. At this time, parent training stands as a particularly integral component in promoting the continued development and skill acquisition of individuals with autism.

REFERENCES

Alpern, G., and Boll, T. (1972). *Developmental profile* Aspen CO: Psychological Development Publication.

Azrin, N. H., Hontos, P.T., and Basalel-Azrin, V. (1979). Elimination of enuresis without a conditioning apparatus: An extension by office instruction of the child and parents. *Behavior Therapy,* 10, 14-19.

Baker, B. and Blacher, J. (2002). For better or worse? Impact of residential placement on families. *Mental Retardation, 40,* 1-13.

Baker, B.L., Blacher, J., and Olsson, M.B. (2005). Preschool children with and without developmental delay: Behaviour problems, parents' optimism and well-being. *Journal of Intellectual Disability Research,* 49, 575-590.

Baker, B.L., Heifetz, L.J., and Murphy, D.M. (1980). Behavioral training for parents of mentally retarded children: One-year follow-up. *American Journal on Mental Deficiency,* 85, 31-38.

Baker, B.L., McIntyre, L.L., Blacher, J., Crnic, K., Edelbrock, C., and Low, C. (2003). Preschool children with and without developmental delay: Behaviour problems and parenting stress over time. *Journal of Intellectual Disability Research, 47*, 217-230.

Belchic, J.K., and Harris, S.L. (1994). The use of multiple peer exemplars to enhance the generalization of play skills to the siblings of children with autism. *Child and Family Behavior Therapy,* 16, 1-25.

Berkowitz, B.P., and Graziano, A.M. (1972). Training parents as behavior therapists: A review. *Behaviour Research and Therapy,* 10, 297-317.

Bouma, R. and Schweitzer, R. (1990). The impact of chronic childhood illness on family stress: A comparison between autism and cystic fibrosis. *Journal of Clinical Psychology,* 46, 722-730.

Boyd, B. A. (2002). Examining the relationship between stress and lack of social support in mothers of children with autism. *Focus on Autism and Other Developmental Disabilities,* 17, 208-215.

Bristol, M.M., Gallagher, J.J., and Holt, K.D. (1993). Maternal depressive symptoms in autism: Response to psychoeducational intervention. *Rehabilitation Psychology,* 38, 3-10.

Celiberti, D.A., and Harris, S.L. (1993). Behavioral intervention for siblings of children with autism: A focus on skills to enhance play. *Behavior Therapy,* 24, 573-599.

Coe, D.A., Matson, J.L., Craigie, C.J., and Gossen, M.A. (1991). Play skills of autistic children: Assessment and instruction. *Child and Family Behavior Therapy*, 13, 13-40.

Colletti, G. and Harris, S.L. (1977). Behavior modification in the home: Siblings as behavior modifiers, parents as observers. *Journal of Abnormal Child Psychology,* 5, 21-30.

Cunningham, C.E., Boyle, M., Offord, D., Racine, Y., Hundert, J., Secord, M., et al. (2000). Triministry study: Correlates of school-based parenting course utilization. *Journal of Consulting and Clinical Psychology,* 68, 928-933.

Donovan, A.M. (1988). Family stress and ways of coping with adolescents who have handicaps: Maternal perceptions. *American Journal on Mental Retardation, 92,* 502-509.

El-Ghoroury, N.H., and Romanczyk, R.G. (1999). Play interactions of family members towards children with autism. *Journal of Autism and Developmental Disorders,* 29, 249-258.

Farmer-Dougan, V. (1994). Increasing requests by adults with developmental disabilities using incidental teaching by peers. *Journal of Applied Behavior Analysis*, 27, 533-544.

Friedrich, W.N. and Friedrich, W.L. (1981). Psychosocial assets of parents of handicapped and nonhandicapped children. *American Journal on Mental Deficiency,* 85, 551-553.

Freud, S. (1959). Analysis of a phobia in a five-year-old boy. In *Collected papers, Vol. 3.* NY: Basic Books.

Gill, M.J. and Harris, S.L. (1991). Hardiness and social support as predictors of psychological discomfort in mothers of children with autism. *Journal of Autism and Developmental Disorders,* 21, 407-416.

Guerney, B.G. (Ed.). (1969). *Psychotherapeutic agents: New roles for non-professionals, parents and teachers*. NY: Holt, Rinehart, and Winston.

Hanline, M.F. (1991). Transitions and critical events in the family life cycle: Implications for providing support to families of children with disabilities. *Psychology in the Schools, 28,* 53-59.

Hanson, M.J., Lynch, E.W., and Wayman, K.I. (1990). Honoring the cultural diversity of families when gathering data. *Topics in early Childhood Special Education,* 10, 112-131.

Harris, S.L. (1983). *Families of the developmentally disabled. A guide to behavioral intervention.* NY: Pergamon Press.

Harris, S.L. (1986). Brief report: A 4- to- 7 year questionnaire follow-up of participants in a program for parents of autistic children. *Journal of Autism and Developmental Disorders,* 16, 377-383.

Harris, S.L. (1987). Parents as teachers: A four to seven year follow-up of parents of children with autism. *Child and Family Behavior Therapy,* 8, 39-47.

Harris, S.L., Alessandri, M., and Gill, M.J., (1991). Training parents of developmentally disabled children. In J.L. Matson and J.A. Mulick (Eds.), *Handbook of mental retardation (2nd ed.)* (pp. 373-381). Elmsford NY: Pergamon.

Harris, S.L., and Romanczyk, R.G. (1976). Treating self-injurious behavior of a retarded child by overcorrection. *Behavior Therapy,* 7, 235-239.

Harris, S.L., Wolchik, S.A., and Milch, R.E. (1982). Changing the speech of autistic children and their parents. *Child and Family Behavior Therapy,* 4, 151-173.

Harris, S.L., Wolchik, S.A., and Weitz, S. (1981). The acquisition of language skills by autistic children: Can parents do the job? *Journal of Autism and Developmental Disorders,* 11, 373-384.

Hart, B., and Risley, T. R. (1980). In vivo language intervention: Unanticipated general effects. *Journal of Applied Behavior Analysis,* 13, 407-432.

Hastings, R.P., and Brown, T. (2002). Behavior problems of children with autism, parental self-efficacy, and mental health. *American Journal on Mental Retardation,* 107, 222-232.

Hastings, R.P. and Johnson, E. (2001). Stress in UK families conducting intensive home-based behavior intervention for their young child with autism. *Journal of Autism and Developmental Disorders,* 31, 327-36.

Heifetz, L.J. (1977). Behavioral training for parents of retarded children: Alternative formats based on instructional manuals. *American Journal of Mental Deficiency,* 82, 194-203.

Heller, T., Markwardt, R., Rowitz, L., and Farber, B. (1994). Adaptation of Hispanic families to a member with mental retardation. *American Journal on Mental Retardation*, 99, 289-300.

Hemsley, R., Howlin, P., Berger, M., Hersov, L., Holbrook, D., Rutter, M., et al. (1978). Treating autistic children in a family context. In M. Rutter and E. Schopler (Eds.), *Autism: A reappraisal of concepts and treatment* (pp. 379-411). NY: Plenum.

Holden, G.W., Lavigne, V.V., and Cameron, A.M. (1990). Probing the continuum of effectiveness in parent training: Characteristics of parents and preschoolers. *Journal of Clinical Child Psychology,* 19, 2-8.

Holmes, N., Hemsely, R., Rickett, J., and Likierman, H. (1982). Parents as co therapists: Their perceptions of a home-based behavioral treatment for autistic children. *Journal of Autism and Developmental Disorders,* 12, 331-342.

Howlin, P.A. (1981a). The effectiveness of operant language training with autistic children. *Journal of Autism and Developmental Disorders,* 11, 89-103.

Howlin, PA. (1981b). The results of a home-based language training programme with autistic children. *British Journal of Disorders of Communication,* 16, 73-88.

Howlin, P.A. Marchant, R., Rutter, M., Berger, M., Hersov, L., and Yule, W. (1973). A home-based approach to the treatment of autistic children. *Journal of Autism and Childhood Schizophrenia,* 3, 308-336.

Ingersoll, B. and Dvortcsak, A. (2006). Including parent training in the early childhood special education curriculum for children with autism spectrum disorders. *Journal of Positive Behavior Interventions,* 8, 79-87.

Ingersoll, B., and Schreibman, L. (2006). Teaching reciprocal imitation skills to young children with autism using a naturalistic behavioral approach: Effects on language, pretend play, and joint attention. *Journal of Autism and Developmental Disorders,* 36, 487-508.

Koegel, R.L., Bimbela, A., and Schreibman, L. (1996). Collateral effects of parent training on family interactions. *Journal of Autism and Developmental Disorders,* 26, 347-359.

Koegel, R.L., Glahn, T.J., and Nieminen. G.S. (1978). Generalization of parent training results. *Journal of Applied Behavior Analysis,* 11, 95-109.

Koegel, R.L., and Koegel, L.K. (2005). *Pivotal response treatment for autism.* Baltimore: Brookes Publishing Co.

Koegel, R.L., Koegel, L.K., and Schreibman, L. (1991). Assessing and training parents in teaching pivotal behaviors. *Advances in Behavioral Assessment of Children and Families,* 5, 65-82.

Koegel, R.L., Russo, D.C., and Rincover, A. (1977). Assessing and training teachers in the generalized use of behavior modification with autistic children. *Journal of Applied Behavior Analysis,* 10, 197-205.

Koegel, R.L., Schreibman, L., Britten, K.R., Burke, J.C., and O'Neill, R.E. (1982). A comparison of parent training to direct child treatment. In R.L. Koegel, A. Rincover, and A.L. Egel (Eds.), *Educating and understanding autistic children* (pp. 260-279). San Diego CA: College Hill.

Koegel, R.L., Schreibman, L., Johnson, J., O'Neill, R.E., and Dunlap, G. (1984). Collateral effects of parent training on families with autistic children. In R.F. Dangel and R.A.

Polster (Eds.), *Parent training: foundations of research and practice* (pp 358-378). NY: Guilford Press.

Koegel, R.L., Symon, J.B., and Koegel, L.K. (2002). Parent education for families of children with autism living in geographically distant areas. *Journal of Positive Behavioral Interventions,* 4, 88-103.

Kozloff, M. (1973). *Reaching the autistic child. A parent training program.* Champaign IL: Research Press.

Kwai-sang Yau, M. and Li-Tsang, C. W. P. (1999). Adjustment and adaptation in parents of children with developmental disability in two-parent families: A review of the characteristics and attributes. *British Journal of Developmental Disabilities,* 45, 38-51.

Laski, K.E., Charlop, M.H., and Schreibman, L. (1988). Training parents to use the natural language paradigm to increase their autistic children's speech. *Journal of Applied Behavior Analysis,* 21, 391-400.

Lau, A.S. (2006). Making the case for selective and directed cultural adaptations of evidence-based treatments: Examples from parent training. *Clinical Psychology: Science and Practice,* 13, 295-310.

Leyser, Y. (1994). Stress and adaptation in Orthodox Jewish families with a disabled child. *American Journal of Orthopsychiatry,* 64, 376-385.

Lindsley, O.R. (1966). An experiment with parents handling behavior at home. *Johnstone Bulletin,* 9, 27-36.

Lobato, D., and Tlaker, A. (1985). Sibling intervention with a retarded child. *Education and Treatment of Children,* 8, 347-364.

Lovaas, O.I., Koegel, R.L., Simmons, J.Q., and Long, J.S. (1973). Some generalization and follow-up measures on autistic children in behavior therapy. *Journal of Applied Behavior Analysis,* 3, 131-165.

MacDonald, J.D., Blott, J.P., Gordon, K., Spiegel, B., and Hartmann, M. (1974). An experimental parent-assisted treatment program for preschool language delayed children. *Journal of Speech and Hearing Disorders,* 39, 395-415.

Mansell, W. and Morris, K. (2004). A survey of parents' reactions to the diagnosis of an autistic spectrum disorder by a local service: Access to information and use of services. *Autism,* 8, 387-407.

McGee, G.G., Krantz, P. Mason, D., and McClannahan, L.E. (1983). A modified incidental-teaching procedures for autistic youth: Acquisition and generalization of receptive object labels. *Journal of Applied Behavior Analysis,* 16, 329-338.

McGee, G G., Krantz, P., and McClannahan, L.E. (1985). The facilitative effects of incidental teaching on preposition use by autistic children. *Journal of Applied Behavior Analysis,* 18, 17-31.

McGee, G.G., Krantz, P.J., and McClannahan, L.E. (1986). An extension of incidental teaching procedures to reading instruction for autistic children. *Journal of Applied Behavior Analysis*, 19, 147-157.

Midence, K. and O'Neill, M. (1999). The experience of parents in the diagnosis of autism. *Autism,* 3, 273-285.

Moes, D.R. and Frea, W.D. (2000). Using family context to inform intervention planning for the treatment of a child with autism. *Journal of Positive Behavior Interventions,* 2, 40-46.

Moes, D.R. and Frea, W.D. (2002). Contextualized behavioral support in early intervention for children with autism and their families. *Journal of Autism and Developmental Disorders,* 32, 519-533.

Moore, B. L., and Bailey, J.S. (1973). Social punishment in the modification of pre-school child's "autistic-like" behavior with a mother as therapist. *Journal of Applied Behavior Analysis,* 6, 497-507.

Mowrer, O.H., and Mowrer, W.M. (1938). Enuresis – A method for its study and treatment. *American Journal of Orthopsychiatry,* 8, 436-459.

National Autistic Society (2007). Early Bird Introduction. Retrieved 21 November 2007 from National Autistic Society website via http://www.nas.org.uk/nas/jsp/polopoly.jsp?d=10

Nordquist, V.M., and Wahler, R.G. (1973). Naturalistic treatment of an autistic child. *Journal of Applied Behavior Analysis,* 6, 79-87.

O'Dell, S. L. (1974). Training parents in behavior modification: A review. *Psychological Bulletin,* 81, 418-433.

Olley, J. G., Robbins, F. R., Morelli-Robbins, M. (1993). In E. Schopler. M.E. Van Bourgondien, and M.S. Bristol (Eds). *Preschool issues in autism.* (pp. 223-245). NY: Plenum.

Olsson, M.B. and Hwang, C.P. (2001). Depression in mothers and fathers of children with intellectual disability. *Journal of Intellectual Disability Research,* 46, 535-543.

Patterson, G. R., and Brodsky, M. (1966). Behavior modification for a child with multiple problem behaviors. *Journal of Child Psychology and Psychiatry,* 7, 277-295.

Patterson, G.R., McNeal, N., Hawkins, N., and Phelps, R. (1967). Reprogramming the social environment. *Journal of Child Psychology and Psychiatry,* 8, 181-195.

Powell, T.H., Salzberg, C.L., Rule, S., Levy, S., and Itzkowitz, J.S. (1983). Teaching mentally retarded children to play with their siblings using parents as trainers. *Education and Treatment of Children,* 6, 343-362.

Pumroy, D.K. (1965, September). *A new approach to treating parent-child problems.* Paper presented at the meeting of the American Psychological Association, Chicago IL.

Prieto-Bayard, M. and Baker, B. (1986) Parent training for Spanish-speaking families with a retarded child. *Journal of Community Psychology,* 14, 134-143.

Rabkin, J.G. and Streuning, E.L. (1976). Life events, stress and illness. *Science,* 194, 1013-1020.

Rogers, C. (1951). *Client-centered therapy: Its current practice, implications and theory.* Boston: Houghton Mifflin.

Sallows, G.O., and Graupner, T.D. (2005). Intensive behavioral treatment for children with autism: Four-year outcome and predictors. *American Journal on Mental Retardation,* 110, 417-438.

Salzberg, C.L., and Villani, T.V. (1983). Speech training by parents of Down syndrome toddlers: generalization across settings and instructional contexts. *American Journal of Mental Deficiency,* 4, 403-413.

Sanders, M.R., Markie-Dadds, C., Tully, L.A., and Bor, W. (2000). The Triple P-Positive Parenting Program: A comparison of enhanced, standards, and self-directed behavioral family intervention for parents of children with early onset conduct problems. *Journal of Consulting and Clinical Psychology,* 68, 624-640.

Sanders, M.R., Mazzucchelli, T.G., and Studman, L.J. (2004). Stepping Stones Triple P: The theoretical basis and development of an evidence-based positive parenting program for families with a child who has a disability. *Journal of Intellectual and Developmental Disability,* 29, 265-283.

Sanders, M.R., Plant, K., and McHale, M. (2002, June). *Reducing care-giving stress in families with a developmentally disabled child.* Paper presented at the Third International Conference on Child and Adolescent Mental Health, Brisbane, Australia.

Scorgie, K., Wilgosh, L., and McDonald, L. (1998). Stress and coping in families of children with disabilities: An examination of recent literature. *Developmental Disabilities Bulletin,* 26, 22-42.

Schopler, E. (1978). Changing parental involvement in behavioral treatment. In M. Rutter and E. Schopler (Eds.), *Autism. A reappraisal of concepts and treatment* (pp. 413-421). NY: Plenum.

Schreibman, L., O'Neill, R.E., and Koegel, R.L. (1983). Behavioral training for siblings of autistic children. *Journal of Applied Behavior Analysis,* 16, 129-138.

Shapiro, J. and Simonsen, D. (1994). Educational/support group for Latino families of children with Down syndrome. *Mental Retardation,* 32, 403-415.

Shapiro, J., and Tittle, K. (1986). Psychosocial adjustment of disabled and nondisabled children. *American Journal of Orthopsychiatry,* 56, 289-302.

Smith, M.J., and Ryan, A. (1987). Chinese-American families of children with developmental disabilities: An exploratory study of reactions to service providers. *Mental Retardation,* 25, 345-350.

Smith, T. (1993). Autism. In T.R. Giles (Ed.), *Effective psychotherapies* (pp. 107-13). New York: Plenum.

Smith, T., Groen, A.D., and Wynn, J. W. (2000). Randomized trial of intensive early intervention for children with pervasive developmental disorder. *American Journal on Mental Retardation,* 105, 269-285.

Smith, T., McAdam, D., and Napolitano, D. (2007). Autism and applied behavior analysis. In P. Sturmey and A. Fitzer (Eds.), *Autism spectrum disorders: Applied behavior analysis, evidence, and practice* (pp. 1-29). Austin, TX: Pro-Ed.

Sosne, J.B., Handleman, J.S., and Harris, S.L. (1979). Teaching spontaneous-functional speech to autistic children. *Mental Retardation,* 17, 241-245.

Stimbert, V.E., Minor, J.W., and McCoy, J.F. (1977). Intensive feeding training with retarded children. *Behavior Modification,* 1, 517-530.

Sundberg, M.L. and Partington, J.W. (1998). *Teaching language to children with autism or other developmental disabilities*. Pleasant Hill, CA: Behavior Analysts, Inc.

Sundberg, M.L. and Partington, J.W. (1999). The need for both DT and NE training for children with autism. In P.M. Ghezzi, W.L. Williams, and J.E. Carr (Eds.), *Autism: Behavior Analytic Approaches*. Reno, NV: Context Press.

Swenson-Pierce, A., Kohl, F.L., and Egel, A. (1987). Siblings as home trainers: A strategy for teaching domestic skills to children. *Journal of the Association for Persons with Severe Handicaps,* 12, 53-60.

Tonge, B., Brereton, A., Kiomall, M., MacKinnon, A., King, N., and Rinehart, N. (2006). Effects on parental mental health of an education and skills training program for parents of young children with autism: A randomized controlled trial. *Journal of the American Academy of Child and Adolescent Psychiatry,* 45, 561-569.

Tymchuk, A.J. (1979). *Parent and family therapy*. NY: Spectrum.

Wahler, R.G., and Fox, J.J. (1980). Solitary toy play and time out: A family treatment package for children with aggressive and oppositional behavior. *Journal of Applied Behavior Analysis,* 13, 23-39.

Weber, H. (1936). An approach to the problem of fear in children. *Journal of Mental Science,* 82, 136-147.

Weiss, M.J. (2002). Hardiness and social support as predictors of stress in mothers of typical children, children with autism, and children with mental retardation. *Autism,* 6, 115-130.

Weitz, S. (1982). A code for assessing teaching skills of parents of developmentally disabled children. *Journal of Autism and Developmental Disorders, 12,* 13-24.

Wikler, L. (1986). Periodic stresses of families of older mentally retarded children: An exploratory study. *American Journal on Mental Deficiency,* 90, 703-706.

Whittingham, K., Sofronoff, K., and Sheffield, J.K. (2006). Stepping Stones Triple P: A pilot study to evaluate acceptability of the program by parents of a child diagnosed with an Autism Spectrum Disorder. *Research in Developmental Disabilities,* 27, 364-380.

Wulff, S.B. (1985). The symbolic and object play of children with autism: A review. *Journal of Autism and Developmental Disorders,* 15, 139-148.

In: Behavioral Theories and Interventions for Autism
Editor: Phil Reed
ISBN 978-1-60741-165-9
© 2009 Nova Science Publishers, Inc.

Chapter 11

Training Professionals and Paraprofessionals to Implement Interventions for Children with Autism Spectrum Disorders

***Jennifer B.G. Symon**[*,1]**, Daniel Openden**[2]*
***and Michelle Bush Jacoby**[1]*
[1]California State University, Los Angeles, USA
[2]Southwest Autism Research and Resource Center, USA

Diagnostic criteria for Autism Spectrum Disorders (ASD) include impairments in three major areas: social interaction, communication, and repetitive/restrictive behaviors (*Diagnostic and Statistical Manual of Mental Disorders,* 4th ed., text rev.; American Psychiatric Association, 2000). While there are common challenges, ASDs affect individuals uniquely, generating a wide range in skills, deficits, and severity of symptoms. As a result, working with this population is ever-changing, exciting, and challenging. With increasing prevalence, more and more children with ASD and their families need appropriate, individualized support. Professionals and paraprofessionals working with these children, as well as families, require specialized training. Without specialized interventions, children with ASD experience challenges during academic and social activities in the school, home, and community.

A wide array of services for individuals with ASD can be implemented in school, home, and community settings. Educational settings for these children vary considerably with respect to the least restricted environment and can range from special educational schools to general education classrooms with or without additional supports. The needs of children with ASD vary greatly between them making placement options unique to each situation. Many students with ASD are placed in special day classes (SDC) on a special educational school or

* Please address correspondence to: Jennifer B. G. Symon, PhD., BCBA, Assistant Professor, Coordinator, Programs in Autism, California State University Division of Special Education and Counseling, 5151 State University Drive, Los Angeles, CA 90032, U.S.A.

on a general educational school. In both cases the classrooms have small student to teacher ratio and all the students are diagnosed with special needs. Assistants and paraprofessionals work with the teacher(s) to support all or individual students. It is common with these types of placements to for students with ASD to be grouped together with the idea that they have similar needs and receive instruction from teachers specifically trained in ASD. In practice, however, the children's needs may vary and the staff may not be provided with specialized training. When students are placed in SDC, all support services are provided individually or in small group instructions within the special needs settings.

Other students with ASD are placed in general educational settings for all or a portion of the school day alongside their typically developing peers. In these cases, any additional support services (e.g., speech therapy, occupational therapy) may be provided directly within the routines of the general educational setting or may be provided through "pull-out" services. The students may be included in the general educational setting for certain curricular activities while educated in a special education class for other activities. For those who are fully included in general educational settings, the goal for these students is to access and to participate in the curriculum with peers across academic and extracurricular activities throughout the day as much as possible. Regardless of the educational setting, ranging from a SDC to general education classroom, many students with ASD require one-on-one assistance to participate (referred to as paraprofessionals or one-to-one aides).

In addition to the school settings, services are commonly provided in home and community settings for students with ASD. Home and community programs typically consist of one-to-one intervention therapists who work on specified target goals with the child such as communication, play, and social behaviors. They may include parent education training, vocational and self-help skills and are often provided up to 40 hours per week. Young children under the age of three years often receive home support in lieu of a school setting while older children receive some home support in addition to their educational support to address specific skills and/or to reduce challenging behavior.

Specialists making up an educational team can include occupational, speech, and physical therapists, along with general and special education teachers, school psychologists, and counselors. In addition, paraprofessionals, behavior analysts, and consultants may provide individualized support. Training programs for each of these specialists vary in terms of the type and amount of training provided that specifically focuses on supporting those with autism spectrum disorders. Because of the unique needs of individuals with ASD, training needs to be comprehensive and adequately target interventions specific to this population of learners. Many difficulties arise in developing interventions for students with ASD within general education classrooms as a result of the large range of cognitive strengths and weaknesses students with ASD demonstrate, the social dysfunction related to the disorder, and a lack of training for school based personnel (Rogers, 2000; Simpson, de Boer-Ott, and Smith-Myles, 2003; Williams, Johnson, and Sukhodolosky, 2005).

Several problems seem to be common when providing support to children with ASD. First, many training programs do not provide adequate specialized training specific to working with children with ASD (Grey, Honan, McClean, and Daly, 2005; Scheuermann, Webber, Boutot, and Goodwin, 2003). In addition, the skill set needed to successfully support students with ASD has not been clearly defined nor consistent across states. Rather, many teachers have been hired on emergency credentials in classrooms without knowledge specific to teaching students with ASD because of the high numbers of students with ASD and teacher shortage (Scheuermann et al., 2003). While teacher training programs may provide excellent strategies and knowledge to support diverse learners, many teacher training programs in special education provide only minimal knowledge and strategies in supporting students with ASD in classrooms. The classroom teacher is ultimately responsible for the education of the child with ASD in his or her classroom, yet may not feel adequately equipped to handle the specific behavioral and social communication challenges that students with ASD present. For instance, teachers often are not trained to develop and implement augmentative communication systems (Howlin, Gordon, Pasco, Wade, and Charman, 2007), are not equipped to teach through routines (Tate, Thompson, and McKerchar, 2005) and not prepared to create and implement behavioral interventions (Grey et al, 2005), all of which are commonly needed when working with students with ASD.

Likewise, paraprofessionals and teaching assistants are often placed in classrooms as one-to-one aides to support children with ASD in a variety of educational settings (e.g., general education classroom, special day class). However, these paraprofessionals may receive minimal or no autism-specific training prior to gaining the responsibility to support the student with ASD (Giangreco, Edelman, and Broer, 2001a; Giangreco, Edelman, Luiselli, and MacFarland, 1997; Riggs and Mueller, 2001). Furthermore, the quality and quantity of on-the-job in service training can be inadequate or not specific to the challenges that children with ASD present. On-the-job in service training should, at a minimum, include evidenced-based practices. Some strategies have minimal evidence to support their efficacy, yet they are presented in training programs without teaching how to discriminate best practices. It is important that professionals and paraprofessionals alike understand the importance of discriminating, selecting, and implementing evidence-based practices with this population.

Specialists such as speech and language pathologists, occupational therapists, physical therapists, school administrators and psychologists gain knowledge and expertise in their area of work; however most of their training is not often specific to supporting students with ASD. With the dramatic increase of children diagnosed with ASD across the U.S. as high as 1 in 150 (CDC, 2007), nearly every specialist will have students with ASD on his or her caseload at some point in his/her career. Thus, it is essential to provide adequate training that is specific to educating this population across disciplines.

Training Specific to Autism Spectrum Disorders

The following issues are not specific to ABA approaches but are important when designing and implementing any intervention program for individuals with ASD. Regardless of the type of program provided, these areas are most likely needed for many types of programs.

Teacher and Specialist Training

To effectively support students with ASD, team members must receive on-going training in addition to any appropriate pre-service or in-service training. For all team members working in any capacity to support individuals with ASD (e.g., general or special education teacher, occupational therapist, speech and language pathologist, behavior analyst), this implies a clear understanding of the three core areas that designate the diagnosis of ASD (i.e., communication delay, social delay, restricted range of interests and repetitive behaviors). It also means understanding the broad spectrum of skills and needs individuals with ASD display. Having this base knowledge of ASD will help ensure that the core deficits are consistently addressed and targeted in interventions across all educational settings. Educational goals for students with ASD must include targeting the core deficits of language, social communication, and behavioral needs. Every individualized curriculum must identify and develop specific goals to address the child's needs beyond a focus on core academics. Considering social skills and communication delays constitute the core deficits of ASD, there should be functional goals to address each student's ability to access the curriculum including facilitation of social interactions and fostering independence through behavioral management systems. Training programs for teachers, behavior analysts, and therapists must provide skills in designing supports to improve functioning in these areas. (Grey, et al., 2005; Scheuermann et al., 2003).

Children with ASD demonstrate unique challenges and training must provide skills and strategies to support students with varying levels of communication, social skills, and behavior challenges. Examples of social goals for students with ASD might include sharing toys or materials, initiating toward or responding to peers, maintaining a conversation, greetings, participating with peers in structured play or in academic lessons. By creating routines and teaching across settings, young children can learn a variety of skills such as communication, social, and adaptive behaviors (Lucyshyn, Horner, Dunlap, Albin and Ben, 2002; Wetherby and Woods, 2006). These routines provide consistency and predictability (McNamara and Humphry, 2007) while make learning meaningful (Alcock, 2007) and motivating (Koegel, Koegel, Harrower, and Carter 1999). Opportunities to target these skills can be presented throughout the school day, at home, or in the community. Table 11.1 and Table 11.2 present many examples of targeted communication and social goals for individuals with ASD across a variety of settings. Table 11.1 provides examples for a young child or a child with more severe symptoms while Table 11.2 presents examples for an older child or adolescent or an individual with less severe symptoms. The examples in these tables can be adapted for those who support an individual with ASD and can be tailored to the specific routines or activities the individual will follow in a typical day.

In addition to understanding the core symptoms of ASD, those supporting students with ASD must be aware and familiar with a variety of teaching strategies. With the growing research base on interventions in autism, training in evidence-based practices should be on-going, provided regularly, and include an in-vivo component that focuses on correct implementation of intervention procedures. Considering the variability between individuals with ASD, those supporting students with ASD will need to learn a variety of techniques and how to appropriately apply them into treatment settings (including natural environments such as general education classrooms). For example, many children with ASD respond well to visual supports, including picture schedules, which may help them learn daily routines (Brown and Mirenda, 2006; Dettmer, Simpson and Myles, 2000; Massey and Wheeler, 2000; McClannahan and Krantz, 1999; Myles, 2005). In these cases, professionals should know how to create and teach the individual with ASD to use visual supports as well as develop a plan for fading them to respond to more naturalistic cues.

Table 11.1. Functional Goals targeting core social and communication deficits targeted across the school, home, and community settings for a young child with ASD

Daily School Activities	Communication	Social
Arrival	Teacher stands at bus door and says, "Good morning, Oscar!" She does not move to let him off until he greets her verbally or waves.	Oscar opens the classroom door and holds it open for the other kids.
Free play	At the beginning of free play, teacher shows Oscar a picture list of play options and asks, "What would you like to play?" Oscar must either point or verbally indicate his choice before he can begin free play.	Oscar loves the trains. He must work with another child to build the tracks before the teacher will hand out the trains. The train set is designated as at least a 2 person activity; Oscar may not play with them alone.
Circle time	Teacher shows a picture of a bus and a picture of a spider. Oscar says, either "Wheels on the Bus", or "Itsy Bitsy Spider." Class sings the chosen song.	Oscar loves music. Teacher instructs children to choose a friend for a partner dance. She will immediately start the song when Oscar chooses a partner.
Outdoor play	Teacher presets bubbles (Oscar's favorite activity) in easy view, but out of reach. Oscar must approach teacher and verbally ask her for a ball.	Oscar loves to be pulled in the red wagon. He must take turns by first pulling another child before he is allowed to sit in the wagon.
Lunch/Snack	Teacher asks, "Would you like chocolate or white milk?" She then waits for him to say "I want [blank] milk, please," prompting or modeling if necessary.	Peers request placemats from Oscar. Oscar distributes one to each child for mealtime.
Table top activity	Teacher holds up several colors of paper for a hand writing activity. Oscar points to the one he would like.	Teacher places the can of Oscar's favorite markers between him and another child. Oscar must share the markers by using one at a time.
Getting Ready for School	Mom holds up two shirts. Oscar verbally indicates his choice. If an article of clothing feels uncomfortable, Oscar will say, "This feels scratchy."	Mom asks Oscar for help preparing breakfast or cleaning up a spill.
Breakfast	Mom shows Oscar bread and the cereal box, "Would you like toast or cereal for breakfast." Oscar verbally indicates which he would like.	His sister says, "Oscar, please pass me the ______." Mom does not serve Oscar his food until he has complied with his sister's request.
Chores	While showing pictures of the chores, Mom says, "Before using the computer, are you going to put your clothes in the hamper, or help me take out the trash." Oscar verbally makes his choice.	Mom approaches a door near Oscar with her arms full, and exaggerates her difficulty opening it. She then waits for Oscar to offer to help. If he does not, she prompts him.
Play Time	Mom purposefully stands in Oscar's way. Oscar says, "Move, please." Mom immediately moves out his way.	Mom sets a time when Oscar begins his turn on the computer. When the timer goes off, Oscar gets off the computer so his brother can have his turn.

Table 11.1. (Continued)

Daily School Activities	Communication	Social
Car Rides	Mom opens the door and then waits for Oscar to say, "Help me," to undo his seat belt.	Oscar and his brother take turns choosing the CD.
Bedtime	Dad shows Oscar 2 books, Oscar verbally chooses one and together they read the book Oscar selected.	Dad makes sure the bathroom door is closed even if no one is in there. He prompts Oscar to knock on the door before entering, to see if anyone is using it.
Grocery Store	Mom gives Oscar a list with pictures of preferred food items. Mom tells Oscar that when he sees one of these items, he should say, "Here." He then gets to put it in the cart.	Oscar hands the money to and receive the change from the cashier.
Restaurant	Mom takes him to restaurants that have menus with pictures (or makes her own picture menu). Oscar orders from the waitress by pointing to the picture of the food he wants.	When waitress serves Oscar his food, mom prompts him to say, "Thank-you." He may not eat until he does.
At the Park	When another child is using the piece of equipment Oscar wants to use, Mom prompts him to ask, "My turn, when you're done?"	When another child falls, brings this to Oscar's attention, and says, "Uh-oh, that little boy fell down." She then prompts him to help the boy up or ask, "Are you okay?"
Public Library	Oscar names or points to the book he chooses to read. He verbalizes "turn the page" when he is ready to turn.	Oscar will hand the books to the librarian to check out, and say, "Thank-you," when she gives them back.

Other students with ASD may benefit from self-management behavioral programs to increase independence in classroom settings and reduce reliance on adult support (Apple, Billingsley, and Schwartz, 2005; Boettcher, 2004; Koegel, Koegel, and Hurley, 1992; Newman and Ten Eyck, 2005). Here, team members must be proficient at creating and implementing self-management programs that can benefit the child with ASD.

Specialized training in ASD should also include knowing how to successfully support students with ASD in a variety of classrooms and educational settings. Training for professionals should include teaching skills in conducting appropriate standardized assessment tools (e.g., language, adaptive functioning skills) and non-standardized assessments (e.g., language sample, functional behavioral assessment, social skills), modifying and adapting the core curriculum, developing behavioral intervention programs, and maintaining an on-going evaluation system. Aside from these critical skills, using best practices requires that team members remain current on understanding and being familiar with evidence-based best practices.

Table 11.2. Functional Goals targeting core social and communication deficits targeted across the school, home, and community settings for an older child or adolescent with ASD

Daily School Activities	Communication	Social
Homeroom	When teacher calls out role, Amy will answer with an appropriate, "Here."	Teacher says, "Hello, Amy." Amy will make eye contact and return the greeting.
Math Class	Amy will raise her hand to answer a question or make a comment related to the lesson rather than call out.	Extra protractors are available for students who do not have their own. Amy will pass these and other materials out to peers who need them.
Independent work	Amy will walk up to the teacher and quietly ask for a break if she is becoming overwhelmed or frustrated. Teacher will then say, "Yes Amy, you may go get a drink of water."	If Amy has questions about an assignment, she will ask her neighbor for help before going to the teacher.
Art class	When the students have finished a piece, they will break into pairs to discuss their artwork. Amy will talk about hers for at least 2 minutes.	When her peer talks about her piece, Amy will make at least one compliment.
Lunch	If someone is in her way, Amy will say, "Excuse me," to get past.	Amy will greet familiar peers as she sits down to eat with them.
Getting Ready for School	Amy explains her day's schedule to her mom.	Amy will greet her family members good morning.
Running Errands	Mom tells Amy the errands they need to run; Amy tells mom the order she would like to do the errands.	Amy will respond with a verbal or nonverbal to the employees at the stores.
Homework	When she is finished, Amy will verbally ask her mom to check her work.	If Amy becomes frustrated with her work, she will take a five minute break to prevent a melt down. She will use a timer to self-monitor this break.
Free Time	While Amy is watching television, Mom will sit down and ask what has happened so far. Amy explains the story line so far.	While Amy is doing her own thing, Mom will periodically call her name. Amy will stop what she is doing and respond to her name. Mom will ask a simple question or make an excuse for calling her.
Dinner	Amy will tell at least three things she did during her day, before she can leave the table.	During dinner conversation, Amy will comment on or ask a question about something mom or dad says at least 3 times before she can leave the table.

Table 11.2 (Continued).

Daily School Activities	Communication	Social
Sports Team	Amy asks coach for clarification, "Can you repeat the directions," when she does not understand what she is to do.	Amy will clap or cheer for peers when appropriate.
Grocery Store	At the deli counter, Amy will verbally ask for the cold cuts she would like.	Amy will respond to social greetings from familiar adults in the store.
Restaurant	Amy independently orders her food verbally.	When served her food, she will make eye contact with the waitress and say, "Thank-you."
Library	When Amy has trouble finding a book, Mom will prompt her to go to the reference desk and ask for help.	While waiting in line to check out books, Amy will remain an appropriate distant from the other people in line.
Neighbor's House	Mom will ask Amy to go to neighbor's house to borrow something. Amy will verbally explain to the neighbor that her mother would like to borrow _____.	Amy will say, "Hello" when the neighbor answers the door, and "good –bye" before she leaves.

nterventions that have maintained the strongest empirical base with a variety of individuals with ASD have been those based on procedures of Applied Behavior Analysis (ABA) (Howard, Sparkman, Cohen, Green, and Stanislaw, 2005; Luiselli and Hurley, 2005). ABA has been used to effectively reduce challenging behaviors (e.g., Smith, Eikeseth, Klevstrand, and Lovaas, 1997), increase functional social language (Koegel, Koegel, and Brookman, 2005; McGee, Morrier, and Daly, 1999), teach augmentative communication systems (Bondy, Tincani, and Frost, 2004; Tincani, Crozier, and Alazetta, 2006), develop self-management programs (Apple et al., 2005; Koegel et al., 1992; Newman and Ten Eyck, 2005; Wilkinson, 2005), and reduce self-stimulatory behaviors (Conroy, Asmus, Sellers, and Ladwig 2005; Koegel and Koegel 1990; Lee, Odom, and Loftin, 2007). Teachers (Grey, et al., 2005; Kohler, Anthony, Steigner, and Hoyson, 2001; Noell, Duhon, Gatti, and Connell, 2002), family members (Dunlap, Newton, Fox, Benito, and Vaughn, 2001; Dunlap and Fox, 1999; Frea and Hepburn, 1999; O'neal, Reeb, Korte, and Butter, 2006) and therapists have all been effective at incorporating the scientific principles of ABA into instruction in a variety of settings such as school classrooms, playgrounds, homes, and community settings (Wolery, Barton, and Hine, 2005). Because ABA has such a strong empirical basis and has been successfully implemented with individuals with ASD for decades, providing training in ABA is likely to improve teaching and enhance child gains. As stated, many programs rely extensively on intervention procedures that have yet to be reliably supported in the research literature, yet are often used in treatment programs for children and adults with ASD. Ideally, a collaborative effort between specialists and behavior analysts could allow for more rapid learning and skill acquisition.

Paraprofessional and Home-Based Instructor Training

Paraprofessionals and home-based instructors often play critical roles in supporting students with ASD both in classroom and home settings. Specifically, a burgeoning number of inclusive school programs include the support of one-to-one paraprofessionals in the general education classrooms (Boomer, 1994; Giangreco, Broer and Edelman 2002). Likewise, home-based programs rely on therapists to provide individual assistance for those with ASD. Many agencies that provide in home support prepare the therapists with on-going training and supervision for program implementation. Unfortunately, however, in educational classrooms, paraprofessionals do not have the benefit of working alongside a trained special education teacher (Giangreco, Yuan, McKenzie, Cameron, and Fialka, 2005). Therefore, paraprofessionals may spend more direct time interacting with a child with ASD than any other support provider (Boomer, 1994; Giangreco and Broer 2005; Marks, Schraeder, and Levine, 1999; Scheuermann et al., 2003; Young and Simpson, 1997). While teacher(s) and other specialists are ultimately responsible for the education of students with ASD, paraprofessionals' responsibilities may include assisting with the implementation of behavioral intervention programs, facilitating social interactions, modifying and adapting lessons, and collecting data (Giangreco et al., 2002; Marks et al., 1999; Scheuermann et al., 2003). It is clear, then, that paraprofessionals likely impact the way in which interventions are delivered and subsequently affect child progress. Therefore, it is critical that paraprofessionals be considered core members of interdisciplinary teams that receive adequate training for supporting students with ASD.

As discussed previously, training provided for paraprofessionals is often minimal and deficient (Giangreco et al., 2005; Giangreco et al., 2002; Giangreco et al., 2001b; Giangreco et al., 1997; Riggs and Mueller, 2001), even though both the Individuals with Disabilities Education Act (IDEA) and the No Child Left Behind Act of 2001 (NCLB) specifically address paraprofessional training requirements. Many times, paraprofessionals are not provided with any training or even a clear understanding of their role in the classroom (Riggs and Mueller, 2001). This is particularly troubling considering data suggests that, without proper training, paraprofessionals may be more harmful than helpful for students with disabilities (Giangreco et al., 1997, Giangreco et al., 2005). Thus, in addition to training that is specific to ASD (discussed in the previous sections), it is simultaneously important that training specific to paraprofessionals be provided (Giangreco, Edelman, and Broer, 2003). Like home therapists, paraprofessionals need on-going pre-service, on-the-job, and inservice training to meet students' needs (Trautman, 2004).

First, it is important that paraprofessionals have their job expectations specifically defined (Trautman, 2004). The primary role of the paraprofessional is to provide assistance so that the student may independently have access to and make meaningful benefit from the general education curriculum. To some extent, then, the paraprofessional's "job" is to lose their job. That is, the paraprofessional's goals are to transfer instruction to the teacher, independence to the child, and assistance to the student's peers so that the paraprofessional is no longer needed in the classroom. In doing so, the student can become increasingly independent by receiving instruction from the teacher with assistance from his/her peers, similar to educational programming for typically developing students.

Although paraprofessionals are considered one-to-one support providers for students with ASD, proximity to the student must be a key consideration. Titles such as "one-to-one aide," "shadow," or even "velcro aide" are often misleading with respect to best practices for students with ASD and can lead paraprofessionals into hovering over students (Giangreco et al. 2005; Giangreco and Broer 2005). Thus, paraprofessionals will often ride the bus to school, be seated right next to, and be the only one eating lunch with the student with ASD. If the goal of the paraprofessional is to increase independence for the child, though, it is important that the paraprofessional instead appear to be a classroom assistant (as opposed to a student with ASD's personal assistant). To do so, the paraprofessional should provide support as needed. At times, the paraprofessional may be seated away from the student with ASD and roam through all of the desks in the classroom. Essentially, the paraprofessional is looking and waiting for times when the student with ASD requires additional assistance. If additional assistance is necessary, the paraprofessional may approach the student's desk, quickly and unobtrusively to provide the assistance necessary, and should then move away from the child. If assistance is not or is no longer required, the paraprofessional may be assisting other students, thereby maintaining the perception that the paraprofessional is a classroom assistant.

In addition to providing academic assistance for the student with ASD when necessary, paraprofessionals should also identify times when the teacher and peers may assist the child (Giangreco et al., 2005; Broer, Doyle, and Giangreco, 2005). During independent seat work, for instance, the teacher may also be circulating the classroom and assisting students, including the student with ASD. Similarly, peers (particularly those seated next to the student with ASD) may be helpful at providing assistance. The role of the paraprofessional can be to demonstrate ways classmates can assist each other. For example, where appropriate, the paraprofessional should look for opportunities for the child with ASD to request assistance from or work with his/her peers (Young and Simpson, 1997). Likewise, there are often times when a student with ASD may be able to assist a typically developing student. By identifying such opportunities, paraprofessionals simultaneously provide opportunities for social interaction (Broer et al. 2005; Koegel et al., 2006).

An important benefit of including students with disabilities in general education classrooms is the opportunities to learn from and socially interact with typically developing peers. For students with ASD, though, improving social interactions with peers is a critical component of comprehensive programming (National Research Council, 2001). Interestingly, paraprofessionals tend to feel responsible only for the academic and behavioral needs of students (Marks et al., 1999). While these needs are important, targeting social interactions may be a primary goal for students with ASD and paraprofessionals are in an optimal position to assist with the implementation of social interventions delivered throughout the school day. Therefore, like in home interventionists, paraprofessionals in the classroom should be trained in a number of social facilitation strategies, including developing sharing exchanges, seeking assistance from peers, engaging children in mutually reinforcing games and activities, implementing buddy systems, teaching appropriate pragmatic behaviors and "small talk," and priming (Koegel et al., 2006). Most importantly, though, is that paraprofessionals are able to use these strategies to identify and create opportunities for social interaction through the school day.

FIDELITY OF IMPLEMENTATION

Consistency in program implementation is another essential factor for promoting successful program implementation. Research findings have shown success using various intensities of early ABA intervention models for home and school based programs (Reed, Osborne, and Corness, 2007). Literature also suggests using a consistent, singular, intensive behavioral approach (Howard et al., 2005).

In a study comparing an intensive behavior analytic treatment to two eclectic treatments of different intensities, Howard and colleagues (2005) showed that the intensive behavior analytic treatment group had higher mean standard scores on all dependent measures than the eclectic treatment groups and that these scores were all statistically significant with the exception of motor skills. In either case, using a combination of strategies or a consistent ABA approach it is likely that staff motivation and commitment to the interventions may have contributed to the positive effects of the programs.

Another possible explanation for the observed differences between the intensive behavior analytic treatment group and the eclectic treatment groups (Howard et al, 2005) is that the integrity of intervention was maintained in the intensive behavior analytic group. The eclectic groups, on the other hand, implemented a number of interventions without demonstrating fidelity with any one approach. The importance of implementing treatment with fidelity and measuring fidelity of implementation, then, is critical to effectively delivering intervention.

There are two major considerations for measuring fidelity of implementation. First, while it is critical that parents, professionals, and paraprofessionals use evidence-based practices, it may be even more important for teams to measure and evaluate correct implementation of these interventions. Most evidence-based treatments, particularly those using ABA principles, have been manualized wherein intervention procedures are thoroughly delineated and described.

Treatment manuals should be consulted prior to delivering an evidence based intervention to ensure proper implementation. Further, many treatment manuals include fidelity of implementation measures that may be used to systematically evaluate correct implementation.

A second consideration for measuring fidelity of implementation is that behavior analysts often develop intervention plans and train other professionals and/or paraprofessionals to implement the plan effectively. In these cases, fidelity of implementation tools can be developed and individualized to measure the integrity of intervention programs. Creating and tracking professionals' and paraeducators' use of the designated strategies will most likely lead to accurate and consistent interventions. Those creating and collecting data with a fidelity of implementation tool should construct a datasheet that can be adapted to a variety of teaching situations. The fidelity of implementation tool should also include the extent to which strategies that have been identified as the most critical to the intervention program are implemented correctly. Table 11.3 provides one example of a team-made fidelity of implementation form that could be used by teachers, paraeducators, or other team members working with students with ASD.

Table 11.3. Example of a Fidelity of Implementation tool to ensure consistency and accuracy of program

Child's Name:
Date:
Staff Name:

	Use of Visual Schedule:	Each time you provide an opportunity for communication Circle X if child communicates independently or Circle A if child communicates with your assistance	Each time you facilitate social interaction (name activity)
Arrival	☐	X X X X X X X X X A A A A A A A A A	
Circle Time	☐	X X X X X X X X X A A A A A A A A A	
Independent work	☐	X X X X X X X X X A A A A A A A A A	
Mealtime	☐	X X X X X X X X X A A A A A A A A A	
Group work	☐	X X X X X X X X X A A A A A A A A A	
Recess	☐	X X X X X X X X X A A A A A A A A A	
	☐	X X X X X X X X X A A A A A A A A A	

COLLABORATION

Another critical factor in successfully supporting students with ASD is effective collaboration between team members. Special education laws and reauthorizations call for parent-professional collaboration with parents included in the assessment, goal development, and intervention processes for their children's educational programming. The Individuals with Disabilities Educational Act (IDEA, 1990), its predecessors (Education of the Handicapped Act, 1975; Education of the Handicapped Act Amendments, 1986) and reauthorization acts (IDEA Amendments, 1997; Individuals with Disabilities Improvement Act, 2004) have consistently included parents as valued and essential team members. Likewise, collaboration between team members, such as specialists, psychologists, and teachers, provides consistency toward a shared vision. Moreover, a core value and key component of Positive Behavior Support (PBS) is a systems level approach to behavior change (Carr et al., 2002; Sailor, 1996). Rather than a more limited focus on the behavior changes of individuals, PBS recognizes the rapid effects of viewing the child within a context and the need to support the context in addition to the individual. The context is most commonly a school or home setting. Therefore, those who interact with the child in these settings must be included into the assessment, intervention, and evaluation of the plan. This requires close collaboration. A strong body of literature has demonstrated positive effects when collaboration between team members was implemented as a key component of intervention (e.g. Safran and Safran, 2001; Schwartz, Sandall, McBride, and Boulware, 2004).

Effective collaboration is an on-going process and a developed skill that requires training and strong communication. Training programs should include a focus on collaboration where professionals learn strategies and models to effectively collaborate with other team members and establish working partnerships with families. For instance, the team members should predetermine their roles in terms of planning, preparing, modifying, adapting, and delivering instructions. Who will be responsible for adapting the lesson to meet a particular student's needs? Who will be expected to collect data on prosocial or disruptive behaviors? Who will provide specific instructions to facilitate the child's social interactions with peers? If these tasks are not assigned in advance, then the team members frantically attempt to create these supports during the instruction time. In this case, the child may not receive the benefits of individualized support. Likewise, if the team members are not on the same page in terms of how instruction and support are to be delivered, they may not be following the IEP goals consistently or may miss teaching opportunities. Good collaboration requires a strong commitment from all team members which can ultimately enhance the quality of the program.

Aside from providing strong evidence of effectiveness, good collaboration benefits the target individual as well as the team members. For the target individual, collaborative efforts can lead to consistent expectations which likely reduce problem behavior. For the team members, working together to achieve common goals can allow more efficient service delivery, a diffusion of responsibility, and a heightened sense of empowerment.

Educational team members should receive training and support to learn how to collaborate effectively. Like any relationship or partnership, collaboration requires open-mindedness and compromise. While various collaborative models have been developed (Ozonoff, Rogers, and Hendren, 2003; Safran and Safran, 2001; Schwartz et al., 2004; Simpson et al., 2003), gaining buy-in from all team members is a first step toward success (Dunlap, Hieneman, and Knoster, 2000). Each team member should have the opportunity to express his or her primary goals and concerns for the individual with ASD and should understand his or her role in the process of service delivery. The purpose of team meetings can range and may include aspects such as creating shared visions, sharing information, or joint planning (Schwartz et al., 2004).

Commonly reported reasons for lack of collaboration are time restriction and differing viewpoints. Special education teachers, when asked about their concerns of support providers for children with ASD, indicated that collaboration and lack of training prior to being assigned into their classroom were particularly troubling (Desmone, 2006). Family members, teachers, professionals, and specialists may share or disagree on goals for the child. They may share or have differing opinions as to how to reach these goals. It is important that each team member be treated with dignity and that their strengths and input be respected. For instance, parents can provide the team with values that may influence the type of goals that are addressed and can provide the team with an accurate history of past interventions that have been successful or unsuccessful with their child. Specialists may provide innovative evidence-based interventions that they work on individually with the child to demonstrate gains in skills. Sharing this expertise with the family or classroom teachers may increase opportunities for more rapid learning and generalization of skills.

Successful collaboration requires gaining buy-in from all team members, scheduling and holding regular meetings, communicating effectively, problem-solving, negotiating conflict, sharing strategies, and efficiently coordinating the efforts of numerous adults across multiple settings. Once target goals and intervention plans are agreed upon, the challenge becomes ensuring these strategies are implemented consistently and appropriately across settings and personnel. Students with ASD depend on structure and consistency across settings and people to acquire and generalize academic and social skills (Scheuermann et al., 2003). Over the last decade, researchers and other professionals have developed many collaborative frameworks in an attempt to essentially teach teaming skills (Hunt, Doering, Hirose-Hitae, Maier, and Goetz 2001; Hunt, Soto, Maier, Liboiron, and Bae, 2004; Schwartz et al., 2004; Wiggins and Damore, 2006.). Table 11.4 provides an example of a form used before, during, and/or after a team-meeting to focus and guide intervention plan discussion. To plan for the meeting, each team member completes the form based on his or her individual knowledge of the student's needs.

Table 11.4. Example of form to help collaborative team manage specific interventions and supports across settings and personnel

Setting Activity	Student Need	Modification/ Accommodation/Strategy	Materials	Personnel	Expected outcome

Setting Activity: description of the activity, setting, or event where student needs support.
Student Need: specific definition of the skill the child is having difficulty with during that time.
Modification/Accommodation/Strategy: description of support strategy to be implemented.
Materials: list materials needed for strategy, if any, and who shall create/ provide them (e.g., picture schedule, task organizer, etc.)
Personnel: person or people responsible for implementing the intervention.
Expected Outcome: description of expected student behavior as a result of intervention.

During the meeting, team members can learn from each other's strategies, gain a broader view of student needs and possible supports, and create a comprehensive plan. When the meeting is over, there is now a record for accountability of how, when, where, and by whom each intervention strategy will be implemented. At future team meetings, the form can be a tool to assess intervention efficacy and promote discussion of necessary adjustments.

Strategies: Focus on Evidence-Based Intervention Practices

Successful strategies to improve training and support are essential to address the growing needs of these children and their educational team members. The amount of training for those working with children with ASD varies significantly between programs, schools, and agencies. Some staff, teachers, and professionals receive extensive training, are well informed, and experienced in evidence-based practices while others have little to no specialized training in ASD. Interventionists working in specialized schools for children with ASD (e.g., Fred Keller School, The May Institute) often participate in on-going staff development while home-program therapists receive on-going supervision. However, there are not established criteria to determine the skill level to work with children with ASD, therefore, the type and amount of training for team members ranges tremendously.

Ideally, professionals and paraprofessionals would have a thorough understanding of the needs of children with ASD and would receive considerable training in how to implement evidence-based interventions. One way to improve the knowledge and training of professionals entering the field is through personnel preparation projects wherein professionals complete university coursework and field-based supervision *while* beginning their careers. Without such programs, though, most students receive training in a single discipline and then are expected to determine ways to coordinate with professionals from other disciplines once they begin their professional careers. Families, then, often lack the benefits of a truly comprehensive, integrated program. That is, a child may receive an in-home program that is quite different from his school program and conflicts with his speech and occupational therapy programs. Another training and collaborative model is for community-based intervention centers to provide integrated services. The reality, however, is that many professionals and paraprofessionals begin working with children with ASD with very little training on how to develop and deliver a quality program and have little training in how to collaborate with other agency or school personnel. Thus, many school districts have increased the number of in-service trainings on ASD in hopes of providing staff the skills they need to improve educational outcomes. However, didactic in-service training may be limited with respect to changing the behaviors of professionals and paraprofessionals and their approach to teaching children with ASD.

Below, we have presented one example of a pre-service training model and one example of a collaborative community-based organization which have each addressed the issues discussed previously to promote effective interventions for those with ASD.

PRE-SERVICE TRAINING MODEL: PROJECT PASS

Project PASS (Preparing Autism Spectrum Specialists) is a Personnel Preparation training program at the California State University, Los Angeles and funded through the United States Department of Education. Project PASS provides specialized knowledge, skills, and strategies for supporting individuals with ASD. Each year at the university, masters level students from a variety of disciplines including special education, early childhood special education, school counseling, school psychology, speech and hearing, marriage and family therapy, rehabilitation counseling, curriculum and instruction, and transition support services receive specialized training in ASD in addition to their focus area. Participant students earn a University certificate in autism in addition to their Master of Arts or Master of Science degree. Many participants are working toward earning certification as Board Certified Behavior Analysts (BCBA). Participants' knowledge and skill levels in ABA and ASD vary greatly prior to their participation in the program. All participants have at least some experience supporting individuals with ASD on their caseloads and plan to continue to work in the field for a minimum of two years upon completion of the program.

The university autism certificate includes a four-course sequence. Required coursework provides a foundation of Applied Behavior Analysis, including conducting Functional Behavior Assessments, characteristics and strategies of ASD, and functional communication training. Included in the coursework are characteristics of ASD, common challenges for families, assessment of skills, evidence-based strategies for intervention, collaborative practices and evaluation. Through literature searches, writing literature reviews, and class presentations, students become familiar with the current research and literature in a selected area of intervention related to supporting those with ASD. Examples of topics include, but are not limited to, improving communication skills, peer-mediated strategies, reducing behaviors maintained by automatic reinforcement, parent education, improving social interactions, ABA interventions, augmentative and alternative communications, visual support, self-management, interventions in inclusive settings, and intervention outcomes for young children with ASD.

In addition to the classroom experience, participants must demonstrate their knowledge and skills through a ten-week fieldwork placement course. Participants serve a variety of roles in their fieldwork positions based on their training area. For instance, those in the school psychology Master of Science program typically have positions as School Psychology interns. Special Education credential and Master of Arts students work as special education teachers while participants earning BCBA supervision hours might work in local agencies delivering services in home and community settings. Within their professional training area, each student demonstrates skills in assessments of social skills, communication, and behaviors and then develops and implements intervention programs for individuals with ASD. Through coursework and fieldwork, students learn how to collect data, create data sheets, measure progress, and maintain on-going evaluation for program review. A tenure-track faculty member and Board Certified Behavior Analyst with expertise in ASD supervises the fieldwork. On-campus and on-site supervision takes place throughout the fieldwork course. Table 11.5 details the percentage of participants who received training in PASS target skills and the percentage who demonstrated those skills during the fieldwork component.

Table 11.5. PASS Outcome Evaluation: Percentage of participants receiving training and demonstrating mastery levels in fieldwork placements

	% Students Trained in Skills	% Students Demonstrated Skills
Assessment	100%	100%
Applied Behavior Analysis	100%	100%
Natural Language Paradigm (e.g., PRT)	94%	74%
Structured Teaching (e.g., DTT)	82%	63%
Use of Visual Support	91%	78%
Development of Communication Goals/Intervention	100%	91%
Development of Social Goals/Intervention	100%	94%
Development of Play Goals/Intervention	94%	84%
Data Collection	100%	97%
Cultural/ Contextual fit	100%	100%

After completing the course sequence, participants of the PASS project attend a two-week summer institute on ASD. This institute consists of a 10-day training with specialists from various universities and research centers including experts from the University of California, Santa Barbara Koegel Autism Center; Emory University Autism Center; University of California, San Diego and the Child and Adolescent Services Research Center (CASRC); Division of Child and Adolescent Psychiatry, Lucile Packard Children's Hospital at Stanford; Yale University Child Study Center; The University of British Columbia; University of California, Los Angeles, Autism Evaluation Clinic; Center for Autism and Related Disorders (CARD), and the National Institute of Mental Health Pediatric and Developmental Neuropsychology. Presentation topics include: advocacy and legal issues for those with ASD; early intervention approaches; ABA interventions including Discrete Trail Training; Natural Language ABA Interventions (i.e., Pivotal Response Treatment, Incidental Teaching); visual supports; augmentative communication; improving play skills; diagnosis and the medical model; family support; collaboration; and transition services. Each day of the institute consists of presentation along with an active learning component for students to gain strategies for application to their work.

Creating a multidisciplinary team is a goal of the training program. By accepting students from various disciplines to participate in a training cohort, participants gain insight and experience from each other. Sharing their knowledge and experience from their training areas creates learning opportunities that are often not provided with homogeneous training programs.

COMMUNITY-BASED COLLABORATIVE MODEL: SARRC

Southwest Autism Research and Resource Center (SARRC) is a nonprofit, community-based organization dedicated to autism research, intervention, education and outreach for children and young adults with ASD and their families. In addition to undertaking clinical and pharmaceutical trials and engaging in collaborative genetic research, SARRC provides a comprehensive model of service delivery for children with ASD and their families. The SARRC intervention model, however, is a unique approach to providing comprehensive services in that it integrates disciplines a priori. That is, a collaborative team made up of highly trained professionals from various disciplines employed within a single agency is in place prior to the start of assessment and intervention (as opposed to pulling together professionals that are currently working with children from various service providers and disciplines). Therefore, integrating services and providing a comprehensive intervention plan is at the forefront of every child's program.

It should be noted that SARRC is not the only community-based center that implements a comprehensive intervention model wherein services are integrated across disciplines. For instance, the Social Communication, Emotional Regulation, and Transactional Support (SCERTS®) Model has been well described by a group of distinguished researchers in the fields of speech and occupational therapy (Prizant, Wetherby, Rubin, Laurent, and Rydell, 2006). These models tend to be the exception rather than the norm; however, there is great interest in replicating these models throughout the United States and internationally to further build the capacity for communities to support families with children with ASD.

The SARRC intervention model is committed to best practices that rely on evidence-based practices and intervention characteristics. In its attempt to integrate services, then, the SARRC model relies on a framework of core intervention components that span across programs. These include Applied Behavior Analysis (ABA); Pivotal Response Treatment (PRT) (Koegel and Koegel, 2006; Koegel, Openden, Fredeen, and Koegel, 2006); early intervention; parent education and training; services and programs implemented across the lifespan; and capacity building methods that support children with ASD across environments (e.g. home, school, and community). According to Simpson and colleagues, only four approaches, including Applied Behavioral Analysis (ABA), Discrete Trial Training (DTT), Pivotal Response Training (PRT), and Lifeskills and Education for Students with Autism and other Pervasive Behavioral Challenges (LEAP) are scientifically validated for practice and all four are based on Applied Behavior Analysis (ABA) (Simpson, 2005; Simpson, de Boer-Ott, Griswold, Myles, Byrd, Ganz, Cook, Otten, Ben-Arieh, Kline, and Adams, 2005). SARRC's intervention model relies extensively on the science and procedures of ABA in each of its programs with a particular focus on a functional approach to communication, social interaction, and problem behavior and a commitment to data-based decision making. Relatedly, each program integrates PRT (one of the four ABA treatments Simpson and colleagues identified as scientifically validated for practice) to ensure consistency across programs. Also, because PRT is a naturalistic behavioral intervention, it can be readily implemented throughout the day and across home, school, and community environments (another core intervention component of the SARRC model). Similar to other comprehensive approaches (see National Research Council, 2001), the SARRC intervention model attempts to begin intervention as early as possible and trains parents to be primary intervention agents. Next, SARRC's intervention model commences when children with ASD are first identified, continues through the preschool and formal schooling years, and transitions with the child into adult services. Finally, SARRC aims to build capacity in schools and communities by providing intervention in these contexts and providing training for staff such that they are better able to support children with disabilities.

The SARRC intervention model consists of a number of disciplines that each subscribe to the framework of intervention components described above. Each of these disciplines includes a number of programs that make up the model. Oversight, training, and supervision of the model is provided by the Clinical Services Director, a Ph.D. level Board Certified Behavior Analyst with expertise in Applied Behavior Analysis, Pivotal Response Treatment, Positive Behavior Support, parent training, and service delivery. Intervention staff include behavior analysts, preschool teachers, speech and language pathologists, occupational therapists, and music therapists. The model begins with JumpStart™, a parent empowerment program for families of newly diagnosed children that teaches parents how to develop and implement individualized home-based early intervention ABA programs. JumpStart™ has been associated with a decrease in depression and increased sense of empowerment among parents and improvement in child functioning (Brautigam, et al., 2007). Once families complete the JumpStart™ program, they enter SARRC's in-home parent training program where parents are trained to implement PRT throughout the day and across settings with their children. The SARRC intervention model also includes an on-site inclusive preschool modeled after evidence-based preschool programs for children with ASD such as Walden (McGee et al. 1999; National Research Council, 2001) and Learning Experiences: An Alternative Program for Preschoolers and Parents (LEAP) (Strain and Hoyson, 2000). Thus, there is consistency across early intervention programs beginning in the home and continuing in a school-based environment. These programs are further supplemented with speech therapy, occupational therapy, and music wherein ABA methodology, namely PRT, is integrated into therapy and activities that primarily address social communication.

As children with ASD transition from preschool to Kindergarten, SARRC's intervention model includes a school-based consultation program. School-based services have a particular focus on supporting students in inclusive education programs and/or transitioning students from special education to general education placements. Further, training and consultation services aim to build the capacity for schools and districts to independently support the social, academic, and behavioral needs of children with ASD in inclusive programs by designing interventions with the whole school as the unit of analysis (Horner, Todd, Lewis-Palmer, Irvin, Sugai, and Boland, 2004).

Similarly, the SARRC intervention model aims to build capacity into the community with a focus on systems change to improve community environments. Specifically, intervention is implemented in inclusive after-school community programs and summer camps wherein children with ASD gain opportunities to access these programs and interact with typically developing peers. By providing intervention within community activities, these programs incorporate strategies and techniques for including children with disabilities into their programs.

Finally, services in the SARRC intervention model continue into adulthood with the Opus West Vocational and Life Skills Academy. The academy represents the next phase of education and training programs for individuals with ASD. These programs provide youth and adults, ages 13 and up, with instruction and practicum opportunities related to pre-vocational, vocational, life, and leadership skills development. Additionally, the academy is a hub of support for communities, businesses, and families.

All of SARRC's intervention staff are housed in the same building, making it relatively easy to communicate and collaborate across programs. As mentioned, the SARRC intervention model is an interdisciplinary approach; therefore, supervision is provided both within and across programs. First, regular supervision is provided between each discipline lead (e.g. preschool director) and their staff (e.g. preschool teachers) along with weekly supervision provided between each discipline lead and the Clinical Services Director. Next, weekly group supervision is held for each of the discipline leads (e.g. speech and language pathologist, occupational therapist, in-home parent training program managers) and provided by the Clinical Services Director to exchange data, graphs, videotapes, and determine programming decisions. Thus, ongoing supervision and coordination across programs ensures that families with children with ASD receive a comprehensive, integrated approach to intervention that addresses each of the child's needs.

FUTURE DIRECTIONS

In 1995, the American Psychological Association Division 12 Task Force on Promotion and Dissemination developed the first official list of empirically supported treatments with two critical issues in mind: identifying efficacious treatments and the methods used for training and dissemination of these treatments. Similar work specific to ASD interventions would likely improve the development and delivery of efficacious interventions. That is, with the increasing number of children diagnosed with ASD, our better understanding of ASD as a spectrum disorder with great variability in symptoms across children, and the number of interventions available, the field will need to systematically identify both interventions that are most effective for children with ASD as well as effective mechanisms for training large numbers of parents, professionals, and paraprofessionals. Further, as new treatments are developed and tested, it will also be necessary to develop new models for training and dissemination.

There is some literature that has been concerned with identifying empirically supported treatments for ASD (e.g. National Research Council, 2001; Simpson, 2005; Simpson et al., 2005). More recently, the National Autism Center (2007) has convened a panel of well-established autism researchers for the purpose of producing a set of standards for identifying research-based intervention for children with ASD called the National Standards Project (2007). These documents are critical for helping parents, professionals, and paraprofessionals identify interventions that are efficacious. However, it will also be necessary to identify and/or develop methods for effectively training those who work with children with ASD to implement these interventions with fidelity.

As discussed above, pre-service training models are one way of disseminating evidence-based practices to professionals who are entering the field. In these models, though, it is essential to utilize faculty that have expertise in delivering evidence-based practices. One way to do so may be to create partnerships between research and teaching universities such that doctoral students who earn their degrees at research universities—and particularly those students who learn to implement and investigate interventions—have opportunities to become faculty members at teaching universities. These partnerships would likely improve the quality of education professionals entering the field receive as they would be taking courses and learning from those with expertise in evidence-based practices specific to ASD.

There is also a need to develop and systemically investigate models for providing effective training in evidence-based practices. Not surprisingly, improving translational research to close the research-to-practice gap has been a priority of federal funding agencies (see National Institutes of Health; Institute of Education Sciences). In a randomized clinical trial under real world conditions, Openden (2005) examined the efficacy and effectiveness of training groups of parents to implement Pivotal Response Treatment (PRT) within a parent education workshop. Significant differences between the treatment and waitlist control groups were found on each of the parent and child variables, including correct implementation of the procedures and improvements in functional verbalizations produced by the children with ASD. The training model was adapted for training teams of intervention providers towards province-wide dissemination and implementation of PRT for young children with ASD in Nova Scotia, Canada (Bryson et al., 2007). Similar models of training may be developed to disseminate intervention broadly to large numbers of professionals and paraprofessionals working with children with ASD in homes and schools.

Finally, intervention and training models that are specifically designed to be implemented in schools should be developed. Many interventions for children with ASD have been designed to be implemented in clinics or homes and often are implemented one-on-one with the child. These interventions may be easily adapted for special education classrooms where there are plenty of opportunities for individualized teaching and support. However, more and more children with ASD are being included in general education classrooms and interventions do not always transfer as easily into these settings. The problem is that many evidence-based interventions have been developed, studied, and tested when implemented between an adult and a child. Thus, many evidence-based interventions for children with ASD are either poorly implemented or not implemented at all due to the difficulty of implementing them in inclusive classrooms. Thus, there is a need to develop school-based models of intervention that can be readily implemented in general education classrooms. Indeed, school-based models may not only benefit children with ASD, but also typically developing students. Further, the development of school-based models of intervention that can be readily implemented in classrooms and widely disseminated to schools may be the most effective way of providing quality intervention to reach and benefit large numbers of children with ASD.

REFERENCES

Alcock, S. (2007). Playing with rules and routines: Children making mealtimes meaningful and enjoyable. *Early Years An International Journal of Research and Development,* 27, 281-193.

American Psychiatric Association (2000). *Diagnostic and statistical manual of mental disorders* (4th ed., text revision). Washington, DC: Author.

Apple, A.L., Billingsley, F. and Schwartz, I.S. (2005). Effects of video modeling alone and with self-management on compliment-giving behaviors of children with high-functioning ASD. *Journal of Positive Behavior Interventions,* 7, 33-46.

Boettcher, M.A. (2004). *Teaching social conversation skills to children with autism through self-management: An analysis of treatment gains and meaningful outcomes*. Dissertation Abstracts International: Section B: The Sciences and Engineering, 65(6-B), 3135.

Boomer, L.W. (1994). The utilization of paraprofessionals in programs for students with autism. *Focus on Autistic Behavior,* 9, 1-8.

Bondy, A., Tincani, M., and Frost, L. (2004). Multiply controlled verbal operants: An analysis and extension to the Picture Exchange Communication System. *Behavior Analyst,* 27, 247-261.

Brautigam, S.E., Stephens, S.M., Ober-Reynolds, S., Bay, R.C., Kirwan, J., Jones, J., McIntosh, R., Treulich, K., Grebe, T., and Melmed, R. (2007). *Impact of parental depression on outcomes of children with autism: An evaluation of the SARRC Jumpstart program*. Paper presented at the International Meeting for Autism Research, Seattle, WA.

Broer, S.M., Doyle, M.B., and Giangreco, M.F. (2005). Perspectives of students with intellectual disabilities about their experiences with paraprofessional support. *Exceptional Children,* 71, 415-430.

Brown and Mirenda, P. (2006). Contingency mapping: Use of a novel visual support strategy as an adjunct to Functional Equivalence Training. *Journal of Positive Behavior Interventions,* 8, 155-164.

Bryson, S.E., Koegel, L.K., Koegel, R.L., Openden, D., Smith, I.M, and Nefdt, N. (2007). Large scale dissemination and community implementation of pivotal response treatment: Program description and preliminary data. *Research and Practice for Persons with Severe Disabilities*, 32, 142-153.

Carr, E.G., Dunlap, G., Horner, R.H., Koegel, R.L., Turnbull, A.P., Sailor, W., Anderson, J.L., Albin, R.W., Koegel, L.K., and Fox, L. (2002) Positive behavior support: Evolution of an applied science. *Journal of Positive Behavior Interventions,* 4, 4-16, 20.

Centers for Disease Control and Prevention (CDC). Prevalence of autism spectrum disorders: Autism and developmental disabilities monitoring network, 14 sites, United States 2002. *Morbidity and Mortality Weekly Report* 2007; 56(SS01): 12-28.

Conroy, M.A., Asmus, J. M., Sellers, J.A., and Ladwig, C.N. (2005). The use of antecedent-based intervention to decrease stereotypic behavior in a general education classroom: A case study. *Focus on Autism and Other Developmental Disabilities,* 20, 223-230.

Desmone, M. C. (2006). *The special education teachers' concerns regarding the use of Therapeutic Staff Support (TSS) in the school setting.* Dissertation Abstracts International: Section A: Humanities and Social Sciences 66(9-A), 3265.

Dettmer, S., Simpson, R.L., and Myles, B.S. (2000). The use of visual supports to facilitate transitions of students with autism. *Focus on Autism and Other Developmental Disabilities,* 15, 163-169.

Dunlap, G., Newton, J.S., Fox, L., Benito, N., and Vaughn B. (2001). Family involvement functional assessment and positive behavior support. *Focus on Autism and Other Developmental Disabilities,* 16, 215-221.

Dunlap, G., Hieneman, M., and Knoster, T. (2000). Essential elements of inservice training in positive behavior support. *Journal of Positive Behavior Interventions,* 2, 22-32.

Dunlap, G., and Fox, L. (1999). A demonstration of behavioral support for young children with autism. *Journal of Positive Behavior Interventions,* 1, 77-87.

Education for All Handicapped Children Act of 1975, Pub. L. 94-142.

Education of the Handicapped Act Amendments of 1986, Pub. L. 99-457.

Frea, W.D., and Hepburn, S.L. (1999). Teaching parents of children with autism to perform functional assessments to plan interventions for extremely disruptive behaviors. *Journal of Positive Behavior Interventions,* 1, 112-116.

Giangreco, M.F., and Broer, S.M., (2005). Questionable utilization of paraprofessionals in inclusive schools: Are we addressing symptoms or causes? *Focus on Autism and Other Developmental Disabilities,* 20, 10-26.

Giangreco, M.F., Broer, S.M., and Edelman, S.W., (2002). That was then, this is now! Paraprofessional supports for students with disabilities in general education classrooms. *Exceptionality,* 10, 47-64.

Giangreco, M.F., Edelman, S.W., and Broer, S.M., (2001a). Respect, appreciation, and acknowledgment of paraprofessional who support students with disabilities. *Exceptional Children,* 67, 485-498.

Giangreco, M.F., Edelman, S.W., and Broer, S.M., (2003). Schoolwide planning to improve paraeducator supports. *Exceptional Children,* 70, 63-79.

Giangreco, M. F., Edelman, S. W., Broer, S. M., and Doyle, M. B. (2001b). Paraprofessional support of students with disabilities: Literature from the past decade. *Exceptional Children,* 68, 45-64.

Giangreco, M.F., Edelman, S.W., Luiselli, T.E., and McFarland, S.Z.E. (1997). Helping or hovering: Effects of instructional assistant proximity on students with disabilities. *Exceptional Children,* 64, 7-18.

Giangreco, M.F., Yuan, S., McKenzie, B., Cameron, P., and Fialka, J. "Be careful what you wish for…" Five reasons to be concerned about the assignment of individual paraprofessionals. *Teaching Exceptional Children,* 37, 28-34.

Grey, I.M., Honan, R., and McClean, B. and Daly, M. (2005). Evaluating the effectiveness of teacher training in Applied Behaviour Analysis. *Journal of Intellectual Disabilities*, 9, 209-227.

Horner, R.H., Todd, A.W., Lewis-Palmer, T., Irvin, L. K., Sugai, G., and Boland J.B. (2004). The School-Wide Evaluation Tool (SET): A research instrument for assessing school-wide positive behavior support. *Journal of Positive Behavior Interventions,* 6, 3-12.

Howard, J.S., Sparkman, C.R., Cohen, H.G., Green, G., and Stanislaw, H. (2005). A comparison of intensive behavior analytic and eclectic treatments for young children with autism. *Research in Developmental Disabilities,* 26, 359-383.

Howlin, P., Gordon, R.K., Pasco, G., Wade, A., and Charman, T., (2007). The Effectiveness of Picture Exchange Communication System (PECS) training for teachers of children with autism: A pragmatic, group randomized controlled trial. *Journal of Child Psychology and Psychiatry,* 48, 473-481.

Hunt, P., Doering, K., Hirose-Hatae, A., Maier, J., and Goetz, L. (2001). Across program collaboration to support students with and without disabilities in a general education program. *Journal of the Association for Persons with Severe Handicaps,* 26, 240-256.

Hunt, P., Soto, G., Maier, J., Liboiran, N., and Bae, S. (2004). Collaborative teaming to support preschoolers with severe disabilities who are placed in general education early childhood programs. *Topics in Early Childhood Special Education,* 24, 123-142.

Individuals with Disabilities Education Act of 1990, Pub. L. No. 101-476.

Individuals with Disabilities Education Act Amendments of 1997, Pub. L. No. 105-17,§ 601, 111 Stat. 39; § 614, 111 Stat. 81-88; § 615, 111 Stat. 88-99; § 681, 111 Stat. 146-152.

Individuals with Disabilities Education Improvement Act of 2004, Pub. L. No. 108-446, § 601,118 Stat. 2649.

Koegel, R.L., Klein, E.F., Koegel, L.K., Boettcher, M.A., Brookman-Frazee, L., and Openden, D. (2006). Working with paraprofessionals to improve socialization in inclusive settings. In R.L. Koegel and L.K. Koegel (Eds.), *Pivotal Response Treatments for Autism: Communication, Social, and Academic Development* (pp. 189-198). Baltimore: Brookes.

Koegel, R.L., and Koegel, L.K. (1990). Extended reductions in stereotypic behavior of students with autism through a self-management treatment package. *Journal of Applied Behavior Analysis,* 23, 119-127.

Koegel, R.L., and Koegel, L.K. (2006). *Pivotal response treatments for autism: Communication, social, and academic development.* Baltimore: Brookes.

Koegel, L.K., Koegel, R.L., and Brookman, L.I. (2005). Child initiated interactions that are pivotal in intervention for children with autism. In E.D., Hibbs and P.S., Jensen (Eds.) *Psychosocial treatments for child and adolescent disorders: Empirically based strategies for clinical practice* (2nd ed., pp. 633-657). Washington, DC: American Psychological Association.

Koegel, L.K., Koegel, R.L., Harrower, J.K., and Carter, C.M. (1999). Pivotal Response Intervention I: Overview of Approach. *Journal of the Association for Persons with Severe Handicaps,* 24, 174-185.

Koegel, L.K., Koegel, R.L. and Hurley, C. (1992). Improving social skills and disruptive behavior in children with autism through self-management. *Journal of Applied Behavior Analysis,* 25, 341-353.

Koegel, R.L., Openden, D., Fredeen, R.M., and Koegel, L.K. (2006). The Basics of Pivotal Response Treatment. In R.L. Koegel and L.K. Koegel (Eds.) *Pivotal Response Treatments for Autism: Communication, Social, and Academic Development* (pp. 3-30). Baltimore: Brookes.

Kohler, F., Anthony, L., Steighner, S., and Hoyson, M. (2001). Teaching social interaction skills in the integrated preschool: An examination of naturalistic practices. *Topics in Early Childhood Special Education,* 21, 93-103.

Lee, S.H., Odom, S.L., and Loftin, R. (2007). Social engagement with peers and stereotypic behavior of children with autism. *Journal of Positive Behavior Interventions,* 9, 67-79.

Luiselli, J.K. and Hurley, A.D. (2005). The significance of applied behavior analysis in the treatment of individuals with autism spectrum disorders (ASD). *Mental Health Aspects of Developmental Disabilities,* 8, 128-130.

Lucyshyn, J. M., Horner, R. H., Dunlap, G., Albin, R. W., and Ben, K. R. (2002). Positive Behavior Support with Families (pp. 3-43). In J.M. Lucyshyn, G. Dunlap, and R.W., Albin (Eds.) *Families and Positive Behavior Support: Addressing problem behavior in family contexts.* Batimore, MD, Paul H. Brookes Publishing.

Macy, M.G. and Bricker, D.D. (2007). Embedding individualized social goals into routine activities in inclusive early childhood classrooms. *Early Childhood Development and Care,* 177, 107-120.

Marks, S.U., Schrader, C., and Levine, M. (1999). Paraeducator experiences in inclusive settings: Helping, hovering, or holding their own. *Exceptional Children,* 65, 315-330.

Massey, N.G., and Wheeler, J.J. (2000). Acquisition and generalization of activity schedules and their effects on task engagement in a young child with autism in an inclusive preschool classroom. *Education and Training in Mental Retardation and Developmental Disabilities,* 35, 326-335.

McClannahan, L.E. and Krantz, P.J. (1999). *Activity schedules for children with autism: Teaching independent behavior.* Bethesda, MD: Woodbine House.

McGee, G.G., Morrier, M.J., and Daly, T. (1999). An incidental teaching approach to early intervention for toddlers with autism. *Journal of the Association for Persons with Severe Handicaps,* 24, 133-146.

McNamara, P. and Humphry, R. (2007). Now this is what you do: Developing structured routines. *Occupation, Participation and Health,* 27, 88S-89S.

Myles, B.S. (2005). *Children and Youth with Asperger syndrome: Strategies for success in inclusive settings*. Thousand Oaks, CA: Corwin Press.

National Autism Center (2007). National Standards Project. Retrieved April 1, 2007 from http://www.nationalautismcenter.org/about/national.php.

National Research Council, Committee on Educational Interventions for Children with Autism, Division of Behavioral and Social Sciences and Education. (2001). *Educating children with autism*. C. Lord and J. P. McGee (Eds.), Washington, D.C.: National Academy Press.

Noell, G.H., Duhon, G.J., Gatti, S.L., and Connell, J.E. (2002). Consultation, follow-up, and implementation of behavior management interventions in general education. *School Psychology Review,* 65, 315-328.

Newman, B. and Ten Eyck, P., (2005). Self-management of initiations by students diagnosed with autism. *Analysis of Verbal Behavior,* 21, 117-122.

O'Neal, B.J., Reeb, R.N., Korte, J.R., and Butter, E.J. (2006). Assessment of home-based behavior modification programs for autistic children: Reliability and validity of the behavioral summarized evaluation. *Journal of Prevention and Intervention in the Community,* 32, 25-39.

Openden, D. (2005). *Pivotal Response Treatment for multiple families of children with autism: Effects of a 4-day group parent education workshop.* Unpublished dissertation.

Ozonoff, S., Rogers, S.J., and Hendren, R.L. (2003). *Autism Spectrum Disorders: A research review for practitioners*. Washington, DC: American Psychiatric Publishing, Inc.

Prizant, B.M., Wetherby, A.M., Rubin, E., Laurent, A.C., and Rydell, P.J. (2006). *The SCERTS model: A comprehensive educational approach for children with autism spectrum disorders (Vols. 1-2).* Baltimore, MD: Paul H. Brookes Publishing.

Reed, P., Osborne, L.A., and Corness, M. (2007). Brief Report: Relative Effectiveness of Different Home-based Behavioral Approaches to Early Teaching Intervention. *Journal of Autism and Developmental Disabilities*, 37, 1815-1821.

Riggs, C. and Mueller, P. (2001). Employment and utilization of paraeducators in inclusive settings. *Journal of Special Education,* 35, 54-74.

Rogers, S.J. (2000). Interventions that facilitate socialization in children with autism. *Journal of Autism and Developmental Disorders,* 30, 399-409.

Safran, J.S., and Safran, S.P. (2001). School based consultation for Asperger syndrome. *Journal of Educational and Psychological Consultation,* 12, 385-395.

Sailor, W. (1996). New Structures and Systems Change for Comprehensive Positive Behavioral Support. In L.K. Koegel, R.L. Koegel, and G. Dunlap (Eds.) *Positive Behavioral Support: Including People with Difficult Behavior in the Community* (pp. 163-206). Baltimore: Brookes.

Scheuermann, B., Webber, J., Boutot, E.A., and Goodwin, M. (2003). Problems with personnel preparation in autism spectrum disorders. *Focus on Autism and Other Developmental Disabilities,* 18, 197-206.

Schwartz, I.S., Sandall, S.R., McBride, B.J., and Boulware, G. (2004). Project DATA (Developmentally Appropriate Treatment for Autism): An inclusive school-based approach to educating young children with autism. *Topics in Early Childhood Special Education,* 24, 156-168.

Simpson, R.L. (2005). Evidence-based practices for students with autism spectrum disorders. *Focus on Autism and Other Developmental Disorders,* 20, 140-149.

Simpson, R.L., de Boer-Ott, S.R., Griswold, D.E., Myles, B.S., Byrd, S.E., Ganz, J.B., Cook, K.T., Otten, K.L., Ben-Arieh, J., Kline, S.A., and Adams, L.G. (2005). *Autism spectrum disorders: Interventions and treatments for children and youth.* Thousand Oaks: Corwin Press.

Simpson, R.L., de Boer-Ott, S.,R., and Smith-Myles, B. (2003). Inclusion of learners with autism spectrum disorders in general education settings. *Topics in Language Disorders,* 23, 116-133.

Smith, T., Eikeseth, S., Klevstrand, M., and Lovaas, O.I., (1997). Intensive behavioral treatment for preschoolers with severe mental retardations and pervasive developmental disorder. *American Journal on Mental Retardation,* 102, 238-249.

Strain, P.S., and Hoyson, M. (2000). The need for longitudinal intensive social skill intervention: LEAP follow-up outcomes for children with autism. *Topics in Early Childhood Special Education,* 20, 116-122.

Tate, T.L.., Thompson, R.H., and McKerchar, (2005). Training teachers in an infant classroom to use embedded teaching strategies. *Education and Treatment of Children,* 28, 206-221.

Tincani, M., Crozier, S., and Alazetta, L. (2006). The Picture Exchange Communication System: Effects on manding and speech development for school-aged children with autism. *Education and Training in Developmental Disabilities,* 41, 177-184.

Trautman, M.L. (2004). Preparing and Managing Paraprofessionals. *Intervention in School and Clinic,* 39, 131-138.

Wetherby, A.M., and Woods, J.J. (2006). Early social interaction project for children with Autism Spectrum Disorders beginning in the second year of life: A preliminary study. *Topics in Early Childhood Special Education,* 26, 67-82.

Wiggins, K.C., and Damore, S.J. (2006). “Survivors” or “friends”? A framework for assessing effective collaboration. *Teaching Exceptional Children,* 38, 49-56.

Wilkinson, L. A., (2005). Supporting the inclusion of a student with Asperger Syndrome: A case study using Conjoint Behavioural Consultation and self management. *Educational Psychology in Practice,* 21, 307-326.

Williams, S. K., Johnson, C., and Sukhodolsky, D., G. (2005). The role of the school psychologist in the inclusive education of school-age children with autism spectrum disorders. *Journal of School Psychology,* 43, 117-136.

Wolery, M., Barton, E. E., and Hine, J. F. (2005). Evolution of applied behavior analysis in the treatment of individuals with autism. *Exceptionality,* 13, 11-23.

Young, B., and Simpson, R. L. (1997). An examination of paraprofessional involvement in supporting inclusion of students with autism. *Focus on Autism and Other Developmental Disabilities,* 12, 31-39.

In: Behavioral Theories and Interventions for Autism
Editor: Phil Reed

ISBN 978-1-60741-165-9
© 2009 Nova Science Publishers, Inc.

Chapter 12

ACTIVITY SCHEDULES FOR ADULTS WITH AUTISM SPECTRUM DISORDERS

Lynn E. McClannahan*, Gregory S. MacDuff and Patricia J. Krantz
Princeton Child Development Institute, USA

An activity schedule is a set of pictures or words that is used to cue someone to engage in a sequence of activities (McClannahan and Krantz, 1999). For example, one might make a photographic activity schedule for a severely disabled adult with Autism Spectrum Disorder (ASD) to teach him to prepare his own breakfast. Because the young man likes cereal, the instructor decides that will be the initial target. After completing a task analysis, the instructor takes photographs that represent the component tasks, mounts the pictures on a plain background, and places them in a three-ring binder, one photograph per page. The photographs include a picture of hand washing, and pictures of a box of cereal, a bowl, a spoon, a carton of milk, a napkin, a picture of milk being poured on cereal, and a picture of the learner eating cereal.

Let us assume that the man has never before used an activity schedule. Teaching begins with an initial comment such as, "It's time for breakfast." Subsequently, the instructor stands behind the learner and manually guides him to open the schedule book to the first page, point to the photograph of hand washing, and go to a sink and wash his hands. Then he is manually guided to return to his schedule, turn the page, and point to the next picture—a photograph of a box of cereal. Remaining behind him, the teacher guides him to obtain a box of his preferred cereal from a cabinet and put it at his place at the table. Then he is guided to return to his schedule, turn the page, point to the next photograph (a picture of a bowl), obtain a bowl, and place it on the table. This sequence continues until the learner arrives at the last photograph, a picture of himself eating cereal; the instructor manually guides him to be seated at the table, pick up the spoon, and begin to eat.

* Please address correspondence to: Lynn E. McClannahan, Princeton Child Development Institute, 300 Cold Soil Road, Princeton, New Jersey 08540, USA.

After each task in the schedule is completed, if inappropriate behavior was not observed, the instructor places a token (in this case, a coin) on the man's token board and after all tasks are completed, the learner exchanges them for a preferred activity. Initially, tokens are delivered following prompted responses but as the person gains skills, tokens are delivered for responses that are made with lesser assistance and eventually, with no assistance. The man in our example often exchanges his tokens for opportunities to listen to music or watch TV, although he has many other reward choices. For him and other nonreaders, the available rewards are depicted in photographs; choices change over time as a result of frequent reinforcer assessment.

The teacher does not use verbal prompts or gestures because the goal is to help the man *independently* prepare his own breakfast. The target responses are not evoked by others' instructions, but by the same stimuli that are responsible for our own breakfast preparation—for example, time of day, hunger, and the availability of breakfast foods.

When the learner begins to make the relevant responses with less manual guidance, prompts are faded in a most-to-least hierarchy: manual guidance, graduated guidance, spatial fading, shadowing, and decreased proximity of the instructor to the learner. And when he independently obtains and consumes cereal, new photographs are added to the activity schedule and he is taught to pour juice and later, to make buttered toast. As he becomes a more proficient schedule follower, he is taught to use a second activity schedule to make an alternate breakfast—a frozen waffle that he warms in a toaster oven and covers with syrup, and an orange that he peels. Over time, he learns to use activity schedules to prepare several different breakfasts. His breakfast choices are identified by photographs placed on the covers and spines of his activity schedules and each morning he independently selects one of these schedules and uses it to prepare his own breakfast.

Like the young man in this example, many severely disabled adults have learned to use activity schedules to achieve greater independence and to make choices that contribute to a better quality of life. Of course, if the man in our example were a reader, the instructor would create a written activity schedule that included textual cues such as "wash hands," "get cereal," "get bowl," "get spoon," and so on, but the relevant responses would be taught in the same way, beginning with manual prompts that are gradually faded from most to least.

THE EVOLUTION OF ACTIVITY SCHEDULES

The first activity schedules used at the Princeton Child Development Institute (PCDI) were photographic. Photographs were mounted on plain black backgrounds and placed in three-ring binders, one photo per page, and the last photograph depicted a preferred item or activity. Typically, children's first schedules included only three to six pages and most activities were completion-based; that is, an activity was finished when the youngster used all of the component parts (e.g., all pieces were placed in a puzzle, all Lego© blocks were assembled, or all picture cards were sorted into categories). But many activities are time-based (e.g., looking at books, watching videos, playing computer games, riding bicycles); therefore, young people learned to set timers. These skills were taught using photographic activity schedules that displayed timers with color-coded buttons; users matched colored buttons depicted in schedules to colored buttons on timers to set their timers for varying lengths of time (McClannahan and Krantz, 1999, pp. 69-72).

As people became accomplished schedule followers, photographic schedules grew increasingly bulky and unwieldy; eventually, learners had daily schedule books that referred them to many different sub-schedule books. For example, a photo of snack foods in a youth's main schedule cued him to obtain one of several sub-schedules that he used to make preferred snacks, and a picture of exercise equipment cued him to get the sub-schedule he used for his workout in the gym.

For readers, written schedules were initially presented as lists, and students struck through or made checkmarks next to completed items. Lists were later supplanted by written entries in daily planners or appointment books and typically, these entries directed users to more detailed textual cues that were located in notebooks, on clipboards, or in file folders. In response to the written entry "cook" in her daily planner, a teenager might obtain a notebook that contained previously mastered recipes and select a written task analysis for making pasta, chicken and rice, or an omelet. Or she might respond to a written cue in her schedule to select a new recipe to prepare with her teacher's assistance.

More recently, many adolescents' and adults' photographic and written activity schedules have been replaced by personal digital assistants (PDAs) such as BlackBerrys™ or Palms™. For nonreaders, digital photographs are imported to folders on PDAs. For example, a man employed as a hotel housekeeper accesses photographs on his PDA to guide him through a lengthy task sequence that includes making beds, dusting, vacuuming, folding and hanging towels, and cleaning bathrooms. A recent comparison of a person's performance when using a picture schedule presented in a three-ring binder versus using a picture schedule presented on a PDA showed that both formats were associated with high engagement and task completion (Decker, Ferrigno, May, Natoli, Olson, Schaefer, Cammilleri, and Brothers, 2003). Further, PDAs are more portable than photographic schedules and they enhance the social competence of adults with ASD by enabling them to appear more like their typical co-workers.

Less severely disabled readers also use schedules displayed on PDAs, and many use textual cues to add their own written schedules to their handheld devices (see Table 12.1). In this case, as with all other photographic and written schedules, instructors use only manual prompts that are faded to graduated guidance, then spatial fading, shadowing, and finally, to decreased proximity of teacher and learner. Verbal prompts and gestures are never used. Of course, before introducing the written schedule shown in Table 12.1, it is important to teach a person to identify and label items such as "USB cable," "stylus," and "case."

Our data and others' investigations show that schedule-following performance is essentially the same whether readers use textual cues presented on paper or on PDAs (cf. Bellovin, Burck, Tarnoski, Cammilleri, and Brothers, 2003).

Rehfeldt, Kinney, Root, and Stromer (2004) described the construction of computer-based activity schedules created with PowerPoint™, and gave step-by-step instructions on how to prepare closed-ended and open-ended schedules that include photographs, sound, text, and videos. Although lack of portability of computer-based schedules may limit their use in workplaces and other community settings, the same or similar outcomes can be achieved with Microsoft Pocket PCs™ or PalmPilots™.

Table 12.1. A Written Activity Schedule for Adding a Schedule to a Personal Data Assistant (a PalmPilot™)

Tasks	
___	Plug small end of USB Hot Sync cable into Palm Pilot
___	Plug large end of USB Hot Sync cable into computer
___	Double click the *Palm Desktop* icon on the computer
___	Double click *New to Do* icon
___	Type first activity in the title box
___	Click *Add Another*
___	Add each activity and click *Add Another*
___	Click *OK* when finished
___	Turn on Palm Pilot
___	Use stylus to click on the Hot Sync button
___	Click on *Palm Desktop* on top of computer screen
___	Click on *Quit Palm Desktop*
___	Unplug USB cord from computer
___	Unplug USB cord from Palm Pilot
___	Put Palm Pilot in case
___	Put cord in box by computer

Why Use Activity Schedules?

Our research on activity schedules emerged from our concern about the prompt dependence that is so often displayed by people with ASD. By prompt dependence, we mean that a person responds to prompts rather than to the stimuli that are expected to control a response (Touchette and Howard, 1984). At the time of our initial investigation of activity schedules (mid 1980s), discrete-trial teaching was a predominant intervention strategy in our setting as well as elsewhere, and our data indicated that young people in PCDI's intervention programs received verbal prompts from instructors at very high rates.

Because verbal prompts are frequently paired with reinforcement, they may acquire stimulus control (Bickel, Stella, and Etzel, 1984; Schneider and Salzberg, 1982). We have often discussed how the inter-trial latencies and verbal instructions that are key components of discrete-trial teaching may come to signal reinforcement and thus become discriminative stimuli:

"The teacher gives an instruction or asks a question, and the learner attempts (or does not attempt) to follow the instruction, receives (or does not receive) a reward, and waits for the teacher to initiate the next trial...Behavior other than quiet waiting delays the next trial and the next reinforcement opportunity. Therefore, both passive waiting and instructions become discriminative for reinforcement" (McClannahan and Krantz, 1997, p. 271).

In practice, we repeatedly observed this problem. A person who long ago learned to make popcorn passively waited in the kitchen until someone instructed, "Get the popcorn." Another who was a proficient biker stood near the bicycle until a staff member prompted, "Why don't you ride the bike now?" And a student who practiced handwriting every school day sat looking at a worksheet until a teacher said, "It's time to do handwriting." Other researchers have also noted "deleterious relationships between verbal prompts and the potential emergence of spontaneous behaviors" (Reed, undated, p. 19).

In our initial investigation of activity schedules as a means of ameliorating prompt dependence (Knapp, McClannahan, and Krantz, 1986), we used a multiple-baseline design across three students. The teaching procedures included verbal prompts, modeling, and behavioral rehearsal, and as the young people learned to follow photographic activity schedules, verbal prompts were replaced by gestures and the teacher's proximity was gradually faded until she was no longer present in the room. The learners met criterion in the training setting, but probes in a different setting at a different time of day showed that schedule-following skills did not transfer until the teacher instructed. Although two of the participants responded to a single instruction to generalize ("Do your schedule"), the third remained dependent on verbal prompts.

Packages of prompting procedures such as those used in that first study may miscue learners and prevent them from responding to the critical stimuli (cf. Hoogeveen, Kouwenhoven, and Smeets, 1989). Further, the use of multiple types of prompts makes it difficult to determine which components of the treatment package are responsible for the results, and may also result in selective stimulus control (i.e., one type of stimulus blocks the effect of other types). Thus, in our second study (MacDuff, Krantz, and McClannahan, 1993), we assessed the effects of photographic activity schedules taught only with graduated guidance that was delivered from behind a learner and then faded. The data indicated that the three participants (residents of a group home) displayed sustained engagement with scheduled activities, and their independent schedule-following skills generalized to a different sequence of photographs and to new photographs. Similar results were obtained in a third study that used the same prompting procedures (Krantz, MacDuff, and McClannahan, 1993).

In our subsequent research on photographic and written activity schedules, we have continued to use graduated manual guidance, followed by spatial fading (prompts to the hand, then the wrist, then the elbow, and then the shoulder). When a person acquires a correct response chain, the instructor shadows and finally, decreases physical proximity. This most-to-least prompt hierarchy is "errorless"--that is, in contrast to most other teaching procedures, it achieves a very low error rate and prevents errors that might otherwise be embedded in response chains. But if a learner pauses for more than a few seconds, begins to make an error, or engages in inappropriate behavior, manual prompts are reinstated and again faded. All prompts are delivered from behind learners and instructors attempt never to insert any part of their bodies between the learners and their activities or their schedules, because to do so may make their presence more salient, promote prompt dependence, and make it more difficult to fade physical proximity.

Our early uses of activity schedules were directed toward children and adolescents, but as learners matured we modified the content of activity schedules to provide age-appropriate activities for adults with ASD. Today, it is difficult to imagine an intervention program for adults in which schedules do not occupy a prominent position. We are not aware of other procedures that are equally successful in diminishing prompt dependence and promoting independence and choice.

The Participants in PCDI's Adult Life-Skills Program

Prior to 1984, when the first young person with ASD had his twenty-first birthday and completed his schooling at PCDI but needed continuing support, we embarked on the development of a program for adults. It was, and continues to be, an uphill battle to persuade funding agencies of the importance of a seamless transition from adolescence to adulthood, but the benefits of program continuity are worth the effort. Intervention for preschool and school-age children enhances their outcomes in adulthood, and data on adults' repertoires often result in key revisions of the curriculum for children (McClannahan, MacDuff, and Krantz, 2002).

At PCDI, all adults with ASD receive the services of staff members identified as Life-Skills Coaches. They provide job coaching and ensure effective work performance; in addition, they teach a plethora of other relevant skills such as shopping and money management, grooming and health-care skills, menu planning and food preparation, housekeeping, family participation, and use of leisure time. The ratio of learners to staff members is 2 to 1.

Presently, 20 adults (18 men and 2 women), ages 21 to 44, receive services. All have diagnoses of autism. They have been enrolled in PCDI's programs for 17 to 38 years. All of them receive day services; 10 of 20 reside in the Institute's group homes, 5 participate in supervised apartment or supported community-living programs, and 5 live at home with their own families.

Due to serious health issues or low-rate but severe behavior problems, two men work at PCDI, completing contract work for local organizations. The other adults hold jobs in community workplaces. Their positions include word-processing, data-entry, general office work, and employment in food services, hotel housekeeping, and grounds maintenance. All of the adults use photographic or written activity schedules to complete employment-related tasks. As children, four of the adults were participants in our study of the effects of activity schedules on generalization and maintenance of complex response chains (MacDuff, et. al., 1993) and two others participated in our research on parents' use of activity schedules (Krantz, et. al., 1993). Most of the adults have been schedule followers for at least a decade and when new schedules are introduced, their acquisition rates are typically related to the severity of their disabilities.

Six people are non-readers who use photographic activity schedules. Four continue to learn sight words when those words are relevant to their scheduled activities. Sight words are taught via discrete-trial procedures (albeit with trials embedded in their daily activities rather than with massed trials); new sight words are not placed in written schedules until they are mastered. The remaining ten adults are readers who use written activity schedules; their reading grade levels range from kindergarten to fourth grade. They learn new sight words in the context of their schedules and activities.

Because PCDI provides continuity of services to people who continue to need them (from early childhood through adulthood), all of the adults have lengthy histories of schedule-following. However, evidence from other settings suggests that adults with developmental disabilities who have never previously been introduced to activity schedules can achieve impressive benefits from this intervention strategy (cf. Watanabe and Sturmey, 2003; Weiberg-Aurdal, undated).

ADULTS' SCHEDULES: SOME EXAMPLES

It is difficult to identify a skill area in which adults at PCDI do not use schedules, but because all of them have long schedule-following histories, many activities that were once guided by multiple photographs or lengthy written task analyses are now cued by single pictures or words. With few exceptions, the adults routinely manage their own photographic or written schedules—that is, they obtain or create their schedules at the beginning of each day, transport them across activities and settings, and turn pages or check off activities as they are completed. When new skill sets are mastered, new activities are added; schedules are dynamic rather than static.

Personal Hygiene

As children and adolescents, many of the adult participants in PCDI's programs used activity schedules to complete daily hygiene tasks, such as washing face, brushing teeth, taking a shower, and dressing. But standards for appropriate grooming evolve during childhood and adolescence; the tooth-brushing repertoire that was acceptable for a seven-year-old is not appropriate for an adult and as a result, activity schedules are modified to meet new age-related expectations (McClannahan, et.al., 2002). For example, a young child may follow a face-washing schedule that includes washing with soap, rinsing, and drying his face, but a teenager's schedule may include washing with anti-acne soap, rinsing, drying, and applying acne medication.

As children grow up, new schedules are introduced. A teenage boy learns to follow a detailed schedule for shaving (e.g., *get shave cream, get razor, put water in sink, wet face...)* and when it is mastered, tasks are gradually faded until they are replaced with a single word (*shave*). An adolescent girl learns to follow a schedule that pertains to her menstrual cycle.

Young men who recently began work as hotel housekeepers have new items in their dressing schedules—for example, a picture of a name badge or a textual cue (*put on name badge).*

Schedule-following repertoires help people make rapid adaptations to changes in routine. For example, a person who needs seasonal allergy medication quickly learns to take his pill when a cue is added to his morning hygiene schedule. Although some adults continue to need detailed schedules to complete personal care tasks, many now respond to lists of the relevant tasks, or to general textual cues ("Get ready for work"), or they no longer need any cues to complete personal hygiene activities. Some activity schedules have been completely faded without decrements in the target skills that were taught.

Home Living

Like personal hygiene schedules, schedules for completing home-living activities are usually introduced during childhood. Young children learn to be helpful family members by following schedules to set the table or unload the dishwasher, and housekeeping schedules are expanded as they move through adolescence and arrive at adulthood.

Illustrative home-living schedules for adolescents and adults include doing laundry, ironing, washing windows, and cleaning oven and refrigerator. An activity schedule for cleaning a bathroom is typically preceded by several component schedules, such as cleaning sink and shower, cleaning a toilet, washing mirrors and windows, dusting, and mopping. When the component schedules are mastered, the person is prepared to use a schedule to clean the bathroom.

Other home-living schedules include menu planning, making a grocery list, and preparing food. These schedules may be written or pictorial. For example, a non-reader plans menus by selecting pictures from categories such as fruit, vegetables, main dishes, and desserts and placing them on pages that represent days of the week. And when making a grocery list, a non-reader checks cupboard shelves; if there is no salt near the photograph of salt, he removes that picture and places it in a notebook that he will take to the grocery store; the notebook serves as the shopping list.

Food preparation schedules (i.e., recipes) are selected on the basis of learners' preferences, although menu-planning schedules guide them to make selections that result in healthy diets. Successive activity schedules for food preparation become increasingly lengthy and complex and gradually introduce measures such as one-fourth cup and one-half teaspoon; utensils such as grater, sifter, and spatula; and tasks such as whisking, peeling, mincing, and dicing.

Presently, many adolescents and adults prepare entire meals that include entrees such as meatloaf, enchiladas, spaghetti and meatballs, and roast beef, as well as a variety of salads, vegetable dishes, and desserts. Although their cooking repertoires are extensive, only a few have learned to use typical cookbooks or recipes on food containers. For that reason, their "cookbooks" are notebooks that contain photographic or written schedules for preparing previously mastered foods.

Community Participation

Typically, using an activity schedule to learn to make a single purchase (e.g., buying a beverage or a snack) precedes a schedule that teaches grocery or clothing shopping. Similarly, a schedule for placing an order in a fast-food restaurant is often mastered before a schedule for eating in a restaurant is introduced. Calculating tips, using a laundromat, using an automatic teller machine, and using vending machines are also schedules that are frequently used in community settings. A schedule for packing a suitcase has been useful to group home residents who regularly visit their families, as well as for adults who occasionally take vacations with family members, staff members, or friends.

In community settings, written schedules are less likely to call undue attention to people with developmental disabilities, and such schedules are often reduced in size, so that they can be easily carried in a shirt pocket or purse. Photographic schedules displayed on PDAs accomplish the same objective.

Activity schedules for using cell phones deserve special mention because this skill set contributes to the safety of adults with ASD. Learning to call an instructor, a parent, or the agency's main telephone number may be very important if transportation from work to home is delayed, if a person is ill, or if unexpected events occur at a job site when a staff member is not present.

Leisure Skills

Photographic and written activity schedules have been useful in teaching adults to take and print digital photographs, to load and play computer games and view DVDs, to use exercise equipment, and to construct scrapbooks. Schedules have also been helpful in enabling people to independently put on protective equipment relevant to biking and skating, and to set up recreational equipment such as indoor golf putting greens. Recently, activity schedules have also enabled people to send and receive e-mail and to manage e-mail accounts.

Employment

In the best of circumstances, adolescents use activity schedules to acquire repertoires that contribute to their employment opportunities in adulthood. For example, learning to clean a room is a skill set that is important in a person's living environment, but it may also contribute to successful employment as a hotel housekeeper. Activity schedules that teach people to collect and recycle paper and plastics, to inventory custodial supplies, to restock office or cleaning supplies, or to sweep sidewalks and pick up trash on lawns often contribute to their later success in community workplaces.

Adults who have acquired competitive word processing and data-entry skills benefit from schedules that teach other white-collar repertoires, such as filing; using copiers, scanners, and laminators; and taking coffee breaks in office settings. And although some people may need continuous supervision in the intervention setting, activity schedules help to diversify the employment activities that they can perform in-house. In our day-treatment program, we have used activity schedules to teach adults to complete a very broad array of contracted employment tasks, including stringing tennis rackets; assembling rivet kits; assembling and packaging materials as diverse as paint-mixing equipment and toys; doing auto detailing; preparing mailings for insurance companies; and packaging books to be sent to public libraries.

Of course, the effectiveness of an activity schedule is dependent upon on the skillfulness of the instructor who creates the task analysis upon which the schedule is based. For example, tasks and task sequences may be different for an Epson™ scanner than a Xerox™ scanner, and the person who constructs the task analysis must know how to operate the scanner that the learner will use. The job coach who prepares an activity schedule that will be used by a hotel housekeeper must not only know all of the job components, but must also know management's expectations about how beds should be made, how towels should be folded, and where amenities such as soap, shampoo, and shower cap should be placed.

Social Skills

Activity schedules offer an invaluable framework for teaching people with ASD to initiate conversation. At PCDI, a severely disabled man has a photographic activity schedule that includes pictures of potential conversation partners. He also has a file box that contains photographs of conversation topics—for example, pictures of him at an amusement park, in a swimming pool, and at a fast-food restaurant. When he turns a page of his activity schedule and encounters a picture of a conversation partner (a peer or staff member), he selects a picture of a topic, mounts it in his schedule, and then seeks out the depicted recipient. Although he has a very small spoken vocabulary, the schedule enables him to open conversation with brief statements such as, "Roller coasters are fun," "I like to swim," or "McDonalds is great!" His schedule enables him to initiate conversation; without the schedule, his frequency of social interaction is much lower.

Pictures of potential conversation partners or the textual cue "talk" can also be used to cue learners to obtain audiotaped or written scripts, approach interaction partners, and say scripts; subsequently, scripts are gradually faded from end to beginning. Eventually, after many sets of scripts have been introduced and faded, many people learn to engage in spontaneous conversation. The use of these procedures is more fully described in Teaching conversation to children with autism: Scripts and script-fading (McClannahan and Krantz, 2005).

Schedules also provide a useful structure for teaching people to report next activities and recently completed activities. For example, the word "talk" or a photograph of a learner talking to someone appears in a person's activity schedule before and after selected activities. When he encounters this cue, he is guided to obtain an audiotaped or written script, approach someone, and say the script. Scripts that a person might say before beginning the next activity are: "I'll do word processing," "Time for lunch," and "I'm going to walk on the treadmill." Scripts he might use after completing these activities are "I did word processing," "I had lunch," and "I walked for twenty minutes." When such scripts are completely faded and a person continues to talk about word processing, lunch, and walking on the treadmill, new scripts are introduced before and after different activities (e.g., playing a computer game, making a purchase, riding a bicycle).

After several sets of scripts have been introduced and faded, the word "talk" or a photographic cue is inserted in the schedule before and after activities that have never been associated with scripts. If the learner does not discuss these activities, we continue to provide multiple exemplars. If he initiates conversation in the absence of scripts, the "talk" cue temporarily remains in his schedule, but we occasionally remove it and observe whether he interacts in its absence. When he discusses his activities in the absence of the cue, it is permanently removed.

Learning to report next and recently completed activities is a critical skill for adults with ASD, because it makes it possible to fade supervision. If a worker in an office setting says, "I'm going to the copy room" and the data show that he accurately reports next activities, the job coach need not draw co-workers' attention by following him. Or if a group home resident reports, "I'm going to do the laundry," a staff member need not interrupt a teaching activity with others to follow her to the laundry room.

Activity schedules also help adults who live in group homes or supervised apartments learn to entertain guests. A written schedule may contain items such as: *Say "Welcome! Please come in"; take coats; invite guests to sit in living room; ask "Would you like coffee or tea?"; say "Excuse me for a moment"; serve beverages; serve cookies.* We know some adults with ASD who use written schedules to prepare meals for guests and to plan special events with family members and peers.

Daily, Weekly, and Monthly Schedules

Upon their arrival at adulthood, most service receivers at PCDI are familiar with daily activity schedules, and those who use textual cues may have daily schedules that include activities such as *check e-mail, take a photograph and print it, feed the fish, iron work clothing, set the table.* They have also learned to sequence their own activities, and many of them begin each day by removing note cards from a box; each card displays the name of a daily activity. The schedule user arranges the cards in a preferred sequence, and then writes the sequence of activities in a daily planner or types them on a computer and then prints the page (of course, these activities were taught using an activity schedule).

A next step is to teach people to schedule their own weekly and monthly activities. For example, a woman who uses a daily schedule arrives at the textual cue "Plan a weekly activity." She obtains a list of weekly activities, such as *check calendar for birthdays and holidays, make shopping list, do laundry, iron clothes, water plants, call Mom and Dad.*

She selects an activity from the list, writes it in her daily schedule, and draws a line through the activity on the list that she has just transferred to her daily schedule. Her monthly list includes *make haircut appointment, make manicure appointment, call grandmother, clean oven, clean closets, invite someone to dinner.* Although she accomplishes these tasks with paper and pencil, other learners use calendar programs such as Apple Computer's iCal™ program. These skills are taught in the same manner as other schedule-following skills.

Problem Solving Schedules

People in supervised apartments and supported-living programs and people who are employed in community workplaces, like the rest of us, sometimes encounter unanticipated issues—the computer quits, cable television doesn't work, there is an electrical power outage, or there is no water. Some of these problems are potentially serious: a person sustains a deep cut while dicing vegetables, a smoke detector sounds, there is a fire in the kitchen, or a person becomes ill at work when a job coach is not present.

A man who participates in PCDI's supervised apartment program has a notebook that includes these problem-solving schedules. Each written schedule is identified by a tab that identifies a topic (e.g., "Electricity," "Water," "TV"). If his computer freezes or does not work, he has learned to go to the notebook section labeled "Computer" and follow the schedule, which includes textual cues such as: *If computer is on, turn it off, Unplug computer, Plug computer in, Turn computer on. Does computer work? If not, call your Life-Skills Coach.* Another section of the notebook, "Smoke Detector," contains the following schedule: *Get your cell phone, take this notebook, go outside quickly, close the door, stand on the sidewalk near the bike rack, call your Life-Skills Coach.* His Life-Skills Coach knows where to find him, and because she lives in the adjacent apartment building, she can arrive quickly and assess the problem. She also makes practices as realistic as possible; the learner does not know in advance that a pretend "emergency" will occur.

Activity schedules help people with ASD acquire repertoires that will be relevant in the event of real emergencies. Staff members create opportunities for a person to practice following schedules that address life's problems, teach until criteria are met, and regularly assess skill maintenance. Of course, an important aspect of maintenance is that a person always knows where these schedules are kept and can quickly access them.

End Note

Although the foregoing discussion devotes minimal attention to reinforcement procedures they are, of course, essential to the acquisition of schedule-following skills. All of the adults at PCDI have learned to use token reinforcement. People who have not yet acquired these skills are rewarded with: (a) edibles that are dropped in a cup and consumed as soon as schedules are completed; (b) rewards that are programmed as the final activity in a schedule; and/or (c) tangible or activity rewards that are delivered immediately after schedules are completed. However, in our experience, most toddlers, children, and adults with ASD quickly learn to use tokens.

It is also important to note that activity schedules are not intervention strategies to be used in one session per day, or in one setting but not others. They are most effective when they are used to organize a learner's entire day; they provide a framework for instruction. Applied behavior analysis offers many well-documented intervention procedures (e.g. discrete-trial teaching, incidental teaching, video modeling); placing cues for these activities in schedules helps to ensure that people will receive many different instructional strategies that help them learn in many different ways.

Activity Schedules Promote Generalization

There is a body of evidence showing that when activity schedules are taught with graduated guidance, pictures or textual cues become discriminative stimuli that evoke generalized responding. MacDuff, et. al. (1993) demonstrated that after three participants learned to follow picture schedules to complete home-living and leisure activities, their schedule-following skills transferred to a different sequence of photographs and to pictures of two novel leisure activities that were never encountered during teaching. Weiberg-Aurdal (undated) showed that when a developmentally disabled adult was taught to follow lengthy photographic activity schedules to do laundry, make waffles, and make pasta, each successive task was more quickly acquired, with fewer prompts delivered by the trainer.

Table 12.2. Percentage of Tasks Correctly Completed on Pretests with and without Activity Schedules

Participant	Program	Pretest 1—Without Activity Schedule	Pretest 2—With Activity Schedule
Participant 1	Make English muffin pizza	62%	92%
	Make potato-tuna salad	27	52
	Clean a bathroom	8	4
Participant 2	Make potato-tuna salad	0	42
	Dust furniture	0	0
Participant 3	Check personal appearance	0	18
	Clip toenails	0	22
	Make bagel with cream cheese	0	57
Participant 4	Make English muffin pizza	20	36
Participant 5	Set table and make salad	0	40
	Make macaroni and cheese	0	31
	Make soup	0	6
	Make grilled cheese sandwiches	4	40
	Clean mirror and sink	0	7
Participant 6	Set table and make salad	0	19
	Make macaroni and cheese	0	23
	Make soup	7	33
	Make grilled cheese sandwiches	0	33
	Clean mirror and sink	0	14
Participant 7	Make bed	42	71
	Make pasta and sauce	0	38
	Make ziti with cheese	0	52
	Wash face	37	48
	Brush teeth	38	62
Participant 8	Make microwave pizza	0	44
	Make macaroni and cheese	0	70
	Make stuffed shells (pasta)	20	95
	Make microwave lasagna	90	95
	Make salad	85	92
	Make turkey sandwich	70	86
	Make bagel and cream cheese	24	83
	Make ham and cheese sandwich	85	88

During a six-month period at PCDI, we pretested eight participants on every new instructional program that specified a written activity schedule as the intervention procedure (Crognale, Kitson, MacDuff, Zeutenhorst, and McClannahan, 2003). All of the students (7 males and 1 female, ages 12 to 17) had lengthy prior experience with activity schedules. For each new intervention program, two pretests—the first without and the second with an activity schedule—were administered before teaching began. During both pretests, the instructor gave one initial direction to engage in the target repertoire (e.g., "Please clean the bathroom" or "Please make a salad"), after which no prompts were delivered. Pretests ended when a specified amount of time elapsed, when a student ceased to respond for 30 seconds, or when a person requested help. Pretests 1 and 2 were administered for 32 new programs launched for the eight learners.

Percentage interobserver agreement on number of correct responses was calculated by dividing number of agreements by number of agreements plus disagreements and multiplying by 100. Interobserver agreement was obtained on 23 of the 32 programs (72%), and ranged from 85% to 100% for Pretest 1 (mean = 98%) and from 74% to 100% for Pretest 2 (mean = 96%).

On 30 of 32 new programs (94%), the participants' pretest scores were higher when activity schedules were present than when they were absent, and the magnitude of difference ranged from 3% to 75% more tasks correctly completed. These data showed that schedule-following skills generalized to new, never-taught schedules that addressed a variety of activities, and this was true for young people with severe, as well as moderate disabilities. Schedules promote faster acquisition, making it possible to introduce more new curricula.

In practice, we now frequently pretest or conduct baseline probes with, as well as without activity schedules, and we sometimes discover that some programs for adults need not be implemented. For example, a young man who moved from his parents' home to his own apartment achieved criterion scores on pretests when given written activity schedules for cleaning the refrigerator and the oven, and these programs were never introduced. The schedules were added to a notebook in his home, and he continues to successfully use them when these cleaning tasks appear on his weekly or monthly calendar.

Using Activity Schedules to Teach Self Monitoring

Over the course of several years, we noted that some young people who were long-time users of written activity schedules occasionally stopped making check marks or drawing lines through text to indicate that activities were completed; instead, they began to mark plus (+) or minus (-) beside tasks on their schedules. In our setting, when staff members collect observational data, they mark plus and minus to indicate correct and incorrect responses respectively. In some cases, the students' uses of plus and minus appeared unrelated to correctness but in other situations, it appeared that they were attempting to assess their own performance. These observations led us to wonder whether we could teach them to take interobserver agreement as a means of helping them learn to monitor their own correct responses and errors, and we designed a study to investigate that question (Kitson, Connor, Crognale, MacDuff, Young, and McClannahan, 2007).

Method

Participants and setting. Gary, Brad, and Peter, ages 15, 18, and 14, participated in the study. All had received independent diagnoses of autism, and all were experienced users of written activity schedules. The research was conducted in PCDI's school; teaching was conducted in a kitchen, pre- and posttests were conducted in the youths' usual classroom, and follow up was conducted in a copy room.

Dependent variable. The dependent variable was interobserver agreement between student-instructor pairs. After student and instructor independently marked their own copies of the written activity schedules, each task was scored as an agreement or disagreement. Agreements were scored only if both members of a pair scored plus or minus; marks other than plus or minus, and the absence of marks, were scored as disagreements.

Activities and schedules. The activities used in the study were selected because they were never previously taught, and because the youths' past performance on other written schedules suggested that there would be many opportunities for them to score both plus and minus. The activity schedule selected for teaching was making apple muffins. The activity schedules used on pre- and posttests were (a) assembling metal frames for hanging Pendaflex™ file folders and (b) taking and printing digital photographs. The written schedule for follow-up was sending a fax.

Experimental design and measurement. A nonconcurrent multiple-baseline across participants was used to assess interobserver agreement between instructor-student dyads. Data collectors used a per-opportunity measure to score each task on a written schedule as correct or incorrect. Subsequently, each task was scored as an agreement or disagreement.

Experimental conditions. During baseline, the instructor gave a student a written activity schedule; each task on the schedule was preceded by a blank. The instructor said, "Let's take data on (name of activity). Mark plus if you do something without help and if you do it correctly." Then the instructor modeled marking plus on an activity schedule that was never used for data collection. Next, the instructor said, "Mark minus if you do something incorrectly or if I help you" and modeled marking minus on the schedule. Subsequently, the instructor gave the student the schedule for a never previously taught activity (making apple muffins) and said, "Let's take data." During the data collection period, the instructor did not interact with the student about data collection, but used graduated guidance when necessary to help him complete scheduled tasks. At the end of the activity, the instructor delivered tokens and praise for correctly completing tasks, but did not mention data collection.

During the teaching condition, the instructor gave the same initial instructions used during baseline, and then student and instructor independently marked their data sheets (i.e., activity schedules). Initially, after each task, the instructor placed her schedule adjacent to the student's schedule. If both student and instructor marked plus on a task the instructor said, "You did (task) correctly and I didn't help you. Good, we both scored plus—we agreed," and gave the student a token. If both members of the pair marked minus, the instructor said, "You didn't do (task) by yourself; I helped you. Good, we both scored minus—we agreed," and delivered a token.

If the student scored plus and the instructor scored minus, the instructor said, "You didn't do (task) correctly" or "I helped you do (task); I scored minus but you scored plus—we disagreed" and removed a token. If the student scored minus and the instructor scored plus, the instructor said, "You did (task) without my help and you did it correctly; you scored minus and I scored plus—we disagreed," and removed a token. During teaching, the instructor continued to use graduated guidance to help the young people complete tasks that they did not independently complete. But tokens and feedback were never delivered for correct performance; they were only delivered for agreements between student and instructor.

After two consecutive sessions during which student and instructor achieved 100% interobserver agreement, the instructor no longer delivered feedback after each task was scored. Instead, at the end of the activity, she collected the student's data sheet and calculated interobserver agreement. The student did not see the data sheet after interobserver agreement was calculated. If agreement was 80% or better, the instructor said, "Good, we agreed," and delivered tokens that were immediately exchanged for a reward. If agreement was less than 80%, the instructor said, "We disagreed; it's time for (next activity)" and did not deliver any tokens. After at least six sessions during which (a) the instructor did not deliver immediate feedback and (b) overall interobserver agreement was consistently above 90%, maintenance began. The maintenance condition was identical to baseline.

Peter's maintenance condition began immediately after he returned from a one-week school recess during which he was ill. Although he met criterion for entering the maintenance condition, the first three data points in this condition showed that overall agreement between Peter and the instructor declined and their nonoccurrence agreement fell to an all-time low. For that reason, he returned to the teaching condition and again met criterion before moving to maintenance.

Follow-up data were collected 10 weeks after Gary's last maintenance session, 10 weeks after Brad's last session, and 7 weeks after Peter's last session. On follow-up, the youths were given a written activity schedule for a new, never-taught task—sending a fax. Follow-up procedures were identical to those used during baseline.

Pre- and post-teaching tests. Once during baseline and once during maintenance, the instructor provided written activity schedules never used prior to the study or in any experimental conditions. These schedules pertained to two new data-collection activities on two never-taught tasks—assembling metal Pendaflex™ frames for hanging file folders and taking and printing a digital photograph. The instructor followed the same procedures used during baseline. The instructor and a second observer recorded the student's performance, after which student-instructor interobserver agreement and instructor-observer interobserver agreement were calculated. These pre- and post-teaching tests assessed whether the student learned to reliably collect data (i.e., whether he learned to self-monitor his correct and incorrect schedule-following responses).

Assessment of the independent variables. On at least two sessions during the teaching condition for each participant, independent observers scored whether the instructor (a) modeled marking plus or minus signs on a sample data sheet, (b) aligned her data sheet and the student's data sheet after each scoring opportunity, (c) provided the specified feedback, and (d) contingently gave or removed tokens. The data indicated that the instructor exhibited these responses on 100% of opportunities for Gary and Brad, and on 99% of opportunities for Peter. Interobserver agreement between independent observers on the integrity of the teaching procedures was 100%.

Interobserver agreement. Percentage overall agreement and percentage nonoccurrence agreement were calculated by dividing number of agreements by number of agreements plus disagreements and multiplying the result by 100. Mean overall agreement between instructor and observer was 100% in baseline and 99% in teaching (range = 98% to 100%). One data point between instructor and observer during Peter's maintenance condition yielded 100% interobserver agreement.

Results

During baseline, all participants had 0% interobserver agreement with the instructor. They either made check marks in the blanks beside tasks on their activity schedules, marked through completed activities, or did not mark their schedules. Mean percentage overall interobserver agreement for student-instructor dyads in the teaching condition was 95% for Gary, 83% for Brad, and 98% and 99% for Peter in his first and second teaching conditions respectively. In maintenance, mean percentage overall agreement was 100% for Gary, 99% for Brad, and 93% and 100% for Peter (see Figure 12.1).

On pretests of taking and printing digital photographs and assembling Pendaflex frames, all three youths had 0% overall interobserver agreement with the instructor. On posttests conducted during maintenance, Gary's overall interobserver agreement scores on Pendaflex frames and digital photos were 100% and 96%, Brad's were 80% and 90%, and Peter's were 100% and 93%.

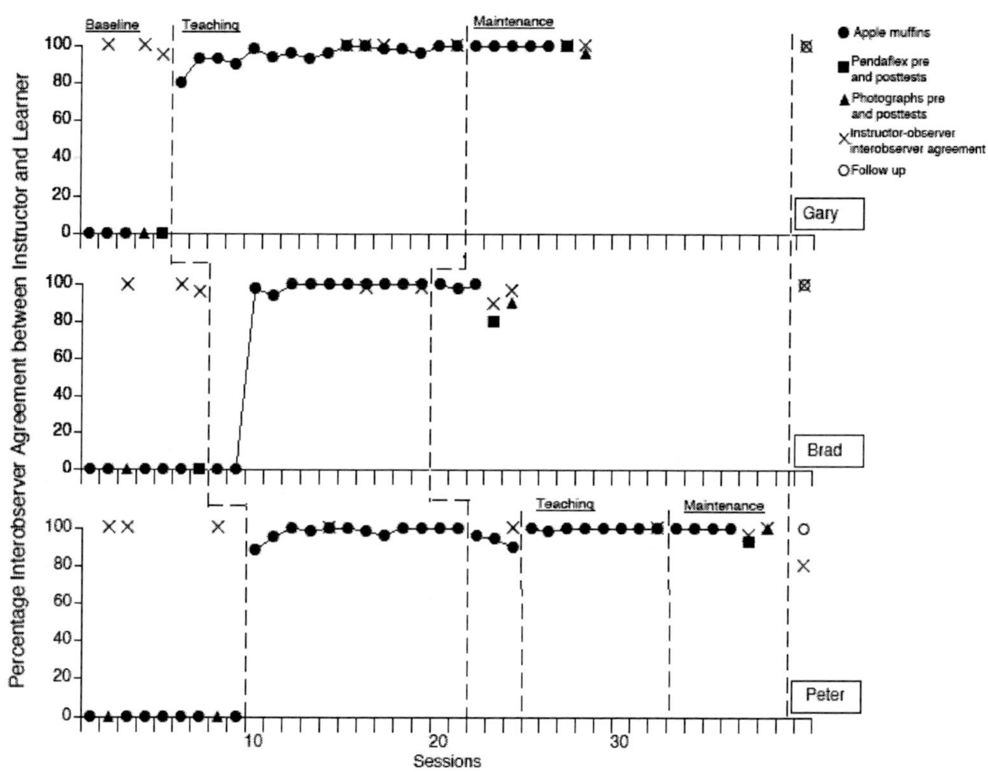

Figure 1. Percentage overall interobserver agreement between instructor and students and between instructor and an observer during baseline, teaching, maintenance, and follow-up. Percentage overall agreement is also shown for pretests during baseline and posttests during maintenance.

Follow-up assessment occurred seven to ten weeks after maintenance ended. Using the never-taught activity schedule for sending a fax, all three participants achieved 100% overall interobserver agreement with the instructor.

Mean overall percentage nonoccurrence interobserver agreement during teaching was 76% for Gary (range = 36% to 100%), and 78% for Brad (range = 0% to 100%). Means in Peter's two teaching conditions were 91% (range = 67% to 100%) and 99% (range = 98% to 100%). In his two maintenance conditions, mean nonoccurrence agreement was 54% (range = 44% to 62%) and 100%. At follow-up, percentage nonoccurrence agreement was 100% for all three participants.

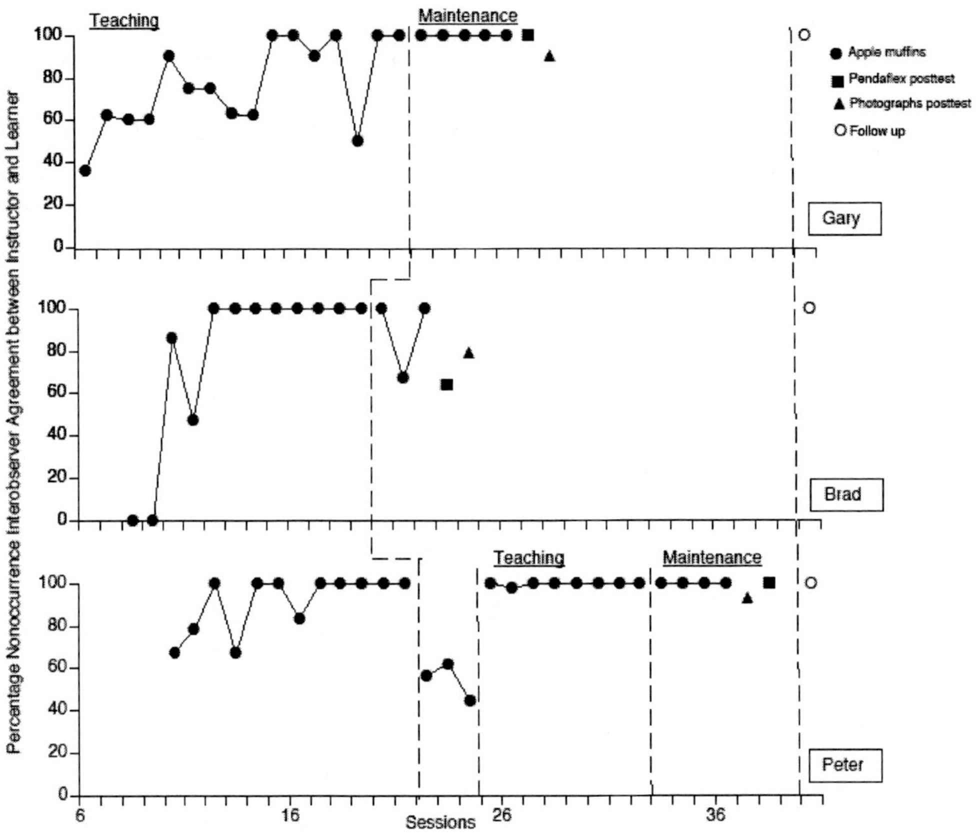

Figure 2. Percentage nonoccurrence interobserver agreement for each student-instructor dyad during teaching, maintenance, and follow-up. Because Peter's nonoccurrence interobserver agreement scores declined during his first maintenance condition, he returned to teaching.

Discussion

We embarked on this investigation to determine whether people with lengthy histories of using written activity schedules could be taught to take interobserver agreement with an instructor. The participants' levels of interobserver agreement during maintenance, posttests, and follow up show that they correctly scored their own responses as correct or incorrect—that is, they engaged in self-monitoring.

Nonoccurrence interobserver agreement was calculated for every scheduled task on which either or both members of a dyad scored a response as incorrect. During teaching, all three participants' percentage nonoccurrence agreement showed an ascending trend as they learned to correctly score errors as well as correct responses. Data on nonoccurrence agreement are important because it may be easier for people to tact correct versus incorrect performance. A correct response may occur because a task was previously mastered or because the person had some prior experience about how to complete it. For example, the participants in this study had prior experience with tasks such as "Get the ___," "Put ___ away," or "Tell the teacher you are finished with __." Such tasks would be more easily recognizable as correct.

During maintenance, posttests, and follow-up, the youths did not receive item-by-item feedback on their interobserver agreement with the instructor, as they did during the initial phase of the teaching condition. Thus, they received less information about their data collection activities than nonhandicapped observers typically receive after they collect data. It would be interesting to know how the participants' nonoccurrence agreement scores compare with staff members' scores on similar data-collection tasks. It was noteworthy that at follow-up, all participants achieved 100% interobserver agreement with the instructor, but instructor and observer obtained 80% interobserver agreement on Peter's follow-up assessment (two items that Peter and the instructor scored minus were scored plus by the observer).

During the weeks between maintenance and follow-up, none of the students was asked to obtain interobserver agreement with the instructor. But when presented with a new written activity schedule for ironing clothing, Brad spontaneously took data on his own performance and he and the instructor had 100% interobserver agreement. These anecdotal data, as well as posttest and follow-up data, indicate that self-monitoring correct and incorrect responses generalized to new tasks.

All of the participants in this study had lengthy experience with activity schedules; we think it unlikely that novice schedule users would be equally successful in self-monitoring their schedule-following skills. It should also be noted that activity schedules provide only one avenue for helping people to engage in self monitoring. Other strategies have also produced encouraging results (cf. Kirby, Fowler, and Baer, 1991; Likins, Salzberg, Stowitschek, Lignugaris/Kraft, and Curl, 1989; Maag, Reid, and DiGangi, 1993). Nevertheless, activity schedules appear to be useful tools that help people with ASD learn to self-monitor their correct and incorrect responses during scheduled activities. Future research might examine whether such self-monitoring extends to inappropriate behavior such as stereotypy.

SUMMARY

Activity schedules taught with graduated guidance and a most-to-least prompt fading procedure help people with ASD learn to complete lengthy response chains and foster generalized responding to new activities (MacDuff, et. al., 1993). Schedules have been shown to provide a platform for making choices (McClannahan and Krantz, 1999; Watanabe and

Sturmey, 2003), to increase engagement with appropriate activities (Anderson, Sherman, Sheldon, and McAdam, 1997; Bryan and Gast, 2000), and to decrease disruptive behavior (Krantz, et.al., 1993). In addition, photographic and written activity schedules offer a framework for teaching social interaction skills (Krantz and McClannahan, 1998; McClannahan and Krantz, 2005; Stevenson, Krantz, and McClannahan, 2000).

Teaching adults with ASD to display complex repertoires of long duration is an essential component of preparing them for the world of work. Workers who display sustained on-task and who successfully complete diverse assignments are more likely to retain employment.

Using activity schedules as vehicles to teach choice making is often important to job placement decisions. For example, because one young man in our setting was a competent typist and computer user, we initially assumed that we should help him find employment in an office setting. But before launching a job search, we provided some choices in his activity schedule; he had opportunities to choose word processing tasks or manual labor tasks. It was interesting to note that he consistently chose manual labor, and we identified a job placement that was commensurate with his preferences. He went to work in a hotel laundry, where he performed very well.

Activity schedules also provide a structure for teaching social skills relevant to employment. Adults who learn to report task completion, appropriately take coffee breaks, engage in social interaction with co-workers, ask supervisors for additional work assignments, and monitor their own productivity are more likely to become valued employees. All of these skills can be taught via schedules.

Unfortunately, most of the research literature on activity schedules pertains to children. Our data suggest that photographic and written activity schedules are invaluable tools for adults. We hope that, in the near future, applied researchers will focus on the multiple functions of activity schedules for adults with ASD.

REFERENCES

Anderson, M.D., Sherman, J.A., Sheldon, J.B., and McAdam, D. (1997). Picture activity schedules and engagement of adults with mental retardation in a group home. *Research in Developmental Disabilities*, 18, 231-250.

Bellovin, E.R., Burck, S.E., Tarnoski, J.M., Cammilleri, A.P., and Brothers, K.J. (2003, May). *A comparison of the effects of textual activity schedules on paper versus textual activity schedules of a personal data assistant (PDA).* Poster presented at the First Annual Conference of the Princeton Child Development Institute, Princeton, NJ.

Bickel, W.K., Stella, M.E., and Etzel, B.C. (1984). A re-evaluation of stimulus overselectivity: Restricted stimulus control or stimulus control hierarchies. *Journal of Autism and Developmental Disabilities*, 14, 137-157.

Bryan, L.C., and Gast, D.L. (2000). Teaching on-task and on-schedule behaviors to high-functioning children with autism via picture activity schedules. *Journal of Autism and Developmental Disorders*, 30, 553-567.

Crognale, B. C., Kitson, M.E., MacDuff, M.A., Zeutenhorst, D., and McClannahan, L.E. (2003, May). *Schedule-following repertoires improve pretest performance.* Poster presented at the First Annual Conference of the Princeton Child Development Institute, Princeton, NJ.

Decker, D.M., Ferrigno, T.K., May, D. T., Natoli, C.L., Olson, K.D., Schaefer, M.A., Cammilleri, A.P., and Brothers, K.J. (2003, May). *A comparison of student performance on paper and electronic picture activity schedules*. Poster presented at the First Annual Conference of the Princeton Child Development Institute, Princeton, NJ.

Hoogeveen, F. R., Kouwenhoven, J. A., and Smeets, P. M. (1989). Establishing sound blending in moderately mentally retarded children: Implications of verbal instruction and pictorial prompting. *Research in Developmental Disabilities*, 10, 1-18.

Kirby, K.C., Fowler, S.A., and Baer, D.M. (1991). Reactivity in self-recording: Recording procedure and peer comments. *Journal of Applied Behavior Analysis*, 24, 487-498.

Kitson, M.E., Connor, S.M., Crognale, B., MacDuff, M.A., Young, J., and McClannahan, L.E. (2007). *Does learning to obtain interobserver agreement promote self-monitoring?* Poster presented at the Fifth Annual Conference of the Princeton Child Development Institute, Princeton, NJ.

Knapp, L., McClannahan, L.E., and Krantz, P.J. (1986). *Using photographic activity schedules to program generalization of autistic children's academic and leisure skills.* Unpublished manuscript.

Krantz, P.J., MacDuff, M.T., and McClannahan, L.E. (1993). Programming participation in family activities for children with autism: Parents' use of photographic activity schedules. *Journal of Applied Behavior Analysis*, 26, 137-139.

Krantz, P.J., and McClannahan, L.E. (1998). Social interaction skills for children with autism: A script-fading procedure for beginning readers. *Journal of Applied Behavior Analysis*, 31, 191-202.

Likins, M., Salzberg, C.L., Stowitschek, J.J., Lignugaris/Kraft, B., and Curl, R. (1989). Co-worker implemented job training: The use of coincidental training and quality-control checking on the food preparation skills of trainees with mental retardation. *Journal of Applied Behavior Analysis*, 22, 381-393.

Maag, J.W., Reid, R., and DiGangi, S.A. (1993). Differential effects of self-monitoring attention, accuracy, and productivity. *Journal of Applied Behavior Analysis*, 26, 329-344.

MacDuff, G.S., Krantz, P.J., McClannahan, L.E. (1993). Teaching children with autism to use photographic activity schedules: Maintenance and generalization of complex response chains. *Journal of Applied Behavior Analysis*, 26, 89-95.

McClannahan, L.E., and Krantz, P.J. (1997). In search of solutions to prompt dependence: Teaching children with autism to use photographic activity schedules. In E.M. Pinkston and D.M. Baer (Eds.), *Environment and behavior* (pp. 271-278). Boulder, CO: Westview Press.

McClannahan, L.E., and Krantz, P.J. (1999). *Activity schedules for children with autism: Teaching independent behavior*. Bethesda, MD: Woodbine House.

McClannahan, L.E., and Krantz, P.J. (2005). *Teaching conversation to children with autism: Scripts and script fading*. Bethesda, MD: Woodbine House.

McClannahan, L.E., MacDuff, G.S., and Krantz, P.J. (2002). Behavior analysis and intervention for adults with autism. *Behavior Modification*, 26, 9-26.

Reed, P. (undated). *A quasi-experimental, longitudinal evaluation of prompt dependence during implementation of a standard prompt hierarchy for teaching profoundly learning disabled adults during routine care*. Manuscript submitted for publication.

Rehfeldt, R.A., Kinney, E.M., Root, S., and Stromer, R. (2004). Creating activity schedules using Microsoft® PowerPoint®. *Journal of Applied Behavior Analysis*, 37, 115-128.

Schneider, H.C., and Salzberg, C.L. (1982). Stimulus over-selectivity in a match-to sample paradigm by severely retarded youth. *Analysis and Intervention in Developmental Disabilities*, 2, 273-304.

Stevenson, C.L., Krantz, P.J., and McClannahan, L.E. (2000). Social interaction skills for children with autism: A script-fading procedure for non-readers. *Behavioral Interventions*, 15, 1-20.

Touchette, P. E., and Howard, J. S. (1984). Errorless learning: Reinforcement contingencies and stimulus control transfer in delayed prompting. *Journal of Applied Behavior Analysis*, 17, 175-188.

Watanabe, M., and Sturmey, P. (2003). The effect of choice-making opportunities during activity schedules on task engagement of adults with autism. *Journal of Autism and Developmental Disorders*, 33, 535-538.

Weiberg-Aurdal, E. (undated). *Photographic activity schedules: An aid towards greater independence for people with developmental disabilities*. Unpublished manuscript.

INDEX

B

C

D

F

G

J

K

L

M

N

O

P

Q

R

S

T